Essential Travel Medicine

Essential Travel Medicine

EDITED BY

Jane N. Zuckerman, MD, FRCP, FRCPath, FFPH, FFPM, FFTM

Consultant in Travel Medicine
Honorary Senior Lecturer, UCL Medical School, University College London, UK;
Honorary Consultant, Royal Free London NHS Foundation Trust and Great Ormond Street Hospital for
Children NHS Foundation Trust, London, UK;
Adjunct Professor, College of Public Health, Medical and Veterinary Sciences, James Cook University,
Townsville, Qld, Australia

Gary W. Brunette, MD, MS, FFTM

Chief, Travelers' Health Branch
Division of Global Migration and Quarantine
Centers for Disease Control and Prevention, Atlanta, GA, USA

Peter A. Leggat, AM, MD, PhD, DrPH, FAFPHM, FFPH, FFPM(Hon), FACTM(Hon), FFTM, FACAsM

Professor and Dean, College of Public Health, Medical and Veterinary Sciences, James Cook University,
Townsville, Qld, Australia;
Visiting Professor, School of Public Health, Faculty of Health Sciences, University of the Witwatersrand,
Johannesburg, South Africa;
Conjoint Professor, School of Health Sciences, Faculty of Health, University of Newcastle, NSW, Australia;
Adjunct Professor, Research School of Population Health, College of Medicine, Biology and Environment,
Australian National University, Canberra, ACT, Australia

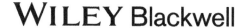

This edition first published 2015 © 2015 by John Wiley & Sons, Ltd

Registered office: John Wiley & Sons, Ltd, The Atrium, Southern Gate, Chichester, West Sussex, PO19 8SQ, UK

Editorial offices: 9600 Garsington Road, Oxford, OX4 2DQ, UK
The Atrium, Southern Gate, Chichester, West Sussex, PO19 8SQ, UK
111 River Street, Hoboken, NJ 07030-5774, USA

For details of our global editorial offices, for customer services and for information about how to apply for permission to reuse the copyright material in this book please see our website at www.wiley.com/wiley-blackwell

Library of Congress Cataloging-in-Publication Data applied for.

A catalogue record for this book is available from the British Library.

ISBN: 9781118597255

Wiley also publishes its books in a variety of electronic formats. Some content that appears in print may not be available in electronic books.

Cover image: Globe-North America ©DNY59 (iStockphoto.com)

Set in 9/12pt, MeridienLTStd by SPi Global, Chennai, India

1   2015

Contents

List of contributors

Michael Bagshaw, MB, BCh, MRCS, FFOM, DAvMed, DFFP, FRAeS
Visiting Professor of Aviation Medicine
Honorary Civilian Consultant Adviser in Aviation Medicine to the Army
King's College London
London, UK;
Cranfield University
Cranfield, UK

Sally S.J. Bell, MB BS, Master in Maritime Medicine
Clinical Quality Consultant
London, UK

Robert Bor, DPhil, CPsychol, CSci, FBPsS, UKCP, Reg FRAeS
Professor, Lead Consultant Clinical, Counselling and Health Psychologist
Royal Free London NHS Foundation Trust;
Director, Dynamic Change Consultants
London, UK

Gary W. Brunette, MD, MS, FFTM
Chief, Travelers' Health Branch
Division of Global Migration and Quarantine
Centers for Disease Control and Prevention
Atlanta, GA, USA

I. Dale Carroll, MD, FACOG, DTM&H, FFTM RCPS (Glasgow)
Medical Director
The Pregnant Traveler
Spring Lake, MI, USA

Ian C. Cheng, BE, BMed, DipOccEnvironHealth, DipAvMed, MPH, FAFOEM, FACAsM
Adjunct Associate Professor
College of Public Health, Medical and Veterinary Sciences
James Cook University
Townsville, Queensland, Australia;
Staff Specialist - Occupational Medicine
Royal North Shore Hospital
Sydney, NSW, Australia

Anna Cristina C. Carvalho, MD, PhD
Researcher in Public Health
Laboratory of Innovations in Therapies, Education and Bioproducts)
Oswaldo Cruz Institute, FioCruz
Rio de Janeiro, Brazil

Eilif Dahl, MD, MHA, PhD
Professor Emeritus, University of Bergen
Norwegian Centre for Maritime Medicine
Haukeland University Hospital
5021 Bergen
Norway

Claire Davies, MRCP, MRCGO, DTM&H, MFTM RCPS (Glasgow)
Medical Team Manager/Travel Health Clinician
InterHealth Worldwide
London, UK

Charles D. Ericsson, MD
Professor of Medicine and Dr. and Mrs. Carl V. Vartian Professor of Infectious Diseases;
Head, Clinical Infectious Diseases
University of Texas Medical School at Houston
Houston, TX, USA

Philip R. Fischer, MD, DTM&H
Professor of Pediatrics
Mayo Clinic
Rochester, MN, USA

Richard C. Franklin, BSc, MSocSc, PhD
Associate Professor, College of Public Health, Medical and Veterinary Sciences
James Cook University
Townsville, Queensland, Australia;
Royal Life Saving Society, Australia

David O. Freedman, MD
Professor of Medicine and Epidemiology
Division of Infectious Diseases
University of Alabama at Birmingham
Birmingham, AL, USA

Joanna Gaines, PhD, MPH
Doctoral Epidemiologist
Travelers' Health Branch
Division of Global Migration and Quarantine
Centers for Disease Control and Prevention
Atlanta, GA, USA

Mark D. Gershman, MD
Medical Epidemiologist
Travelers' Health Branch
Division of Global Migration and Quarantine
Centers for Disease Control and Prevention
Atlanta, GA, USA

Brian D. Gushulak, BSc (Hon), MD
Medical Consultant
Migration Health Consultants, Inc.
P.O. Box 463
Qualicum Beach, BC, Canada

Sean T. Hudson, MBBS, MSc, FAWM, Dip Mtn Med
General Practitioner and Honorary Consultant
Accident and Emergency
Maryport Health Centre
West Cumberland Hospital
Maryport, Cumbria, UK;
Director and Founder, Expedition Medicine
Cumbria, UK

Tomas Jelinek, MD
Medical Director
Berlin Center for Travel and Tropical Medicine
Berlin, Germany

Caroline J. Knox, MBBS MSc MRCGP
General Practitioner, Castlegate Surgery
Cockermouth, Cumbria, UK;
Founder, Expedition Medicine
Cumbria, UK

Tamar Lachish, MD
Senior Doctor, Infectious Diseases Unit and the Internal Medicine Ward
Shaare-Zedek Medical Center
Jerusalem, Israel

Ted Lankester, MA, MB, Bchir, MRCGP, FFTM, RSPSG
Director of Health Services
InterHealth Worldwide
London, UK

Regina LaRocque, MD, MPH
Co-Director, Global TravEpiNet (GTEN) Program
Massachusetts General Hospital;
Assistant Professor of Medicine, Harvard Medical School
Boston, MA, USA

Karin Leder, MBBS, FRACP, PhD, MPH, DTMH
Associate Professor, Head of Infectious Disease Epidemiology Unit
Department of Epidemiology and Preventive Medicine
School of Public Health and Preventive Medicine
Monash University
Melbourne, VIC, Australia;
Head of Travel Medicine and Immigrant Health
Royal Melbourne Hospital at the Doherty Institute for Infection and Immunity
Melbourne, VIC, Australia;
Victorian Infectious Diseases Service
Royal Melbourne Hospital
Parkville, VIC, Australia

Peter A. Leggat, AM. MD, PhD, DrPH, FAFPHM, FFPH, FFPM(Hon), FACTM(Hon), FFTM, FACAsM
Professor and Dean, College of Public Health, Medical and Veterinary Sciences
James Cook University
Townsville, Queensland, Australia;
Visiting Professor, School of Public Health, Faculty of Health Sciences
University of the Witwatersrand
Johannesburg, South Africa;
Conjoint Professor, School of Health Sciences
Faculty of Health
University of Newcastle
Newcastle, New South Wales, Australia;
Adjunct Professor, Research School of Population Health
College of Medicine, Biology and Environment
Australian National University
Canberra, ACT, Australia

Louis Loutan, MD, MPH
Professor, Division of International and Humanitarian Medicine
Department of Community Medicine and Primary Care
University Hospital of Geneva
Geneva, Switzerland

Douglas W. MacPherson, MD, MSc(CTM), FRCPC
Migration Health Consultants, Inc.
Qualicum Beach, BC, Canada;
Associate Professor, Pathology and Molecular Medicine
McMaster University
Hamilton, ON, Canada

Karen J. Marienau, MD, MPH
Medical Consultant and Advisor
St. Paul, MN, USA;
Formerly Division of Global Migration and Quarantine
US Centers for Disease Control and Prevention
Atlanta, GA, USA

Alberto Matteelli, MD
Head of Community Infection Unit
Clinic of Infectious and Tropical Diseases
Spedali Civili Hospital
University of Brescia
Brescia, Italy

Anne E. McCarthy, MD, MSc, FRCPC, DTM&H, FASTMH
Professor of Medicine, University of Ottawa;
Director, Tropical Medicine and International Health Clinic
University of Ottawa
Ottawa, Canada

Sarah L. McGuinness, MBBS, BMedSc, DTMH
Infectious Diseases Registrar
Victorian Infectious Diseases Service
Royal Melbourne Hospital
Parkville, VIC, Australia

Karl Neumann, MD, FAAP, CTM
Clinical Associate Professor of Pediatrics
Weill Medical College of Cornell University, USA;
Clinical Associate Attending Pediatrician
New York Presbyterian Hospital–Cornell Medical Center
New York, (emeritus) USA;
Attending Pediatrician
Long Island Jewish Hospital, USA;
Director
Family Travel and Immunization Clinic of Forest Hills, Queens, USA

Gilles Poumerol, MD
Medical Officer
Travel Health, Information & Communication
Global Capacities Alert & Response
World Health Organization
Geneva, Switzerland

Mark A. Read, PhD
Senior Instructor, Expedition and Wilderness Medicine
Thuringowa Central. Queensland, Australia

Gary Rhodes, PhD
Director, Center for Global Education
Graduate School of Education and Information Studies
University of California at Los Angeles
Los Angeles, CA, USA

Sara Ritchie, MBChB, MRCGP, DFFP, DTM&H, MPH, Dip Derm
Honorary Clinical Fellow in Tropical and HIV Dermatology
University College London Hospitals NHS Foundation Trust London, UK

Edward T. Ryan, MD, FACP, FIDSA, FASTMH
Co-Director, Global TravEpiNet (GTEN) Program
Director, Travelers' Advice and Immunization Center
Massachusetts General Hospital;
Professor of Medicine, Harvard Medical School;
Professor of Immunology and Infectious Diseases, Harvard School of Public Health
Boston, MA, USA

Patricia Schlagenhauf, PhD
Professor, University of Zürich Centre for Travel Medicine
Zürich, Switzerland

Eli Schwartz, MD, DTMH
Professor, Director of the Center for Geographic Medicine
The Chaim Sheba Medical Center
Tel-Hashomer, Israel;
Sackler School of Medicine
Tel-Aviv University
Tel-Aviv, Israel.

Marc T.M. Shaw, DrPH, FRGS, FRNZCGP, FFTM (ACTM), FFTM RCPS (Glasgow), DipTravMed
Adjunct Professor, College of Public Health, Medical and Veterinary Sciences
James Cook University
Townsville, Queensland, Australia;
Medical Director, WORLDWISE Travellers Health Centres
Auckland, New Zealand

David R. Shlim, MD
Medical Director
Jackson Hole Travel and Tropical Medicine
Wilson Medical Center
Wilson, WY, USA

Will Smith, MD
Medical Director, Grand Teton National Park, Teton County Search and Rescue;
Clinical Faculty, University of Washington School of Medicine;
Emergency Medicine, St. John's Medical Center
Jackson, WY, USA

Mark J. Sotir, PhD, MPH
Lead, Surveillance and Epidemiology Team
Travelers' Health Branch
Division of Global Migration and Quarantine
Centers for Disease Control and Prevention
Atlanta, GA, USA

J. Erin Staples, MD, PhD
Medical Epidemiologist
Arbovirus Disease Branch
Division of Vector Borne Diseases
Centers for Disease Control and Prevention
Fort Collins, CO, USA

Kathryn N. Suh, MD, MSc, FRCPC
Associate Professor of Medicine
University of Ottawa;
Division of infectious Diseases
University of Ottawa
Ottawa, Canada

Andrea P. Summer, MD, MSCR
Associate Professor of Pediatrics
Medical University of South Carolina
Charleston, SC, USA

Joseph Torresi, MBBS, BMedSci, FRACP, PhD
NHMRC Practitioner Fellow
Department of Microbiology and Immunology
The Peter Doherty Institute for Infection and Immunity
University of Melbourne;
Associate Professor, Department of Infectious Diseases
Austin Hospital
Melbourne, VIC, Australia

Alfons Van Gompel, MD, DTM
Specialist in Internal Medicine and Tropical Medicine
Associate Professor, Tropical Medicine
Chief Physician of the Medical Services and Travel Clinic of the Institute for Tropical Medicine
Antwerp, Belgium

Francisco Vega-López, MD, MSc, PhD, FRCP, FFTM, RCPSG
Consultant Dermatologist and Honorary Professor
University College London Hospitals NHS Foundation TrustLondon, UK

Abinash Virk, MD
Associate Professor, Internal Medicine
Mayo Medical School
Division of Infectious Diseases
Mayo Clinic
Rochester, MN, USA

Mary J. Warrell, MB BS, FRCP, FRCPath
Honorary Research Associate
Oxford Vaccine Group
University of Oxford;
Centre for Clinical Vaccinology and Tropical Medicine
Churchill Hospital
Oxford, UK

Annelies Wilder-Smith, MD, PhD
Professor in Infectious Diseases
Lee Kong Chian School of Medicine
Nanyang Technological University
Singapore

Claire S. Wong, RN, MSc, FFTM RCPS (Glasgow)
Travel Health Specialist Nurse
WORLDWISE Travellers Health Centres
Auckland, New Zealand

Jane N. Zuckerman, MD, FRCP, FRCPath, FFPH, FFPM, FFTM
Consultant in Travel Medicine;
Honorary Senior Lecturer, UCL Medical School
University College London, London, UK;
Honorary Consultant, Royal Free London NHS Foundation Trust and Great Ormond
Street Hospital for Children NHS Foundation Trust, London, UK;
Adjunct Professor, College of Public Health, Medical and Veterinary Sciences
James Cook University
Townsville, Queensland, Australia

Preface

The discipline of travel medicine continues to develop with established roots and structures worldwide. The necessity for the clinical practice of travel medicine in the prevention of ill health has never been more understood than now, with ever-increasing numbers of people traveling and criss-crossing the world alongside the potential hazards that travelers themselves may be exposed to and also the potential inherent risk to public health and populations internationally as a consequence of travel. Protecting travelers and, concomitantly, communities and populations requires the skill and expertise of travel medicine practitioners whose knowledge base is underpinned by continued professional development. Knowledge and education go hand in hand, with specialist training being an essential element, so enabling best clinical practice in a constantly evolving specialty.

The purpose of this book is to support those studying for a qualification or higher degree in travel medicine, and it is hoped that it will be used alongside and complement travel medicine reference books. This book is designed not only to support postgraduate training in the discipline but also to encourage undergraduate training in travel medicine in the curriculum of multidisciplinary healthcare training programs. It has been written in a style to complement lectures, with easily accessible information on the core topics required to enable the day-to-day clinical practice of travel medicine. Authors from different continents were chosen specifically in order to represent a range of views reflecting clinical practice and training courses that are available in different countries through the world.

It is hoped that this book will become a useful aide for those furthering their knowledge in addition to being a practical guide that will enhance the clinical practice and profile of travel medicine as a specialty. For those new to the growing discipline of travel medicine, an aspiration is that this book will stimulate interest and enthusiasm for the discipline for the next generation of travel medicine practitioners.

Jane N. Zuckerman
Gary W. Brunette
Peter A. Leggat

Acknowledgments

The Editors would like to thank Maria Khan and Oliver Walter of Wiley-Blackwell for their enthusiasm, patience, and commitment that enabled the publication of this new book in travel medicine. In addition, we would like to thank Jennifer Seward and Jasmine Chang, also of Wiley-Blackwell, for all their help in the preparation of this edition. We would also like to thank all the authors for contributing to this book and to supporting the future development of the discipline of travel medicine. In particular, we would like to thank our families for their unfailing support and understanding, specifically Eugene, Tunde, and Pan, without whom this new text-book would not have been realized.

Acknowledgments

SECTION I
Travel medicine

CHAPTER 1

Basic epidemiology of infectious diseases

Mark J. Sotir[1] & David O. Freedman[2]

[1] Centers for Disease Control and Prevention, Atlanta, GA, USA
[2] University of Alabama at Birmingham, Birmingham, AL, USA

Infectious conditions comprise a substantial portion of texts and guidelines related to travel medicine [1,2]. To prescribe optimal pre-travel advice, preventive measures, and education to travelers, travel health providers must be familiar with basic epidemiologic concepts, and also the epidemiology and geographic distribution of relevant infections. As past experience may predict future risk, a traveler-specific risk assessment allows possible measures, advice, and behavior modification to be appropriately prioritized for each traveler.

During the past two decades, the most important and relevant data on travel-related disease have come from surveillance of travelers themselves. Although available Ministry of Health data based on people native to an endemic locale may reflect national or state-level trends and identify the most important diseases to monitor within a country, the risk behaviors, eating habits, accommodations, knowledge of preventive measures, and precise itineraries of travelers can differ greatly from those of local populations. The GeoSentinel surveillance system, a collaborative effort between the International Society of Travel Medicine and the US Centers for Disease Control and Prevention, maintains the largest such surveillance database, with more than 200,000 records from patients with a confirmed or probable travel-related diagnosis. GeoSentinel is a global provider-based network of travel and tropical medicine clinics, which, as of August 2013, has 57 participating clinics on six continents. Details of the standard data collection instrument, diagnostic categories, and patient classification methods used in GeoSentinel have recently been published [3]. The network also facilitates rapid communication, obtains data, and reports on unusual or newly emerging health events in travelers [3].

The most recent surveillance results on travelers published from the GeoSentinel network [4] indicate that Asia (32.6%) and sub-Saharan Africa (26.7%) were the most common regions where illnesses were acquired (Figure 1.1). Three-quarters of travel-related illness was due to gastrointestinal (34.0%), febrile (23.3%), and dermatologic (19.5%) diseases. Malaria, dengue, enteric fever, spotted-fever group rickettsioses, chikungunya, and non-specific viral syndromes remained the most important of the acute systemic febrile illnesses. Falciparum malaria was mainly

Essential Travel Medicine, First Edition.
Edited by Jane N. Zuckerman, Gary W. Brunette and Peter A. Leggat.
© 2015 John Wiley & Sons, Ltd. Published 2015 by John Wiley & Sons, Ltd.

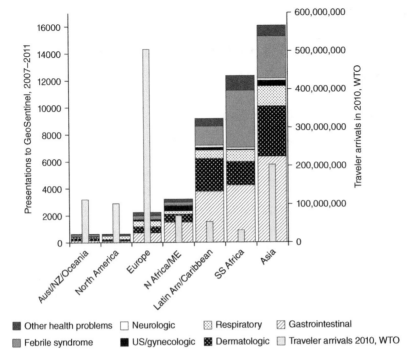

Figure 1.1 Presentations to GeoSentinel by diagnostic category and region (2007–2011), plus 2010 regional WTO traveler arrivals. Left vertical axis shows cumulative number of presentations to GeoSentinel sites by ill returned travelers during 2007–2011 according to syndromic presentation and region of illness acquisition. Right vertical axis (narrow gray bars) shows traveler arrivals in 2010 by region, according to WTO data. WTO, World Tourism Organization; Aust, Australia; NZ, New Zealand, N Africa, North Africa; ME, Middle East; SS Africa, sub-Saharan Africa; GU, genitourinary. Source: Adapted from Leder et al. 2013 [4].

acquired in West Africa, and enteric fever was largely contracted on the Indian subcontinent; leptospirosis, scrub typhus, and murine typhus were principally acquired in South-East Asia. More than two-thirds of dengue infections were acquired in Asia, mostly Thailand, Indonesia, and India; seasonality of dengue varies according to destination. Common skin and soft tissue infections, mosquito bites (often infected), and allergic dermatitis remain the most common dermatologic conditions affecting travelers; of the more exotic infections, hookworm-related cutaneous larva migrans, leishmaniasis, myiasis, and tungiasis are the most important. The relative frequency of many diseases varies with both travel destination and reason for travel, with travelers visiting friends and relatives (VFRs) in their country of origin having both a disproportionately high burden of serious febrile illness (malaria) and very low rates of seeking advice before travel (18.3%). Although the most travel-related illness seen in GeoSentinel clinics comes from Asia, the proportion of travelers who become ill enough to seek specialized care appears to be much higher in travelers returning from Africa or Latin America. Only 40.5% of all ill travelers reported pre-travel medical visits.

Regional surveillance networks such as TropNet, a consortium of European centers, have contributed additional information on large numbers of travelers with dengue, schistosomiasis, leishmaniasis, and in particular malaria [5]. Sentinel event detection has led to notifications of outbreaks of travel-related African trypanosomiasis [6], leptospirosis, and malaria that have been indicative of possible changes in destination-specific risk.

Although GeoSentinel and similar traveler surveillance networks offer many advantages over disease-specific studies or data collated at single centers, they have several limitations. The reported cases represent a sentinel convenience sample of ill returned travelers visiting specialist clinics and do not reflect the experience of healthy travelers or those with mild or self-limited illness who visit primary care practices or other healthcare sites. In addition, referral patterns, patient populations, and travel demographic characteristics are not consistent between sites. Although collecting data exclusively from ill patients does not permit absolute or relative risks to be determined, the available data do show the relative frequency and range of illnesses seen in wide samples of travelers.

Estimates of true incidence and true risk in travelers (often expressed as number of events per 100,000 travelers) have been elusive for a number of reasons. Although a number of approaches to measure risk have been discussed in detail [7], such estimates have been limited in terms of obtaining both an accurate numerator (number of cases of disease) and denominator (number of travelers overall or to a specific destination who are susceptible to infection and illness). Many travelers to a specific location who become infected or ill will have returned to their home country by the time they develop signs and symptoms, so will not be captured by surveillance in the country of exposure, even if reporting is good. Similarly, diseases with short incubation periods may have resolved by the return home and not be captured in the country of origin. A denominator for all travelers to a specific location that could be used to calculate incidence is also generally problematic, and those available are typically estimates provided only at the country or region level and not at the actual destination level [8].

Many of the cited data on incidence of infection in travelers, some of which were published more than three decades ago, are based on extrapolations of small single-site studies or limited data collected from small samples of travelers. Authoritative texts such as the 2014 US CDC Yellow Book [1] often contain tables of global risk estimates that may range from 20–40% of all travelers for travelers' diarrhea to 0.0001% for Japanese encephalitis for all travelers to Asia. Although such numbers are useful as a guide to relative disease risks in large populations, the travel advisor should always seek out the most destination-specific information possible. Unfortunately, for many diseases, such information is only available to the national or, at most, the first geographic administrative level and might apply only to native populations and not to travelers.

A number of factors are important in analyzing epidemiologic data on travel-related diseases or in interpreting published reports. First, the characteristics specific to the disease itself, such as mode of transmission (vector-borne, food-borne, water-borne, environmental exposure), incubation period, signs and symptoms, duration of illness, diagnostic testing, and importance of comorbidities in acquiring and presenting with illness, and clinical outcomes must be considered. Second, the presence, frequency, seasonality, and geographic distribution of the disease need to be assessed, and these might change over time due to outbreaks, emergence or re-emergence in new areas or populations, successful public health interventions, and other factors. Third, as discussed above, travelers represent a unique subset of individuals, hence their exposure might differ compared with that of residents of a destination country.

As a result, along with demographic characteristics, additional travel-specific variables that must be considered would be trip length, destinations (both current and previous), specific travel itineraries (if known), purpose of travel, and type of traveler; preparation before and behaviors during travel also factor into the epidemiology of travel illnesses. Some but not all of these variables are systematically collected by surveillance systems that either focus on travelers, such as GeoSentinel, or collect data on illnesses that affect travelers. In addition, travelers are a heterogeneous group, and because analyses are always composed of samples rather than entire populations, the sample profile must be carefully examined and disclosed. For example, VFRs have consistently represented higher proportions of serious febrile illness, particularly malaria, among travelers [9,10].

Data on the health characteristics and pre-travel healthcare of travelers are important to provide insight into the itinerary, purpose of travel, or existing medical conditions in order to prioritize the most relevant interventions and education. A US-based provider network, Global TravEpiNet (GTEN), systematically collects data from travelers presenting to a consortium of 26 travel and tropical medicine clinics. Of 13,235 travelers seen from 2009 to 2010 in GTEN clinics, India, South Africa, and China were the most common intended destinations for these travelers, with more than one-third of trips occurring in June, July, and August [11]. Travelers seen in sampled GTEN clinics ranged in age from 1 month to 94 years, with a median of 35 years. The median duration of travel was 14 days, although 22% of travelers pursued trips of >28 days, and 3% of travelers pursued trips of >6 months. About 75% were traveling to malaria-endemic countries; of the 72% who were prescribed an antimalarial, 70% of the prescriptions were for atovaquone/proguanil. Of the 87% of travelers who were prescribed an antibiotic for presumptive self-treatment of travelers' diarrhea, a fluoroquinolone or azithromycin was prescribed in almost equal proportions. Vaccines against hepatitis A and typhoid were the most frequently administered. About 38% of travelers were visiting yellow fever-endemic countries, for which they may need a vaccine requiring a higher level of practitioner knowledge. Immunocompromising conditions, such as HIV infection and AIDS, organ transplant, or receipt of immunocompromising medications, were present in 3% of travelers. Although this is a relatively large multicenter sample, GTEN is limited to a subset of specialized travel and tropical medicine clinics in the United States and does not capture travelers who seek pre-travel care from primary care and other providers, and data have only been collected since 2009.

As travel medicine continues to grow with regard to both number of practitioners and subject matter, infectious diseases will remain an important and perhaps an even greater component of the discipline. Likewise, the epidemiology of infectious diseases in travelers will remain important, with surveillance and reporting potentially being enhanced and refined, resulting in more complete and informative data being available to both clinical and public health practitioners and allowing more informed decisions to be made with regard to protecting the health of the traveler.

References

1 Brunette G (ed.) *CDC Health Information for International Travel 2014: The Yellow Book.* New York: Oxford University Press, 2014.

2 World Health Organization. *International Travel and Health 2012.* Geneva: World Health Organization, 2012.

3 Harvey K, Esposito DH, Han P, et al. Surveillance for travel-related disease – GeoSentinel surveillance system, United States, 1997–2011. *MMWR Surveill Summ* 2013; **62**(3): 1–23.

4 Leder K, Torresi J, Libman M, et al. GeoSentinel surveillance of illness in returned travelers, 2007–2011. *Ann Intern Med* 2013; **158**: 456–468.

5 Mühlberger N, Jelinek T, Gascon J, et al. Epidemiology and clinical features of vivax malaria imported to Europe: sentinel surveillance data from TropNetEurop. *Malaria J* 2004; **3**: 5.

6 Jelinek T, Bisoffi Z, Bonazzi L, et al. Cluster of African trypanosomiasis in travelers to Tanzanian national parks. *Emerg Infect Dis* 2002; **8**: 634–635.

7 Leder K, Wilson M, Freedman DO, Torresi J. A comparative analysis of methodological approaches used for estimating risk in travel medicine. *J Travel Med* 2008; **15**: 263–272.

8 Behrens RH, Carroll B. The challenges of disease risk ascertainment using accessible data sources for numbers of travelers. *J Travel Med* 2013; **20**: 296–302.

9 Mali S, Kachur SP, Arguin PM. Malaria surveillance – United States, 2010. *MMWR Surveill Summ* 2012; **61**(SS-2): 1–17.

10 Leder K, Black J, O'Brien D, et al. Malaria in travelers: a review of the GeoSentinel surveillance network. *Clin Infect Dis* 2004; **39**: 1104–1112.

11 LaRocque RC, Rao SR, Lee J, et al. Global TravEpiNet: a national consortium of clinics providing care to international travelers – analysis of demographic characteristics, travel destinations, and pretravel healthcare of high-risk US international travelers, 2009–2011. *Clin Infect Dis* 2012; **54**: 455–462.

CHAPTER 2

Basic epidemiology of non-infectious diseases

Richard C. Franklin & Peter A. Leggat
James Cook University, Townsville, Queensland, Australia

Introduction

Travel can be an exciting mix of new experiences, friends, sights, food, and sensations. It can awaken a person's desire for adventure, but unfortunately it can also be fatal, and although most travel medicine focuses on the exotic, the infectious, and the unusual [1,2], it can be everyday activities, such as driving or living with a disease, that are the cause of tragedy. In this chapter, we explore the basic epidemiology of non-infectious disease while traveling, including illnesses due to travel, deaths, and morbidity while traveling, risk and risk factors, common causes of accidents and prevention strategies, the potential risks befalling children and older travelers, and dental problems encountered while traveling.

Establishing a picture of the modern travelers and their destinations is important for aiding our understanding of what types of non-infectious disease conditions may occur and how interventions might take place. This is part of the travel health risk assessment. Although travel medicine focuses on those traveling outside their country, usually abroad, there is a wider role for the travel medicine specialist in providing advice to all types of travelers, including those undertaking recreational activities close to home. Although an underexplored area, there are more people who travel within their country than those who travel to destinations abroad, yet few of these travelers seek advice about keeping themselves healthy and safe.

In this chapter, a broad definition of travel medicine has been used: travel medicine includes all those who travel (no matter what the distance) and who are exposed to a risk that is outside their normal day-to-day routine or where travel is a common part of their work environment that exposes them to risk where a travel medicine specialist would be an appropriate person from whom to seek advice. This would include the older traveler who is traveling with a caravan around their country and not used to traveling long distances, towing a caravan, or visiting sites that have different hazards from those at home such as caves with bats or waterways. It would also include the person who travels for work and is exposed to risky environments, such as divers or truck drivers traveling into areas where there are tropical diseases and hazards, sometimes lurking just below the water's surface.

Essential Travel Medicine, First Edition.
Edited by Jane N. Zuckerman, Gary W. Brunette and Peter A. Leggat.
© 2015 John Wiley & Sons, Ltd. Published 2015 by John Wiley & Sons, Ltd.

Why do people travel?

The number of people traveling continues to grow, with over 1 billion international tourist arrivals in 2012 [3]; however, each person travels for a different reason, and this places each traveler at a different risk of injury or, for example, a cardiovascular event. Broadly, there are five groups of travel scenarios:
- pleasure – leisure, recreation, and holidays;
- visiting friends and relatives (VFR);
- work related;
- religion;
- medical (including dental).

Even within each of these categories there are different groups of travelers; for example, within the work-related group there are those traveling to conferences, those who will be visiting hostile zones, and those working in the aftermath of a disaster or humanitarian crisis, each bringing its own risks. For the more dangerous work-related travel, the people traveling normally have full occupational medical examinations before traveling. Medical tourism continues to grow as the cost of medical care in developed countries increases, and this has its own risk [4]. There is also a subset of travelers who are seeking death (suicide) [5] as opposed to dark travel where the traveler seeks out sites of morbid fascination [6].

There is also a group who cross over between medical tourism and VFR. This group may travel with a chronic condition, such as cancer, and knowing they are unwell and may not have long to live, seek out relatives, friends, or just their country of birth to spend some of their last remaining time [7].

Travel pattern?

Travel patterns in the 20th and 21st centuries have seen dramatic changes in the way people move around the world and the volume of people traveling. In 2012, over half (52%) of all international travel was by air, 40% was by road, 6% by water and 2% by rail [3]. Although the majority of people travel by air, a recent study of people who died while traveling to the United States found that the majority (62%) of deaths were of people undertaking sea travel (predominately cruise ship passengers) (85%) and air travel (38%), with just one death associated with land travel [8]. These deaths were predominately (70%) from cardiovascular causes, followed by infectious disease (12%) and cancer (6%) [8]. Of the 26 deaths from infectious diseases, 19 also had an underlying chronic disease [8].

Illness due to travel

There are a range of illnesses caused by travel itself, with impact from minor illness to death. Conditions include motion sickness, jet lag, deep venous thrombosis (DVT), altitude sickness, sunburn, dehydration, and alcohol toxicity. See Chapters 3 and 24.

Motion sickness

Anyone can develop motion sickness if enough stimuli are provided [9]. Motion sickness is caused by the brain receiving conflicting sensory information. Risk factors that increase susceptibility include age, gender, people who get migraine headaches and some medications [9]. Approximately two-thirds of people who suffer from migraines are also sensitive to motion [10].

Jet lag

Jet lag is caused when a person's circadian rhythm is out of synchronization with external time cues [11], caused by traveling across three or more time zones [12]. It is estimated that it takes 1 day for each time zone change for the circadian system to realign; however, there is some variability depending on direction; westward is faster [11]. Common complaints include poor sleep, reduced performance, fatigue during the day, and gastrointestinal disturbances [12]. It is also more common in older people. Long-term consequences can include gastrointestinal problems, increased risk of cancer, infertility, and heart disease [11].

Venous thromboembolism

In a meta-analysis, venous thromboembolism (VTE) has been found to be twice as common among travelers than non-travelers. Traveling for longer periods was also found to increase the risk, with an 18–22% increase for every 2-hour increase in travel duration, and travelers were three time more likely to develop DVT or pulmonary embolism [13]. Other factors that have been identified as increasing the risk include age over 40 years, women using oral contraceptive drugs or hormone replacement therapy, obesity, varicose veins on the lower limbs, and genetic thrombophilia [14]. The incidence ranges from 0.2 to 4.8 per 1 million hours of flying [14].

Altitude illness

Altitude illness (sickness) is an issue of significance as more people take up the challenge of reaching new heights. It can occur when people travel above 2500 m and is divided into three syndromes, the most common being acute mountain sickness (AMS) [15]. In a study of trekkers on Mount Kilimanjaro [16], 3% were AMS positive at 2743 m and 47% at 4730 m. There was no difference between those who took a rest day at 3700 m; however, those who were preacclimatized had a significant reduction in AMS. This is consistent with advice that having exposure prior to moving to higher altitude is valuable; also, it is recommended to avoid alcohol, to ascend slowly at a rate of around 500 m each day after 2700 m, and to plan an extra day of acclimatization for every 1000 m [15]. See also Chapter 25.

Death while traveling

There is no definitive source on how many people die each year while traveling, nor do we know what the risk is of suffering death, illness, or injury while traveling.

Estimates of risk vary depending on the country visited and the country of origin (Table 2.1). Some papers only explore particular types of death, such as injury-related death [17]; it does appear, however, that as more people are traveling so are more travelers dying [18,19].

Morbidity while traveling

Our understanding of morbidity amongst travelers is predominately based on data collected in the 1980s [23] and is commonly acquired from insurance data and returning travelers. Unfortunately, common information about what happens to travelers overseas derived from insurance data often excludes pre-existing medical and dental conditions, as this is not covered under their insurance and the information does not include those not insured. We know from Australian data that a significant proportion of travelers require emergency assistance overseas, including for medical and dental problems, requiring medical or hospital treatment or, in a small number of cases, aero-medical evaluation [24]. Common conditions requiring assistance included musculoskeletal disorders (28%), gastrointestinal disorders (15%), dental conditions (14%), and respiratory problems (12%), demonstrating the significant and immediate impact of non-infectious conditions on travelers [24].

Common claims for non-infectious conditions identified in insurance data include musculoskeletal (16%), dental (7%), and cardiovascular (6%) [25]. A recent study exploring common conditions presenting to GeoSentinel clinics from returning travelers included some information on non-infectious conditions (although we note that infectious diseases make up a significant proportion of what is seen within these clinics) [23]. Common non-infectious conditions seen included underlying chronic disease (19/1000 patients), injury (14/1000 patients), neurologic disorders (15/1000 patients), psychologic disorders (12/1000 patients), and cardiovascular disease (8/1000 patients) and make up a very small number of the cases seen post-travel in GeoSentinel clinics [23]. See also Chapter 24.

Risks

Depending on the location where one is traveling, one is more likely to die from non-infectious than infectious causes. For example, in Australia between 2001 and 2003, the most common cause of death was from ischemic heart disease, followed by malignant neoplasms, and nearly one-quarter (23%) of the deaths were from accidents predominately related to transport (14% of all deaths) and drowning (5% of all deaths) [7], and US travelers traveling to Mexico were more likely to die from injuries (51%) than any other cause, followed by circulatory diseases (37%), with motor vehicle accidents and drowning being the most common types of injury event [26]. The type of activities in which a person participates also increases his or her risk of being injured or dying; for example, taking part in aquatic activities increases the risk of drowning, and road travel and the type of vehicle used increase the likelihood of being involved in a road traffic incident.

Table 2.1 Crude rate of traveler deaths and common causes.

Ref.	Population	Time frame	No. of tourist deaths	No. of tourists	Crude rate per 100,000 visitors	Common causes of death
Leggat and Wilks 2009 [7]	Visitors to Australia	2000–2003	1063	34,396,700 (ABS)	0.77	Ischemic heart disease – 26% Malignant neoplasms – 16% Transport injury – 14% Drowning – 5% Suicide – 3%
Tonellato et al. 2009 [17]	Injury deaths of US travelers	2004–2006	2361	114,627,758	0.69	Vehicle accidents – 33% Violent deaths – 34% Drowning – 11% Air accidents – 3% Drug-related – 3% Disasters – 2%
Lunetta 2010 [18]	Finnish residents traveling abroad	1969–2007	6894	2005–2007 = 3,163,000	0.75	Natural causes – 67% Injuries – 27%
Redman et al. 2011 [20]	Scottish travelers	2000–2004	572			Trauma – 20% Non-infectious diseases – 75% Infectious diseases – 2%
Lawson et al. 2012 [8]	International travelers arriving in the USA	1 July 2005 to 30 June 2008	213	137,897,860 (http://tinet.ita.doc.gov/)	0.05	Cardiovascular – 70% Infectious diseases – 12% Cancer – 6% Unintentional injury – 4% Intentional injury – 1%

(continued overleaf)

Table 2.1 (*continued*)

Ref.	Population	Time frame	No. of tourist deaths	No. of tourists	Crude rate per 100,000 visitors	Common causes of death
Pawun et al. 2012 [21]	Visitor to Chiang Mai, Thailand	2010 to 2012	102			Cardiac diseases – 35% Malignant neoplasms – 20% Infectious diseases – 12% Accidents – 4% Suicide – 4% Drug overdoses – 2% Drowning – 1%
MacPherson et al. 2007 [22]	Canadians traveling overseas	1996 to 2004	2410	166,680,000 (http://www.statcan.gc.ca)	0.95–2.79	Natural – 74% Accidental – 18% Suicide – 4% Homicide 4%

Exposure

Although it is difficult to determine if exposure to travel-related disease differs by gender, the reason why male and female travelers present to travel health advisers does vary, with females more likely to present with diarrhea, irritable bowel syndrome, upper respiratory tract infection, urinary tract infection, psychological stressors, oral and dental conditions, or adverse reactions to medication, whereas males are more likely to have febrile illnesses; vector-borne diseases such as malaria, leishmaniasis, or rickettsioses; sexually transmitted infections; viral hepatitis; or non-infectious problems, including cardiovascular disease, acute mountain sickness, and frostbite [27].

Exposure to travel-related disease is not static and changes depending on the activity that the person is undertaking, the location they are visiting, the time of year, how long they are staying in a particular area, and where they are staying. Much is known about risk and transmission of infectious diseases among travelers, including sexually transmitted infections, although again subpopulations such as adolescents are at greater risk [28]. Overseas travel involving British university students found that they were more likely to drink alcohol, use cannabis, and have casual sex during their holiday [28].

Risk taking

The difference between risk taking and perceived risk in travel is not well understood and is influenced by travelers' existing knowledge, beliefs, socio-cultural background, previous experiences, familiarity, and ability to identify and control risk [29]. It is interesting that perception of risk varies little between pre- and post-travel except for accidents, which increase post-travel; however, risks due to exposure to mosquitoes were perceived to be the highest risk [30]. Some risk taking is expected and is part of the reason why people travel [31]. Risk taking is also influenced by many factors, such as time of year, the activities being undertaken, length of stay, age, gender, and where people stay. For example visiting areas where there is snow in the winter would not only imply the presence of low temperatures and thus possible hypothermia, but also skiing-related injuries and the need for advice about using a helmet [32]. However, during summer trekking may be involved and participants should be aware of body-stressing issues, dehydration, and sunburn. It is also interesting that approximately half of travelers in a recent Australian study have participated in one activity with an injury risk in their last overseas trip, and males and those aged 18–24 years were significantly more likely to participate in at least one activity with an injury risk; common activities included motorcycles and/or off road vehicles (24%), water sports other than swimming (23%), and contact sports (8%) [33]. See also Chapters 3 and 5.

High-risk travelers

There are those travelers who are at a higher risk of being ill or sustaining an injury when traveling, and also those with underlying medial and physical conditions that may worsen while traveling [34]. People who may be at higher risk of being injured include those intending to undertake thrill-seeking or risky activities, sports, going to places where there are known risks such as the "full moon festival" [35], and those who have underlying health conditions that may place them at greater risk of injury or death, such as people with cardiovascular or respiratory conditions who undertake scuba diving or snorkeling [36]. It should also be noted that some high-risk activities are excluded under the terms and conditions of travel insurance policies, hence for those intending to undertake these activities, careful consideration of the policy is recommended.

Providing advice to travelers

The challenge for all travel medicine consultants is to have the difficult conversation around what people may do while traveling – most of the time people are interested in having their vaccinations to protect them against infectious disease and do not want to discuss the things that may kill them! There are a range of risky activities that people undertake when they travel: by far the most dangerous is being on the road, followed by being in, on, or around water, which includes scuba diving, boating, and marine creatures. There are a range of other risky activities where people do need to ensure their safety, including hiking around volcanoes, climbing, caving, canyoning, canoeing, being close to wild animals, and thrill-seeking activities such as sky diving, bungee jumping, climbing glaciers, and snow skiing. Associated with a range of these activities is the use of alcohol and drugs, which can increase the risks of injury and trauma. The experience of trauma can, of course, give rise to a risk of infectious disease by exposing travelers to local hospitals and medical facilities in countries where infection control practices may be suboptimal [33].

Road travel

Road travel is by far the most risky activity that any traveler can undertake; it is estimated that 1.3 million people die each year as a result of road traffic injuries [37]. These incidents involve cars, trucks, buses, motorcycles, bicycles, and pedestrians. This risk increases for travelers who visit countries where people drive on the "wrong" side of the road, and this includes pedestrians [38].

Although much of the advice about road travel is what one would call common knowledge and common sense, and should also be used at home, it is valuable to reiterate the key points: wear a seat belt (including in taxis and buses where fitted) and ensure that children are in a safety seat, adhere to speed limits, take breaks at least every 2 hours on long trips, avoid driving at night, pay close attention to the side of the road you are supposed to be driving on if in a country that drives on the opposite side, avoid alcohol and driving, wear a helmet when riding motorcycles and bicycles, do not text while driving, avoid talking on your mobile phone and driving (it is illegal in many countries, including using hands-free devices), avoid overloaded buses and boats, be alert when crossing the road, practice in a safe area before using a vehicle with which you are unfamiliar, and check about any special local road rules (e.g., "hook turns" in Australia; being on the correct side of the road; knowing what to do when a road train is approaching in the outback) [39]. As a final note, relying too heavily on technology such as navigation systems can also be hazardous, as a recent death in Death Valley, USA, demonstrated [40].

Drowning

Drowning is a significant cause of mortality, with an estimated number of drowning deaths of about 350,000 per annum worldwide [37], although many believe that this is an underestimation as often people are buried without any record and those who drown during flooding, cyclones, typhoons, or other natural disasters are never found [41]. From an exposure perspective, drowning has been found to have a higher fatality rate than road traffic accidents [42], and the drowning death rate in tourists is often higher than that in the local population [19].

Many preventive strategies have been proposed to prevent deaths from drowning, and these strategies vary depending on the age of the person, swimming ability, existing medical conditions, and type of body of water, such as rivers, lakes, or oceans [43]. These preventive strategies may be primary, such as encouraging swimming pool fencing legislation in host countries, secondary, such as the presence of lifeguards or wearing of personal flotation devices (PFDs) (or life jackets), and tertiary, such as learning first aid, including cardiopulmonary resuscitation (CPR) [44]. Restricting a child's access to water via the use of barriers is effective for children under the age of 5 years [45]; however, as they become older this method is less reliable. Supervision either by a parent or by trained personnel such as a life saver or lifeguard can also save a life [45]. The use of PFDs is also valuable, but they need to be worn prior to the event and placed in locations that are easy to access. Being able to swim is not a panacea for preventing drowning, but it does increase one's chances of survival. Also, being unprepared to rescue a family member, particularly a child, has been found to be a notable cause of death and is particularly risky for tourists [46].

Alcohol and drowning are commonly found together in adults [47], and the best advice is to try to avoid any activity that involves water, such as swimming, supervising children, or operating water craft, after consuming alcohol [43]. Swimming between the safety flags, particularly at beaches, is important for all tourists, and wearing of personal flotation devices, even when on boats, can also save lives [48].

Scuba diving

Scuba diving is not without its risks, but they are small. It is estimated that the annual death rate per diver ranges from 0.48 per 100,000 student dives to 1.03 per 100,000 non-course dives, with an annual fatality rate ranging from 3.4 to 71 per 100,000 divers. Common triggers of scuba deaths are gas supply problems, entrapment/entanglement, and equipment troubles. Common disabling agents are emergency descent, insufficient breathing gas, and buoyancy problems. Common causes of death are drowning (~70%), cardiac issues (~13%), arterial gas embolism (~12%), trauma (~4%), decompression sickness (~1%), and marine life (~1%). Risk factors include lack of experience, underlying medical conditions (e.g., cardiac-related and diabetes mellitus), rapid ascent, running out of gas, buoyancy problems, obesity, age, use of helium, and maximum dive depth [49].

Ensuring that a person is medically fit to scuba dive is an important consideration for the travel health adviser, and a diving medical examination or referral to a diving medicine specialist should be undertaken. Unfortunately, many older travelers think that they are able to do what they were doing when they were younger, and a diving medical examination assists in establishing that a traveler is medically fit to dive, which can be a moderately strenuous recreational activity for travelers. In host countries, reminding divers about the basic rules of diving is important, such as never to dive or snorkel alone [43]. A recent Australian study has shown that cardiac-related causes of death are common in snorkelers, followed by drowning, and that 57% of deaths were of people with a known history of cardiac disease [36].

Children

Children represent a vulnerable group, and this can be exacerbated when traveling. Deaths of children who travel are more likely to be from injuries such as in road traffic accidents and by drowning, but the risk of infectious diseases is also present. Deaths from injuries are preventable and not inevitable, and many of the risks faced by children when traveling are the same as when adults travel [50].

Common causes of injury death in children include road traffic accidents (in all types of vehicles, while riding bicycles, and also as a pedestrian), drowning, fires and burns, falls, bites and stings, and poisoning [50]. Prevention strategies include adequate supervision, appropriate seating and use of seat belts in vehicles, wearing a helmet, use of personal flotation devices, swimming in areas where lifeguards are present, avoiding areas with open fires, ensuring that a fire is appropriately extinguished and the area allowed to cool, ensuring that children are not able to leave an area when a supervisory adult is indisposed (e.g., using a chain latch on the door), avoiding animals, and keeping medications and chemicals out of reach. The principles of removing the hazard, placing a barrier between the child and the hazard, supervision, and the use of protective equipment will help to ensure the safety of children.

Older travelers

Although age-related causes of death are a concern for the traveler, there is not a hard-and-fast rule about where this occurs; however, it is clear that older travelers are a vulnerable group when it comes to travel [7,20,22,51]. A recent study [51] exploring the travel-related illness of people over 60 years of age found that compared with a younger age group (18–45 years), they undertook shorter trips, were more likely to undertake organized tours, were less likely to seek medical advice, and were more likely to have chronic diseases. Older travelers are exposed to many of the same risks as their younger counterparts, with some expected differences such as transmission of sexual diseases [51]. The increase in premium tours for mature adults, while providing a safer environment, also results in a number of illnesses and injuries [52,53] and is of concern as these travelers may be less likely to seek prior medical advice.

Dental

Dental problems constitute 7–8% of all claims for travel insurance. Common problems for travelers include pre-existing conditions (26%), particularly those requiring prosthodontic conditions, which are normally rejected by insurers [54]. The most common claims for travelers were those requiring conservative (mostly fillings) (30%), endodontic (mostly root canals) (18%), and prosthodontic (26%) treatment, with a small number of these due to trauma. Females (57%) and those over 60 years of age (52%) were more likely to require dental treatment [25,54]. Travelers should be encouraged to visit their dentist prior to departure. See also Chapters 3 and 18.

Sand hazards

Although sand may not be a common hazard that one would normally think about when heading to the beach, there have and continue to be a number of deaths of people who die of asphyxia following entrapment, normally from the collapse of a hole in the sand. A recent study [55] highlighted five cases of teenagers aged 15–19 years who died following the collapse of the holes they were digging. These holes were often 2 m or more deep and represented significant challenges for the extraction and resuscitation of the victims, with sand continuing to fill the holes, the weight of the sand compressing the torso, making breathing difficult, and sand filling the mouth and general airways [55].

Volcanoes and glaciers

Visits to volcanic regions and glaciers are not new; however, as areas that previously would have been available only to adventurers are now available to the tourist, more people are visiting areas where there are potentially significant risks, and volcanoes and glaciers are examples of such areas. For volcanoes, some of the risks include potentially toxic gases (such as carbon dioxide, sulfur dioxide, hydrogen chloride, and methane), seismic activity, lava flows, mudflows, sharp glass-like surfaces, heat, dehydration, and methane explosions [56]. However, although there are deaths associated with visits to volcanoes, it is often the travel to the location that is the most dangerous part [57]. For glaciers, risks of falling, cold, and overuse injuries are common [58].

Conclusion

Non-infectious causes of death are a common cause of mortality among travelers, with road travel and drowning the most common injury-related causes, followed by cardiovascular disease and cancer. Similarly, common non-infectious causes of morbidity among travelers appear to be related to musculoskeletal problems, including trauma, and to cardiovascular disease and other problems. One of the most significant challenges for the travel health adviser is to convey messages of prevention to a population that is more concerned about exposure to infectious diseases.

References

1 Talbot EA, Chen LH, Sanford C, et al. Travel medicine research priorities: establishing an evidence base. *J Travel Med* 2010; **17**: 410–415.
2 Sanford C. Urban medicine: threats to health of travelers to developing world cities. *J Travel Med* 2004; **11**: 313–327.

3 WTO. *UNWTO Tourism Highlights, 2013 Edition.* Madrid: World Tourism Organization, 2013. http://www.e-unwto.org/content/hq4538/fulltext?p=abbec8cc7d304f969e7b8be4a1b5ca45 &pi=0#section=1177583&page=1 (accessed 27 January 2015).

4 Whittaker A, Manderson L, Cartwright E. Patients without borders: understanding medical travel. *Med Anthropol* 2010; **29**: 336–343.

5 Miller DS, Gonzalez C. When death is the destination: the business of death tourism – despite legal and social implications. *Int J Cult Tourism Hospitality Res* 2013; **7**: 293–306.

6 Biran A, Hyde KF. New perspectives on dark tourism. *Int J Cult Tourism Hospitality Res* 2013; **7**: 191–198.

7 Leggat PA, Wilks J. Overseas visitor deaths in Australia, 2001 to 2003. *J Travel Med* 2009; **16**: 243–247.

8 Lawson CJ, Dykewicz CA, Molinari NAM, et al. Deaths in international travelers arriving in the United States, July 1, 2005 to June 30, 2008. *J Travel Med* 2012; **19**: 96–103.

9 Lankau EW. Motion sickness. In: Brunette GW (ed.) *CDC Health Information for International Travel 2012: The Yellow Book.* New York: Oxford University Press, 2012, pp. 67–69.

10 Baloh RW. Neurotology of migraine. *Headache* 1997; **37**: 615–621.

11 Arendt J. Managing jet lag: some of the problems and possible new solutions. *Sleep Med Rev* 2009; **13**: 249–256.

12 Libassi L, Yanni EA. Jet lag. In: Brunette GW (ed.) *CDC Health Information for International Travel 2012: The Yellow Book.* New York: Oxford University Press, 2012, pp. 65–67.

13 Chandra D, Parisini E, Mozaffarian D. Meta-analysis: travel and risk for venous thromboembolism. *Ann Intern Med* 2009; **151**: 180–190.

14 Gavish I, Brenner B. Air travel and the risk of thromboembolism. *Intern Emerg Med* 2011; **6**: 113–116.

15 Hackett PH, Shlim DR. Altitude Illness. In: Brunette GW (ed.) *CDC Health Information for International Travel 2012: The Yellow Book.* New York: Oxford University Press, 2012, pp. 60–65.

16 Jackson SJ, Varley J, Sellers C, et al. Incidence and predictors of acute mountain sickness among trekkers on Mount Kilimanjaro. *High Alt Med Biol* 2010; **11**: 217–222.

17 Tonellato DJ, Guse CE, Hargarten SW. Injury deaths of US citizens abroad: new data source, old travel problem. *J Travel Med* 2009; **16**: 304–310.

18 Lunetta P. Injury deaths among Finnish residents travelling abroad. *Int J Inj Contr Saf Promot* 2010; **17**: 161–168.

19 Morgan D, Ozanne-Smith J, Triggs T. Descriptive epidemiology of drowning deaths in a surf beach swimmer and surfer population. *Inj Prev* 2008; **14**: 62–65.

20 Redman CA, MacLennan A, Walker E. Causes of death abroad: analysis of data on bodies returned for cremation to Scotland. *J Travel Med* 2011; **18**: 96–101.

21 Pawun V, Visrutaratna S, Ungchusak K, et al. Mortality among foreign nationals in Chiang Mai City, Thailand, 2010 to 2011. *J Travel Med* 2012; **19**: 334–351.

22 MacPherson DW, Gushulak BD, Sandhu J. Death and international travel – the Canadian experience: 1996 to 2004. *J Travel Med* 2007; **14**: 77–84.

23 Freedman DO, Weld LH, Kozarsky PE, et al. Spectrum of disease and relation to place of exposure among ill returned travelers. *N Engl J Med* 2006; **354**: 119–130.

24 Leggat PA, Griffiths R, Leggat FW. Emergency assistance provided abroad to insured travellers from Australia. *Trav Med Infect Dis* 2005; **3**: 9–17.

25 Leggat PA, Leggat FW. Travel insurance claims made by travelers from Australia. *J Travel Med* 2002; **9**: 59–65.

26 Guptill K, Hargarten S, Baker TD. American travel deaths in Mexico. Causes and prevention strategies. *West J Med* 1991; **154**: 169.

27 Schlagenhauf P, Chen LH, Wilson ME, et al. Sex and gender differences in travel-associated disease. *Clin Infect Dis* 2010; **50**: 826–832.

28 Vivancos R, Abubakar I, Hunter PR. Foreign travel associated with increased sexual risk-taking, alcohol and drug use among UK university students: a cohort study. *Int J STD AIDS*, 2010; **21**: 46–51.

29 Leggat PA, Franklin R. Risk perception and travelers. *J Travel Med* 2013; **20**: 1–2.

30 Zimmermann R, Hattendorf J, Blum J, et al. Risk perception of travelers to tropical and subtropical countries visiting a Swiss travel health center. *J Travel Med* 2013; **20**: 3–10.

31 Correia A, do Valle PO, Moço C. Why people travel to exotic places. *International Journal of Culture, Tourism and Hospitality Research* 2007; **1**: 45–61.

32 Ruedl G, Pocecco E, Sommersacher R, et al. Factors associated with self-reported risk-taking behaviour on ski slopes. *Br J Sports Med* 2010; **44**: 204–206.

33 Leggat PA, Zwar NA, Hudson BJ. Hepatitis B risks and immunisation coverage amongst Australians travelling to southeast Asia and east Asia. *Trav Med Infect Dis* 2009; **7**: 344–349.

34 Suh KN, McCarthy AE, Mileno MD, Keystone JS. High-risk travellers. In: Zuckerman JN (ed.) *Principles and Practice of Travel Medicine*, 2nd edn. Oxford: Wiley-Blackwell, 2013, pp. 515–530.

35 *How Many People Die at the Full Moon Party?* 29 September 2013. http://holidayguidethailand. com/koh-phangan/how-many-people-die-at-full-moon-party/ (accessed 25 January 2015).

36 Lippmann JM, Pearn JH. Snorkelling-related deaths in Australia, 1994–2006. *Med J Aust* 2012; **197**: 230–232.

37 Lozano R, Naghavi M, Foreman K, et al. Global and regional mortality from 235 causes of death for 20 age groups in 1990 and 2010: a systematic analysis for the Global Burden of Disease Study 2010. *Lancet* 2013; **380**: 2095–2128.

38 Sleet DA, Ballesteros MF. Injuries & safety. In: Brunette GW (ed.) *CDC Health Information for International Travel 2012: The Yellow Book*. New York: Oxford University Press, 2012, pp. 96–103.

39 Peden M, Scurfield R, Sleet D, et al. *World Report on Road Traffic Injury Prevention*. Geneva: World Health Organization, 2004.

40 Clark K. The *GPS: a Fatally Misleading Travel Companion*. Morning Edition, 26 July 2011. Washington, DC: NPR, 2011. http://www.npr.org/2011/07/26/137646147/the-gps-a-fatally -misleading-travel-companion (accessed 25 January 2015).

41 Szpilman D, Bierens JJ, Handley AJ, Orlowski JP. Drowning. *N Engl J Med* 2012; **366**: 2102–2110.

42 Mitchell RJ, Williamson AM, Olivier J. Estimates of drowning morbidity and mortality adjusted for exposure to risk. *Inj Prev* 2010; **16**: 261–266.

43 Cortés LM, Hargarten SW, Hennes HM. Recommendations for water safety and drowning prevention for travelers. *J Travel Med* 2006; **13**: 21–34.

44 Pearn JH, Franklin RC. "Flinging the squaler" lifeline rescues for drowning prevention. *Int J Aquat Res Educ* 2009; **3**: 315–321.

45 Bugeja L, Franklin RC. An analysis of stratagems to reduce drowning deaths of young children in private swimming pools and spas in Victoria, Australia. *Int J Inj Contr Saf Promot* 2013; **20**: 282–294.

46 Franklin RC, Pearn JH. Drowning for love: the aquatic victim-instead-of-rescuer syndrome: drowning fatalities involving those attempting to rescue a child. *J Paediatr Child Health* 2011; **47**: 44–47.

47 Franklin RC, Scarr JP, Pearn JH. Reducing drowning deaths: the continued challenge of immersion fatalities in Australia. *Med J Aust* 2010; **192**: 123–126.

48 Moran K, Quan L, Franklin RC, Bennett E. Where the evidence and expert opinion meet: a review of open-water recreational safety messages. *Int J Aquat Res Educ* 2011; **5**: 251–270.

49 Denoble PJ, Marroni A, Vann RD. Annual fatality rates and associated risk factors for recreational scuba diving 2011. In: Vann RD, Lang MA. *Recreational Diving Fatalities*. Durham, NC:

Rubicon Foundation. http://archive.rubicon-foundation.org/xmlui/handle/123456789/9303 (accessed 25 january 2015).

50 Sleet DA, Balaban V. Travel medicine preventing injuries to children. *Am J Lifestyle Med* 2013; **7**: 121–129.

51 Gautret P, Gaudart J, Leder K, et al. Travel-associated illness in older adults (>60 y). *J Travel Med* 2012; **19**: 169–177.

52 Shaw MTM, Leggat PA. Illness and injury to travellers on a premium seniors' tour to Indochina. *Travel Med Infect Dis* 2009; **7**: 367–370.

53 Bauer I. Australian senior adventure travellers to Peru: maximising older tourists' travel health experience. *Travel Med Infect Dis* 2012; **10**: 59–68.

54 Leggat PA, Leggat F, Kedjarune U. Travel insurance claims made by travellers from Australia for dental conditions. *Int Dent J* 2001; **51**: 267–272.

55 Heggie TW. Sand hazards on tourist beaches. *Travel Med Infect Dis* 2013; **11**: 123–125.

56 Heggie TW. Volcanoes and travel medicine. *Travel Medicine and Infectious Disease* 2010; **8**: 199–200.

57 Heggie TW. Reported fatal and non-fatal incidents involving tourists in Hawaii Volcanoes National Park, 1992–2002. *Travel Med Infect Dis* 2005; **3**: 123–131.

58 Schöffl V, Morrison A, Schöffl I, Küpper T. The epidemiology of injury in mountaineering, rock and ice climbing. *Med Sport Sci* 2012; **58**: 17–43.

CHAPTER 3

Pre-travel health risk assessment

Peter A. Leggat[1] & Jane N. Zuckerman[2]

[1] James Cook University, Townsville, Queensland, Australia
[2] University College London, London, UK

Introduction

International travel can expose travelers to a variety of health, safety, and security risks, which can result in illness, injury, or even death in some situations. Up to 75% of travelers to the tropics and subtropics experience various forms of health impairment or use of medication, even if minor [1]. About two-thirds of travel insurance claims are for medical and dental conditions, but a significant proportion are for loss, theft, and muggings [2]. Mortality among travelers depends on the destination, but fortunately remains relatively uncommon. For example, among Swiss travelers, the mortality rate of travelers going to developing countries is about 0.8–1.5 per 100,000 per month [1]. All travelers should be encouraged to seek a pre-travel health consultation, as the proportion of all travelers obtaining this advice from a qualified travel health practitioner remains relatively low [3,4]. The pre-travel health consultation is defined by several elements designed to educate and prevent travel-related illness. The most important aspect of the pre-travel health consultation is a comprehensive risk assessment, which helps to inform the advice and interventions given to the traveler.

Defining travel-related risk and the risk assessment

A risk assessment is undertaken as part of the pre-travel health consultation for those travelers who seek travel health advice prior to departure. It involves evaluating the risks associated with both the destination and the individual traveling to this destination [5]. Travel-related risk in this context has been defined as [6]:

> The threat of an adverse event affecting a person's health whilst traveling, which interferes with the trip or necessitates the use of health services.

Generally, risk is evaluated on a gradient from no risk, through to low, medium, and high risk. Most risks, in terms of how they can addressed, could generally be

Essential Travel Medicine, First Edition.
Edited by Jane N. Zuckerman, Gary W. Brunette and Peter A. Leggat.
© 2015 John Wiley & Sons, Ltd. Published 2015 by John Wiley & Sons, Ltd.

categorized as preventable, avoidable, manageable, or unexpected [7]. Indeed, in some situations, it may not be possible to address the risks, or not be able to address the risks fully. In undertaking a pre-travel risk assessment, travel health advisers generally focus on the probability of harm and the severity of possible consequences of travel, and balance these with the probability and the severity of possible consequences of any interventions [8]. The purpose of the risk assessment is to help identify travelers at special risk, such as those with underlying medical conditions, pregnant travelers, children or older travelers, and/or those travelers who maybe undertaking travel that has special risks, for example, long-term travelers, adventure travelers, or those undertaking a pilgrimage or going to a high-risk destination [9].

Pre-travel health consultation

As part of the pre-travel consultation, or indeed as part of the during-travel consultation, where the traveler describes his or her itinerary and/or activities, a risk assessment needs to be undertaken, involving evaluation of the risks associated both with the destination and of the individual traveling to this destination. Information on the exact itinerary, including all the destinations to be visited, and particular medical problems of the traveler needs to be obtained in a timely manner, usually 6–8 weeks before travel for most travelers, perhaps longer when travelers are going overseas for long-term employment, placement, or holiday touring. In the clinic setting, although it is preferable that much of this information is obtained well before the traveler presents for their first face-to-face consultation, often this information is elicited at the time of the pre-travel health consultation. It is necessary to establish:

- The traveler's destinations and schedule.
- Which regions the traveler is going to within these countries.
- Activities planned during travel and anticipating likely scenarios for those activities that are not planned.
- Modes of transport.
- Duration of travel.

This information may be obtained by a standardized questionnaire, which may be developed in the context of a travel clinic network, general practice network, or individual travel health advisers. The World Health Organization (WHO) has provided an example of the types of questions to be asked in *International Travel and Health* [5]. Clinic staff can assist by ensuring that this information is obtained as far in advance as possible before the formal consultation.

In the primary care or general/family practice setting, detailed records may be available to assist in assessing the traveler's medical risks for travel. Travel clinics, general practices, and those in the travel industry should make it clear to prospective travelers that they should present early before travel to obtain their travel medicine health, immunizations, and chemoprophylaxis or be referred for specialist advice, such as a pre-travel dental check. This may be best stated in a formal practice policy and promoted in newsletters, on the website, or through other practice communications, so that travelers are aware of these possible requirements.

Establishing the risks

Risk assessment involves an examination of the epidemiologic evidence, relevant policies, and other clinical considerations and may be modified by the traveler's own responses and preferences. Judgments generally pervade any assessment of risk, including the definition of outcomes that matter, the breadth of the effects to be considered, and measures of consequences. For example, epidemiologic evidence is generally too broad to apply to every location that a traveler is going to, and it changes over time or may even be out of date. Judgments therefore need to be made in the risk assessment. Recently published data by Rossi and Genton reinforce the degree of uncertainty that exists in the pre-travel risk assessment, which must also be managed [10]. This is compounded by travelers who may have only a general idea of the destinations they are planning to visit.

The risks of travel that need to be assessed for most travelers include the following:
- destinations and duration of travel;
- modes of travel;
- purpose of travel;
- traveler's medical history, including concurrent medications;
- recommended interventions.

It is important in the clinical practice of travel medicine to establish the risks associated with the destination and the modes of travel in terms of the hazards and the potential exposure to these hazards and to examine the traveler's medical history to establish host risks (susceptibility and coping strategies), which may impact on selection and use of interventions in the pre-travel health consultation. These facets of risk are then weighed against the risks of the recommended interventions. These various facets of risk in the travel health consultation are summarized in Figure 3.1.

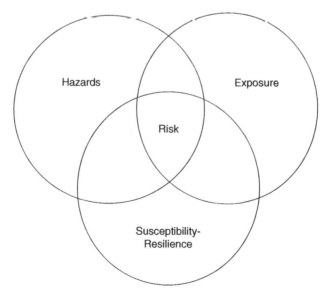

Figure 3.1 Assessment of risk in travel health.

Risks of the destination and duration of travel

The risks associated with the destination and any specific requirements for travel health advice may be obtained from a variety of sources. Online databases have been described for many years as an essential resource for providing the most up-to-date and validated information on the potential risks associated with the destination and for possible key issues to consider in the pre-travel health consultation [11]. Even 20 years ago, 40% of worldwide travel clinics used computerized databases to assist with developing geographically specific recommendations [12]. There are a number of examples of travel health online databases around the world and some examples include:

- Centers for Disease Control and Prevention (CDC), Travel Health site [13].
- TRAVAX [14].

Increasingly, travelers are using the Internet to access information on travel health, so it is important that travel health practitioners keep up-to-date on some of the popular websites visited by travelers for travel health information [15] and on websites directed towards the travel health practitioner [16]. It may be useful to join a travel medicine list server, such as that provided to members of the International Society of Travel Medicine [17], to assist in obtaining advice on difficult destinations or matters, especially those that are not easily resolved by the usual published guidelines and electronic resources.

Published resources are also widely used, such as travel health guidelines covering malaria chemoprophylaxis and travel vaccinations, which are now widely available online. User-friendly guides published by pharmaceutical manufacturers have proved popular amongst general practitioners in previous studies [18]. Regardless of the source, the information obtained needs to be up-to-date and preferably validated by evidence and consensus.

Knowing the destination, in terms of the countries to be visited, can be elicited using questions such as [19]:

- What countries and what parts of these countries are they visiting?
- How long are they going to stay?
- What time of the year are they visiting?
- What are the living conditions?
- What are the current security concerns?
- What activities are they undertaking? Can they walk to the boarding gate? Do they need a diving medical? Can they ascend to altitude? Are they traveling for medical or dental treatment?
- What can the traveler tell you?
- Is there anything special about the destination culturally, legally, or in terms of security?

This needs to be supplemented with further information that may modify their risk, such as [19]:

- Are they traveling alone or as a group?
- What is the traveler's previous travel experience?
- What access is there to appropriate medical and dental care?
- Does the traveler have knowledge about first aid?
- Does the traveler have travel insurance with full coverage?

It is useful to categorize their precise destinations within countries according to the information required for accessing information via online databases. For example, is the traveler going to visit [19]:

- Rural and remote areas and villages and/or have close contact with local people, e.g., healthcare workers.
- Towns and cities, not rural or remote and/or lower-standard accommodation and/or stay over 4 weeks.
- Major cities and tourist resorts and/or medium- to high-standard accommodation and/or reliable water and food sources and/or short-term stays of less than 4 weeks.
- In transit and not exposed to the local environment, e.g., staying in the airplane or short-term stay in a modern airport terminal.

Health and safety risks may be associated only with particular parts or areas of a country and not be a uniform risk throughout a country. In practice, it is virtually impossible to have knowledge of the geographic epidemiology of disease and injury occurrence in every potential destination of travelers and of every country of the world without reference to published guidelines or electronic travel health resources.

Risks of mode of travel

While the majority of the more than 1 billion international travelers travel by airplane and to a lesser extent by road, an increasing number of travelers are choosing to travel by sea, with increasing popularity of cruise ship travel [20]. The risks of the mode of transportation cannot be underestimated. Some travelers may not meet medical guidelines to travel or may need special clearance to fly on commercial aircraft, such as with pre-existing illness, pregnancy, recent surgery, or serious physical or mental incapacity [21], and liaison by travel health advisers with the airline medical departments is usually advisable. Travel health advisers also need to be aware of the potential health effects of modern airline travel. These include the effects of reduced atmospheric pressure, low humidity, closed environment, inactivity, the effects of crossing several time zones on circadian rhythm, alcohol, and the general effects of aircraft motion [21]. These effects can produce conditions such as barotrauma, dehydration, jet lag, motion sickness, claustrophobia and panic attacks, phobias, air rage, and spread of infectious disease and can contribute to the development of deep venous thrombosis (DVT) and venous thromboembolism (VTE) [21]. Concerns have also been raised about the transmission of respiratory tract infections such as severe acute respiratory syndrome (SARS) [22] and tuberculosis [23] through close proximity to infected travelers on commercial aircraft. In an investigation following the 2009 H1N1 avian influenza outbreak, it was found that younger travelers and those on holidays were willing to take more health risks than those who are older or on business trips [24]. However unlikely the risk of transmission of such diseases, the provision of travel health advice and preventive measures for these conditions largely falls to the travel health practitioner.

Although considerable attention has been focused on DVT and VTE, it remains uncertain what the contribution of air travel to the development of this condition among travelers is. What seems to be clear is that the development of DVT and VTE is multifactorial [25]. Although the identification of travelers with predisposing risk factors would seem useful, it is only an option where the risks of side effects of the screening procedure or any interventions do not outweigh the risks of developing DVT after a long-haul flight, which is estimated to be about 1 in 200,000 for travelers on a 12-hour long-haul journey [26]. In the meantime, conservative measures should be recommended, such as in-flight exercises, restriction of alcoholic and caffeinated beverages, and drinking plenty of water. Other preventive measures for some at-risk people, including interventions such as subcutaneous heparin and wearing graduated compression stockings, may need to be considered [27].

People who travel on cruise ships have been exposed to a number of disease risks, including outbreaks of gastrointestinal and respiratory illnesses, with significant attack rates. The CDC [28] has provided information describing recent hygiene inspections of cruise ships visiting US ports. It makes interesting reading for both the traveler and the travel health adviser. Practical considerations for cruise ship travelers include the risks of seasickness and exacerbation of illnesses, which may be difficult to manage at sea.

Accidents and injuries may also befall travelers who may use modes of travel not normally used or undertake activities that they are not used to. This may occur either at their destination or in transit to their destination, such as hiring four-wheel drive vehicles without prior training, unsafe low-cost motor vehicle rentals, motorbike or bicycle riding without helmets, roller-blading, skiing, and the use of unscheduled aircraft or ferries. Accidents will commonly occur, especially in countries where accidents are frequent. Motor vehicle accidents and drowning are common causes of death among travelers [29–33]. Injuries are common causes of travel insurance claims [2]. Travelers need to be certain that they will be covered by their travel or accident insurance if they are driving a vehicle that they are not licensed to operate or if they undertake high-risk recreational or professional sporting activities, including diving. The importance of travel insurance for providing medical assistance and possible aeromedical evacuation where travelers may be exposed to risky modes of transportation cannot be underestimated. In a study of Australian travelers going to Asia, about half of them participated in an activity that had a risk of hepatitis B virus (HBV) infection [3]. HBV vaccination should be considered in all travelers to countries with a moderate to high HBV prevalence (HBsAg $\geq2\%$) and the risk and benefits discussed with the individuals in consultation with the health practitioner. There is no duration of travel without risk of HBV infection; however, travelers with a longer duration of travel (e.g., expatriates) are at greatest risk of HBV infection [34]. Travel health practitioners should provide advice regarding the modes of transmission and the activities that place them at risk of both HBV and HCV infection. This is particularly relevant for those seeking medical or dental treatment abroad.

Risks established from the medical history

Detailed medical information also needs to be obtained from travelers and their records or a referral letter from their usual health provider, which may influence their risks for travel and the advice given to them. A detailed medical history needs to be taken concerning [19]:

- Past travel history, particularly involving any significant medical issues.
- Past medical history, e.g., need for adjusting diabetic treatment.

- Past surgical history, e.g., recent surgery.
- Most recent dental examination.
- Current medications, including the oral contraceptive pill.
- Last menstrual period for females (are they pregnant?).
- Smoking and alcohol history.
- Allergies, including medications and foods.
- Any current illnesses and regular medication.
- Are they traveling alone or with children or with older travelers?
- How fit are they to undertake any proposed exertional activities?

Any pre-existing medical problems will need to be interpreted in the context of official airline policies or travel insurance policies. While airlines have airline policies that may rarely restrict some travelers from flying, most airlines policies have been put in place to assist travelers with various disorders, which can be dealt with much more effectively if they advised in advance to the airlines. Dietary advice for airline travel may also need to be considered, particularly for those travelers with pre-existing conditions, such as diabetes, allergies, or other medical conditions. Allergies among travelers should not be underestimated. It may be possible to arrange special meals on airlines and cruise ships.

Risks of the intervention

Addressing risk in travel medicine is related to modifying risks established in the pre-travel or indeed during the post-travel consultation and is discussed later. Modifying these risks depends largely on preventive interventions, travel health advice and education, and effective management of problems as they arise during or after travel, preferably before they become manifest, for example, through screening and eradication treatment.

The risk of travel may be modified by appropriate preventive measures, including travel health advice and interventions based on:

- Epidemiological evidence.
- Policies/guidelines/consensus statements.
- Availability and use of safety nets, including [19]:
  ○ travel insurance.
  ○ traveling with others.
  ○ access to medical care.
  ○ knowledge of first aid.

A variety of possible interventions may be considered during the pre-travel health consultation. In weighing the foregoing risk assessment against the decision to use an educational intervention, vaccine, or chemoprophylaxis, it is essential to ask the following questions [19]:

- Does the risk of the exposure justify the intervention/cost?
- Can the traveler afford the intervention/cost?
- What do you do if you cannot provide optimal protection because of risks from the medical history or other considerations, such as age of the traveler?

It is important for travel health practitioners to acknowledge that all immunizations, chemoprophylaxis (e.g., antimalarial and drugs to prevent altitude illness), personal insecticide repellents, condoms, and other interventions used by travelers have risks of adverse events or potential side effects, and sometimes serious adverse events. In all instances, it is important to obtain informed consent from the traveler when providing these interventions, and this informed consent may be required to be in written form. There needs to be awareness of current travel health guidelines by travel health practitioners in order to provide the most appropriate advice tailored to the needs of the traveler.

Before employing interventions, valuable background information can be obtained from the traveler concerning their previous experience of travel health interventions to ascertain, for example [19]:

- Tolerability of vaccinations.
- Tolerability of malaria and other chemoprophylaxis.
- Compliance with other preventive and management measures.
- Any other difficulties, problems, or issues that may have arisen during previous travel regarding previous travel health interventions.

In some instances, it may be important to employ screening examinations before employing particular intervention, e.g., glucose-6-phosphate dehydrogenase deficiency before prescribing primaquine or tafenoquine use.

Risk perception

Travelers' responses to pre-travel health advice are influenced by their perceptions of risk, familiarity and concerns about treatments, and the preferred risk management strategies [6]. In terms of risk perception, travelers may confound the likelihood and severity of outcomes and also may be influenced by attributes of the hazard apart from its actual consequences. Familiarity, visibility, and controllability of a hazard all influence the perception of risk [8]. Understanding of the perceptions and also the reality of risk in travel can help travel health practitioners to better prepare travelers for safer and healthier travel.

The presence of pre-existing knowledge and beliefs about diseases and treatments, and their socio-cultural contexts, will already be shaping travelers' perceptions of risk and how they might engage with pre-travel health advice [6]. Noble et al. described various conceptual frameworks, which can be useful in assessing travelers' responses to risks [6]. These frameworks relate traveler's perception of risk and their own ability to respond to it. It has shown that a person's likelihood of taking action in response to a perceived threat to their health is determined by their perceptions of [6]:

- the severity of the threat;
- their susceptibility to the threat;
- the risks, costs, and benefits of taking action; and
- their own ability to undertake the required action successfully.

Travelers are more likely to act to avoid a health threat if they intend to take action following their consideration of the threat and if there are cues to prompt the behavior closer to the time [6]. Noble et al. suggested that there is evidence that travelers' adherence to recommendations may be related to their health beliefs and intentions but that these can be influenced by pre-travel advice [6]. Classically, risk perception can be modified in other ways, for example, by the use of drugs, such as alcohol, which can certainly influence decision-making [35].

Studies have been conducted in a number of groups of travelers to determine their risk perception of travel-related health and safety concerns. For example, students have been reported as having a low risk perception of travel threats and a low corresponding concern for these threats [36]. There has, however, been an increasing focus on the group of travelers visiting friends and relatives (VFR), which has resulted from an increasing number of immigrants to developed countries from less developed countries in Africa, Asia, and Latin America. When these immigrants return to their country of origin as VFR travelers, they are at higher risk of acquiring tropical infections compared with other travelers. Immigrants who return to their country of origin, such as VFR travelers, are more likely to travel to rural areas for long periods of time, to consume contaminated food and beverages, and to have more prolonged, intimate contact with local populations [37]. Consequently, significant rates of morbidity and mortality associated with travel are seen in this specific group of travelers. As a group, they are less likely to seek pre-travel advice or take antimalarial chemoprophylaxis [38]. In terms of assessment, this group of travelers remains a challenge; however, a number of novel approaches have been used [37].

Post-travel consultation

The traveler should also be advised of the possible need for follow-up and management after travel, particularly if going to a high-risk area, if they have any illness upon return, such as fever or persistent or bloody mucous diarrhea [39,40]. It must be impressed upon travelers that, in the event of any illness upon return, they should inform the treating physician of their recent travel and that they have traveled, for example, to a malarious area. This takes the form of a post-travel consultation which can be essential for the well-being of a traveler as well as their family and friends with whom they are in contact (see Chapter 23). It is important when consulting with a traveler with a post-travel health problem that a similar risk assessment to the pre-travel health consultation is undertaken, guided by the presenting features of the illness or injury. As previously alluded to, even travelers who have been seen in the clinic or general practice for pre-travel health advice may need to have the risk assessment re-evaluated if any of the parameters of risk have changed, for example, if they have traveled to a new destination [19].

Post-travel, the risks of travel can be further modified by [19]:
• post-travel screening and interventions;
• malaria treatment; and
• empirical eradication treatment, e.g., deworming treatment.

Effective and early management of post-travel health problems can significantly alter the risks of the conditions encountered and reduce morbidity and mortality to travelers from diseases such as malaria, which may continue to manifest post-travel, as no intervention is necessarily 100% protective. Managing these travel health problems in a timely manner can also reduce the risk to local populations. Additionally, it may assist in reducing the risks to the travelers' own community.

In a study undertaken by Zimmermann et al. [41], who assessed travelers' perception of risk pre- and post-travel and compared this with an expert's opinion, it was interesting that most people did not change their perception of risk from pre- to post-travel, except when an injury had been sustained. Also, depending on age, gender, destination, and region-related travel experience, travelers may perceive the risk differently. It was particularly interesting that men perceived mosquitoes, malaria, and rabies as higher risks than women [41].

Conclusion

Risk assessment is an integral part of the pre-travel, during-travel, and post-travel health consultation. Risk assessment largely determines what health and safety advice and interventions are recommended within the relevant prevailing travel health guidelines. Risk assessment requires time and depends on the available evidence and information, including that given by the traveler. Risk assessment may be assisted by access to online databases and the published literature. Risk assessment of the traveler preferably starts before they enter the consulting room, where travelers may be asked to complete a pre-travel health questionnaire. Travelers should be encouraged to attend a pre-travel health consultation as it provides an opportunity to reduce travel-associated morbidity and mortality.

References

1 Steffen R, DuPont HL, Wilder-Smith A. Epidemiology of health risks in travelers. *Manual of Travel Medicine and Health*, 3rd edn. Hamilton, ON: BC Decker, 2007, pp. 41–49.

2 Leggat PA, Leggat FW. Travel insurance claims made by travelers from Australia. *J Travel Med* 2002; **9**: 59–65.

3 Leggat PA, Zwar NA, Hudson BJ, et al. Hepatitis B risks and immunisation coverage amongst Australians travelling to southeast Asia and east Asia. *Travel Med Infect Dis* 2009; **7**: 344–349.

4 Leggat PA, Leggat FW. Knowledge and acceptance of first aid and travel insurance by hostelers from north and central Queensland, Australia. *J Travel Med* 2002; **9**: 269–272.

5 WHO. *International Travel and Health*. Geneva: World Health Organization, 2012. http://www.who.int/ith (accessed 17 May 2014).

6 Noble LM, Willcox A, Behrens RH. Travel clinic consultation and risk assessment. *Infect Dis Clin North Am* 2012; **26**: 575–593.

7 Zimmer R. The pre-travel visit should start with a "risk conversation." *J Travel Med* 2012; **19**: 277–280.

8 Leggat PA. Risk perception and travelers. *Travel Med Infect Dis* 2006; **4**: 127–134.

9 Simons H, Wong CS, Stillwell A. Travel risk assessment and risk management. *Nurs Pract* 2012; **109**(20): 14–16.

10 Rossi I, Genton B. The reliability of pre-travel history to decide on appropriate counseling and vaccinations: a prospective study. *J Travel Med* 2012; **19**: 284–288.

11 Cossar JH, Walker E, Reid D, Dewar RD. Computerised advice on malaria prevention and immunisation. *BMJ* 1986; **296**: 358.

12 Hill DR, Behrens RH. A survey of travel clinics throughout the world. *J Travel Med* 1996; **3**: 46–51.

13 Centers for Disease Control and Prevention. *Travelers' Health*. http://wwwnc.cdc.gov/travel (accessed 31 March 2014).

14 TRAVAX. Home page. http://www.travax.nhs.uk (accessed 31 March 2014).

15 Leggat PA. Travel medicine online: international sources of travel medicine information available on the Internet for travellers. *Travel Med Infect Dis* 2004; **2**: 93–98.

16 Leggat PA. Travel medicine online: international sources of travel medicine information available on the Internet. *Travel Med Infect Dis* 2003; **1**: 235–241.

17 International Society of Travel Medicine. Homepage. http://www.istm.org (accessed 31 March 2014).

18 Leggat PA, Seelan ST. Resources utilized by general practitioners for advising travelers from Australia. *J Travel Med* 2003; **10**: 15–18.

19 Leggat PA. Risk assessment in travel medicine. *Travel Med Infect Dis* 2006b; **4**: 126–134.

20 United Nations World Tourism Organization. Home Page. http://www.unwto.org (accessed 31 March 2014).

21 Graham H, Putland J, Leggat P. Air travel for people with special needs. In: Leggat PA, Goldsmid JM (eds.) *Primer of Travel Medicine*, 3rd edn. Brisbane: ACTM Publications, 2005, pp. 100–112.

22 Olsen SJ, Chang HL, Cheung TY, et al. Transmission of the severe acute respiratory syndrome on aircraft. *N Engl J Med* 2003; **349**: 2416–2422.

23 WHO. *Tuberculosis and Air Travel*. Geneva: World Health Organization, 2001.

24 Aro AR, Vartti AM, Schreck M, et al. Willingness to take travel-related health risks – a study among Finnish tourists in Asia during the avian influenza outbreak. *Int J Behav Med* 2009; **16**: 68–73.

25 Mendis S, Yach D, Alwan A. Air travel and venous thromboembolism. *Bull World Health Organ* 2002; **80**: 403–406.

26 Gallus AS, Goghlan DC. Travel and venous thrombosis. *Curr Opin Pulm Med* 2002; **8**: 372–378.

27 Zuckerman JN. Recent developments: travel medicine. *BMJ* 2002; **325**: 260–264.

28 Centers for Disease Control and Prevention. *Staying Healthy on a Cruise*. http://www.cdc.gov/features/CruiseShipTravel/ (accessed 31 March 2014).

29 Steffen R. Travel medicine: prevention based on epidemiological data. *Trans R Soc Trop Med Hyg* 1991; **85**: 156–162.

30 Guce CE, Cortes LM, Hargarten S, Hennes HM. Fatal injuries of US citizens abroad. *J Travel Med* 2007; **14**: 279–287.

31 Prociv P. Deaths of Australian travellers overseas. *Med J Aust* 1995; **163**: 27–30.

32 MacPherson DW, Gushulak BD, Sandhu J. Death and international travel-the Canadian experience: 1996–2004. *J Travel Med* 2007; **14**: 77–84.

33 Leggat PA, Wilks J. Overseas visitor deaths in Australia, 2001 to 2003. *J Travel Med* 2009; **16**: 243–247.

34 Johnson DF, Leder K, Torresi J. Hepatitis B and C infection in international travelers. *J Travel Med* 2013; **20**: 194–202.

35 George S, Rogers RD, Duka T. The acute effect of alcohol on decision making in social drinkers. *Psychopharmacology* 2005; **182**: 160–169.

36 Heywood AE, Zhang M, MacIntyre CR, Seale H. Travel risk behaviours and uptake of pre-travel health preventions by university students in Australia. *BMC Infect Dis* 2012; **12**: 43.

37 Fulford M, Keystone JS. Health risks associated with visiting friends and relatives in developing countries. *Curr Infect Dis Rep* 2005; **7**: 48–53.

38 Leder K, Lau S, Leggat PA. Innovative community-based initiatives to engage VFR travelers. *Travel Med Infect Dis* 2011; **9**: 258–261.

39 Ryan ET, Wilson ME, Kain KC. Illness after international travel. *N Engl J Med* 2002; **347**: 505–516.

40 Thielman NM, Guerrant RL. Acute infectious diarrhea. *N Engl J Med* 2004; **350**: 38–47.

41 Zimmermann R, Hattendorf J, Blum J, et al. Risk perception of travelers to tropical and subtropical countries visiting a Swiss travel health center. *J Travel Med* 2013; **20**: 3–10.

CHAPTER 4

Setting up a travel clinic

Marc T.M. Shaw[1] & Claire S. Wong[2]

[1] *James Cook University, Townsville, Queensland, Australia*
[2] *WORLDWISE Travellers Health Centres, Auckland, New Zealand*

Introduction

Travel medicine was described in the first issue of the *Journal of Travel Medicine* in 1991 as a new interdisciplinary field that has the primary goal of keeping travelers alive and healthy [1]. Although the goal of travel medicine remains basically the same, the field has seen some major developments over the last 20 years and is now a medical specialty in its own right. Many of the developments have been driven by the ever-increasing number of international travelers. In 2012, over one billion international tourist arrivals were recorded, an increase of 4% from the previous year [2].

Traditionally, travel health advice has most frequently been provided by part-time practitioners working in a variety of fields, most notably primary care medicine and infectious diseases. Nevertheless, evidence has shown that such advice is not always offered, nor is it always accurate and consistent [3]. Hence there is a need for improvement in the sources of travel health information in this global form of preventive medicine. As a result, increasing numbers of specialist travel medicine services are emerging; a trend that is set to continue as the number of international travelers increases.

As the specialty of travel medicine develops, an effort to define standards of practice and a body of knowledge has been undertaken. The Infectious Diseases Society of America states that although primary care physicians should be able to advise travelers who are in good health undertaking low-risk travel, most travel medicine care should be provided by practitioners who have training in the field, especially for travelers with special health needs [4]. Such guidelines and standards support the rationale for travel advice to be provided in specialist centers and are reinforced by other authorities such as the Faculty of Travel Medicine of the Royal College of Physicians and Surgeons of Glasgow, which recognizes that sections of their guidelines for the practice of travel medicine may be outside the expertise of many primary health practitioners, in which case referral to a specialist should be made [5]. The inference is that specialist centers are in the unique position of being able to provide a dedicated service with advice that is current and of a high standard, delivered by practitioners with experience and training in the field. The key challenge facing travel medicine

Essential Travel Medicine, First Edition.
Edited by Jane N. Zuckerman, Gary W. Brunette and Peter A. Leggat.
© 2015 John Wiley & Sons, Ltd. Published 2015 by John Wiley & Sons, Ltd.

practitioners then is to define the core body of knowledge that transcends the wide spectrum of health perspectives [6].

With this in mind, the first step in setting up a travel clinic is to question whether one has the necessary training and experience to meet the standard expected of a specialist clinic. The United Kingdom's Royal College of Nursing has published a competency document that defines the standard expected of travel medicine practitioners at different levels of experience [7]. Although the focus is on the role of a registered nurse, the guidelines are equally applicable for other disciplines and provide a benchmark to measure competency and training needs.

The underpinning of the pre-travel health consultation is risk assessment and risk management. In order to be able to achieve this, travel medicine providers require a knowledge base derived from the five steps that are the foundation of a traveler's healthy journey [8]:

1 Assessment of their health, and risks to their health, before traveling.
2 Analysis of their anticipated itineraries, with emphasis on infectious and non-infectious disease, and safety and security issues.
3 Provision of appropriate travel health advice for each individual traveler.
4 Recommendation of vaccinations specific to the traveler.
5 Education on the prevention and appropriate self-treatment of travel-related diseases for each traveler.

With these foundation principles in mind, then, let us review the practicalities of setting up a travel clinic. What are the day-by-day elements that travel clinics need for their survival? Ongoing discussion will focus on the "building blocks" of success.

Aims of the clinic

Once the decision to set up a travel clinic has been made, the aims of that clinic need to be considered. A cornerstone of travel medicine is the prevention of communicable disease through proper country-specific health information, including up-to-date routine immunizations. The information given to intending travelers' needs to be academically based yet practical, and it must be correct. Although there is a perception that both vaccinating travelers and administering antimalarial medication are of prime importance at travel health clinics, health education and risk assessment of the upcoming trip need to be the prime focus of all pre-travel consultations [9].

A traveler's health clinic is formed from a continually evolving nidus that will probably refocus from one year to the next, in response to the clinic's growing experience and its knowledge of international events and expectations for safe and healthy travel [7]. The development of policies that enable the efficient running of the clinic is significant to the maintenance of its services [10]. The following aspects will assist.

The basics: "four walls and a space"

The intended location of the clinic will impact on numerous aspects of its function, including the services able to be provided and opening hours. If the clinic is to be free-standing, a visible location is preferable to generate business [6,8]. Clinics hosted within an existing organization may have restrictions on operating hours.

The available space will determine the number of consultation rooms that can be provided and whether travel health products can be offered and displayed. Such attributes need to be targeted to the intended customers of the clinic. Other primary questions that will need to be answered are: Can the clinic be accessed easily? Is parking available? Is public transport to the clinic an option? If post-travel services are to be offered, then is there access to laboratory and radiology facilities?

The legal requirements for operating a travel clinic will vary depending on the country in which the clinic is operating, so it is essential to research these before deciding on a property to ensure that all the requirements for facilities can be met and accommodated. Adequate insurance is a priority and should include not just the buildings and contents, but also professional indemnity and malpractice insurances. Additional insurance policies may also be required by individual clinical staff, usually provided by professional bodies and trade unions.

Equipment: "what's essential and what's not"

Other than a reception area for receiving and parking intending travelers, a clinic needs one or more consulting rooms with a medical plinth that have the capacity for counseling and physical assessment [6,8]. The additional presence of a sink for hand washing, hazardous waste disposal units, sanitation and sterilization units for the clinic, and toilet access for staff and travelers will depend on the clinic's location and its desired range of services.

A large part of any travel clinic's business is the administration of vaccines, which need to be stored in an appropriate refrigerator. Ideally, a commercial pharmacy or vaccine refrigerator should be purchased, which will include temperature recording devices and have automatic defrosting. Information on the handling and storage of vaccines is available from numerous sources, and regional guidelines should be consulted.

Availability and ordering of travel vaccines will vary according to location. The type and number of each vaccine stocked will be guided according to the services that the clinic provides. Demand for vaccines fluctuates in response to seasonal global travel and, until the clinic becomes established, will be difficult to predict. An inventory of vaccines is useful to ensure a minimum supply but will require regular review and will be determined by the delivery times of vaccine suppliers. Yellow fever immunization is a prime travel clinic responsibility, yet in order to be able to administer the vaccine, the clinic and/or clinician must meet the requirements of the national authority.

Computer and Internet access is now vital for the successful operation of any travel clinic. There are numerous computer-based clinic management programs available for the booking of appointments and management of patient records and vaccination recalls. It is best to select one that meets the needs of the prospective clinic, and research is required to determine this.

Setting up a travel clinic checklist

Running a travelers' health clinic can be exciting, as it focuses on the motivation of a generally well-focused population. Table 4.1 gives a simple referral guide to "Top

Table 4.1 Top ten tips.

1	Hypothesize and develop the clinic's aims and objectives
2	Develop and update clinic protocols for all aspects of the clinic's management
3	Develop protocols for pre- and post-travel assessments and examination, travelers with special concerns (e.g., the pregnant traveler, children and travel, travelers with medical conditions, the altitude traveler, the adventure traveler)
4	Maintain vaccine storage and regular cold chain assessment
5	Regularly review clinic protocols in dealing with emergencies
6	Consider a "one-stop shop" that has travel health-related products to complement available clinical services
7	Produce essential resources, and information sources, for the clinic
8	Originate clinic patients' advice publications
9	Develop communication links with pharmaceutical and other companies that provide products for the clinic
10	Develop clinic auditing tools, to assess clinic and personnel performance

Source: Shaw 2006 [3]. Reproduced with permission of Elsevier.

Ten Tips" in setting up a travel clinic. This is intended as a "get the show on the road" essential check-list to clear away the detritus of thought and permit concentrated focus on a clinic's development.

Many travel clinics have two main components: (i) a clinical service, which is supplemented by (ii) a merchandise service, each with particular roles [11]. The instituting of the practice within the clinic is dependent upon a number of building blocks, each of which contributes to the presentation of the clinic to a wider traveling public. These are as follows:

1 The setting up of legal documents to cover the business arrangements of the clinic:
   i. Seek advice regarding any local or national guidelines regarding the establishment of travel clinics.
   ii. Take out appropriate insurances for buildings and contents (including the vaccines) and ensure that all clinicians have indemnity insurance to cover their practice at the clinic.
   iii. Find out about the local regulations regarding the administration of yellow fever vaccination.

2 Staffing:
   i. Define the clinicians' role, whether this be doctor, nurse, or pharmacist.
   ii. Define the clinicians' scope of practice.
   iii. Define the roles of the non-clinical staff.
   iv. Develop and define training programs for the clinic staff, clinical and non-clinical.

3 Equipment and supplies, the basis of which will be:
   i. Consultation room furniture.
   ii. Vaccine refrigerator.
   iii. Product displays.
   iv. Information handouts for travelers.
   v. Computer equipment, Internet access, electronic medical records.

    vi. Emergency equipment. It is crucial that the clinic has equipment to deal with medical emergencies such as anaphylaxis. National guidelines on emergency equipment supplies will vary, but the following is an example of a basic anaphylaxis kit:

       a) adrenaline 1:1000 and dosage chart

       b) needles and syringes

       c) oral airways – adult and pediatric

       d) oxygen

       e) bag-valve-mask resuscitator or one-way valve pocket mask, including pediatric and adult sizes and oxygen tubing

       f) access to a telephone and emergency response team

4 Suppliers are the clinic's lifeblood. Make friends with them!

    i. Contact vaccine suppliers.

    ii. Set up accounts with suppliers of medical equipment such as needles, syringes, and plasters.

    iii. Order necessary stationery items.

    iv. Aim to offer a range of travel health products for sale to complement the travel consultation.

5 Policies and procedures. The development of clinic policies that enable the efficient running of the clinic are significant to the maintenance of its services [12]:

    i. Develop policies for health and safety, including needlestick injuries.

    ii. Devolve responsibility for cold chain maintenance and vaccine ordering to an appropriate staff member.

    iii. Find out the appropriate protocol for the reporting of vaccine adverse events.

    iv. Develop in-house policies for confidentiality, documentation, etc., as appropriate.

    v. Decide whether to offer off-site vaccine administration services and research any legal requirements to do so.

6 Marketing is a travel clinic's survival. Determine a point-of-difference with other clinics and other businesses, and then market this. Professional advice at the outset would be advised.

    i. Decide on a brand; make it appropriate and reflective of the services offered.

    ii. Identify target groups such as travel agents, retail outlets, primary care providers, sports bodies, school groups – and then make initial and regular contact.

    iii. Attend any business networking meetings.

7 Training is the lifeblood of the clinic, so:

    i. Ensure that staff are adequately trained to perform to their roles.

    ii. Make arrangements to meet any mandatory updates required for medical or nursing registration, e.g., CPR training.

    iii. Consider any continuing professional development requirements and how these will be met, including conference and study day attendance.

8 Resources are the brains of the clinic. They are what gives the clinic credibility and what will make it endure. Start to build up clinic resources in the following way:

    i. Ensure that the clinic has the necessary resources (see below) for start-up, including atlases and reference books.

    ii. Consider whether to subscribe to a travel medicine resource for updated country-specific guidance.

    iii. Consider providers of specialist clinical advice should they be required.

    iv. Make contact for referral to laboratory/radiology services or other specialist services.

9 Audit of all aspects of a clinic will maintain skills and preserve standards. This is an essential part of clinic growth and will usually be linked to the maintenance of professional standards. The following are to be considered in evolving audit tools, again specific for each clinic:

    i. Develop a protocol for audit of the clinic and the services provided.

    ii. Decide how to measure quality assurance.

    iii. Adhere to any national audit requirements.

10 The need to have good financial backing for the clinic requires essentials such as:

    i. A sound business plan detailed from good pre-set-up research.

    ii. Good budgeting advice, including anticipated start-up fees and the need to prepare for any unexpected costs.

    iii. Factored staff salaries and ongoing costs until the clinic is viable.

    iv. A good accountant.

Information resources

An essential requirement for any travel health clinic is to establish reliable and up-to-date information sources [6,8]. These should preferably be web-based travel medicine resources and therefore reliable Internet access is required. The publications of the World Health Organization (WHO) and the US Centers for Disease Control and Prevention (CDC) serve as official references for local standards of practice for many countries and are sound primary resources for any clinic progress. Nevertheless, there is an expectation that the travel health practitioner will develop and maintain expertise in the specialty of travel and tropical medicine. The extent of this field is best explored by assessing the International Society of Travel Medicine's *Body of Knowledge* [13].

The *Body of Knowledge* is the scope and extent of knowledge required for health professionals working in the field of travel medicine, and major content areas include the following:

1 global epidemiology of health risks to the traveler;

2 vaccinology;

3 malaria prevention;

4 pre-travel counseling that is designed to maintain the health of the traveling public;

5 post-travel assessment of ill returning travelers.

In addition, any travel health advisory service needs to be authoritative, in order to maintain credibility. Access to global travel, tropical, community, safety and security, and environmental health resources is essential. There is an expectation and, indeed, a responsibility of the clinical staff to access regularly professional and consumer information that is relevant to intending travelers. This needs to include updates on disease epidemiology and outbreaks, individual country yellow fever certificate requirements, global disease and malaria maps, and safety and security advice. Table 4.2 lists six sections of six primary resources that all those setting up

Table 4.2 "6 × 6": essential travel medicine resources in setting up a travel clinic.

Type	Resources
Governmental and professional travel health information sites	CDC, US Centers for Disease Control and Prevention www.cdc.gov/travel/index.htm Health Canada/Santé Canada www.hc-sc.gc.ca Health Protection, Scotland. TRAVAX, Scottish Centre for Infectious and Environmental Health www.travax.scot.nhs.uk International Society for Infectious Diseases ProMED-mail www.promedmail.org International Society of Travel Medicine www.istm.org National Travel Health Network and Centre, England and Wales www.nathnac.org World Health Organization www.who.int
Medical and academic organizations	Bangkok Hospital for Tropical Diseases, Mahidol University, Thailand www.tm.mahidol.ac.th/clinic James Cook University, Queensland, Australia www.jcu.edu.au/school/sphtm Liverpool School of Tropical Medicine www.liv.ac.uk/lstm/lstm.html London School of Hygiene and Tropical Medicine www.lshtm.ac.uk Royal College of Physicians and Surgeons of Glasgow, Scotland; Faculty of Travel Medicine www.rcpsg.ac.uk University College Medical School http://www.ucl.ac.uk/infection-immunity/research/travel
Disease-specific sites	All the Virology on the WWW www.virology.net Hepatitis (viral) www.cdc.gov/ncidod/diseases/hepatitis Malaria Foundation www.malaria.org Human and Animal Rabies www.who.int/GlobalAtlas/ Typhoid and paratyphoid fever www.netdoctor.co.uk/travel/diseases/typhoid.htm World Health Organization; Tropical Diseases www.who.int/topics/tropical_diseases/en/

Table 4.2 (*continued*)

Type	Resources
Specific interest, expedition and adventure, traveler resources	Cruise Ship Medicine http://www.acep.org/Content.aspx?id=24928 Fit For Travel (NHS, UK-based) www.fitfortravel.nhs.uk International Association for Medical Assistance to Travellers, IAMAT www.iamat.org Royal Geographical Society www.rgs.org High Altitude Medicine Guide www.high-altitude-medicine.com/ Wilderness Medicine Society www.wms.org
Safety and security sites	Australian Department of Foreign Affairs & Trade www.dfat.gov.au British Foreign and Commonwealth Office www.fco.gov.uk/travel CIA World Factbook https://www.cia.gov/library/publications/the-world-factbook/index.html FearFree Safety and Security Management www.fearfree.co.nz/ International Crisis Group www.crisisgroup.org/ US State Department www.travel.state.gov/travel/travel_1744.html
Vaccines and pharmaceuticals	British National Formulary www.bnf.org/bnf/ Centers for Diseases Control and Prevention; Vaccine Immunization Statements www.cdc.gov/vaccines/hcp/vis/index.html Institute of Medicine (Immunization Safety Review Committee) www.iom.edu/imsafety NIH Online Vaccine Resource www.niaid.nih.gov/publications/vaccine/pdf/undvacc.pdf National Network for Immunization Information www.immunizationinfo.org/ Vaccines www.vaccines.org

a travel health clinic will find useful. Travel health advisers in general practice tend to use resources produced within their own countries rather than accessing international guidelines, although specialized travel clinics will likely use both country-developed and international resources [14].

Conclusion

Travel medicine and health encompass a wide sphere of disciplines. As a unique and growing specialty, it has become necessary to establish standards of practice. Such standards need to be considered from the setting up of a travel clinic and need to permeate through all aspects of the practice, clinically and non-clinically. Appropriate and defined standards of practice, once in place, will ensure the longevity of the travel clinic.

References

1 Steffen R, DuPont HL. Travel medicine: what's that? *J Trav Med* 1991; **1**: 1–3.
2 World Tourism Organization. *International Tourism Receipts Grew by 4% in 2012*. Press release PR13033, 15 May 2013. http://media.unwto.org/en/press-release/2013-05-15/international-tourism-receipts-grew-4-2012 (accessed 28 January 2015).
3 Shaw MTM. Running a travel clinic. *Trav Med Infect Dis* 2006; **4**: 109–126.
4 Hill DR, Ericsson CD, Pearson RD, et al. The practice of travel medicine: guidelines by the Infectious Diseases Society of America. *Clin Infect Dis* 2006; **43**: 1499–1539.
5 Chiodini JH, Anderson E, Driver C, et al. Recommendations for the practice of travel medicine. *Trav Med Infect Dis* 2012; **10**: 109–128.
6 Virk A, Jong EC. Management of a travel clinic. In: Zuckerman JN (ed.) *Principles and Practice of Travel Medicine*, 2nd edn. Oxford: Wiley-Blackwell, 2013, pp. 37–44.
7 Chiodini J, Boyne L, Stillwell A, Grieve S. *Travel Health Nursing: Career and Competence Development*. London: Royal College of Nursing, 2012.
8 Shaw MTM. Expectations from a travel health professional. In: *Travel Medicine Guide*, 7th edn. *Auckland: MIMS (NZ)*, 2013, pp. 1–6.
9 Hoveyda N, Behrens R. More travel advice and fewer vaccinations are needed. *BMJ* 2003; **326**: 52.
10 Leggat PA, Heydon JL, Menon A. A survey of general practice policies on travel medicine. *J Travel Med* 1998; **5**: 149–152.
11 Leggat PA, Ross M, Goldsmith JM. Introduction to travel medicine. In: Leggat PA, Goldsmith JM (eds.) *Primer of Travel Medicine*, 3rd edn. Brisbane: ACTM, 2005, pp. 3–21.
12 Leggat PA, Seelan ST. Resources utilized by general practitioners for advising travelers from Australia. *J Travel Med* 2003; **10**: 15–18.
13 International Society of Travel Medicine. *Body of Knowledge*. Dunwoody, GA: ISTM. http://www.istm.org/bodyofknowledge (accessed 28 January 2015).
14 Hill DR. Starting, organising and marketing a travel clinic. In: Keystone JS, Kozarsky PE, Freedman DO, et al. (eds.) *Travel Medicine*, 2nd edn. Philadelphia, PA: Mosby Elsevier, 2008, pp. 13–28.

CHAPTER 5

Travel medicine resources

Peter A. Leggat[1], Gary W. Brunette[2], Gilles Poumerol[3], & Jane N. Zuckerman[4]

[1] James Cook University, Townsville, Queensland, Australia
[2] Centers for Disease Control and Prevention, Atlanta, GA, USA
[3] World Health Organization, Geneva, Switzerland
[4] University College London, London, UK

Introduction

Travel medicine is a continually evolving specialty which, by virtue of its very essence, requires practitioners to be up-to-date with respect to risk of exposure to disease and, importantly, security risks amongst others. Accessing information on outbreaks of disease, guidance on best practice, official governmental recommendations, and seeking consular advice or emergency healthcare services abroad can be found readily on the Internet. This chapter aims to provide comprehensive information on available essential travel medicine resources that can be invaluable in supporting the clinical practice of travel medicine.

Professional organizations

The International Society of Travel Medicine (ISTM) (http://www.istm.org/) has over 3000 members in 80 countries and is the largest organization of professionals dedicated to the advancement of the specialty of travel medicine. There are also regional and national travel medicine bodies situated Asia, Pacific, Europe, Africa and North and South America, all of which are listed on the ISTM website.

Other professional societies have a tangential interest in travel medicine. Foremost is the American Society of Tropical Medicine and Hygiene (ASTMH) (http://www.astmh.org), which has a subgroup called the American Committee on Clinical Tropical Medicine and Travelers' Health (ACCTMTH).

There are also a number of important regional groups, which focus on travel medicine or aspects of travel medicine, including, but not exhaustively:

- Faculty of Travel Medicine, Royal College of Physicians and Surgeons of Glasgow (http://www.rcpsg.ac.uk/travel-medicine/about-ftm.aspx)
- Faculty of Travel Medicine, The Australasian College of Tropical Medicine (http://www.travelmedicine.org.au and site for travelers http://www.welltogo.org.au)

- Asia-Pacific Travel Health Society (http://www.apths.org)
- Travel Medicine Society of Ireland (www.tmsi.ie).
   For a fairly comprehensive list of national travel medicine societies, the ISTM website provides a list and details of more than 20 national travel medicine societies worldwide (http://www.istm.org/WebForms/NonIstmLinks/national/default.aspx).
   Other professional organizations that focus on aspects of travel medicine include:
- Wilderness Medical Society (WMS) (http://www.wms.org)
- Infectious Diseases Society of America (IDSA) (http://www.idsociety.org)
- International Society for Infectious Diseases (ISID) (http://www.isid.org)
- Aerospace Medical Association (AsMA) (http://www.asma.org)
- Royal Geographical Society (RGS) Expedition Medical Cell (http://www.rgs.org/OurWork/Fieldwork+and+Expeditions/Specialist+Advice/Medical+Cell/Expedition+Medical+Cell.htm)
- Faculty of Expedition and Wilderness Medicine, Australasian College of Tropical Medicine (http://www.tropmed.org)
- Royal Society of Tropical Medicine and Hygiene (http://www.rstmh.org/)
- Royal College of Nursing Public Health – Travel Health (https://www.rcn.org.uk/development/practice/public_health/topics/travel_health)
- American Travel Health Nurses Association (http://www.athna.org/).

Professional journals

There are two major journals in the field of travel medicine, both of which publish peer-reviewed original articles, reviews, and consensus papers:
- *Journal of Travel Medicine* is published six times per year by ISTM (https://www.istm.org/WebForms/Members/MemberResources/publications/jtm/default.aspx)
- *Travel Medicine and Infectious Disease* is published by Elsevier (http://www.travelmedicinejournal.com/home).
   Most of the other professional organizations mentioned above publish their own journals:
- *American Journal of Tropical Medicine and Hygiene* (ASTMH) (http://www.ajtmh.org)
- *Wilderness and Environmental Medicine* (WMS) (http://wemjournal.org)
- *Journal of Infectious Diseases* (IDSA) (http://jid.oxfordjournals.org)
- *Clinical Infectious Diseases* (IDSA) (http://cid.oxfordjournals.org)
- *International Journal of Infectious Diseases* (ISID) (http://www.ijidonline.com)
- *Aviation, Space, and Environmental Medicine* (AsMA) (http://www.asma.org/publications/asem-journal).
   Other journals of interest include:
- *British Medical Journal* (http://www.bmj.com/)

- *The Lancet* (http://www.thelancet.com/)
- *The Lancet Infectious Diseases* (http://www.thelancet.com/journals/laninf/issue/current)
- *Vaccine* (http://www.journals.elsevier.com/vaccine/).

Travel medicine textbooks

Many textbooks are available of the subject of travel medicine; some of the more notable recently published textbooks are:

- *Travel Medicine: Expert Consult*, 3rd edn. Eds. Jay S. Keystone, David O. Freedman, Phyllis E. Kozarsky, Bradley A. Connor, and Hans D. Nothdurft. Philadelphia, PA: Saunders Elsevier, 2013.
- *Principles and Practice of Travel Medicine*. Ed. Jane N. Zuckerman. Oxford: Wiley-Blackwell, 2013.
- *Wilderness and Travel Medicine*, 4th edn. Eric A. Weiss. Seattle, WA: Adventure Medical Kits, 2012.
- *Manual of Travel Medicine*, 3rd edn. Eds. Allen Yung, Karin Leder, Joseph Torresi, et al. Research, VIC: IP Communications, 2011.
- *Travel and Tropical Medicine Manual*, 4th edn. Eds. Elaine C. Jong and Christopher Sandford. Philadelphia, PA: Saunders Elsevier, 2008.
- *Manual of Travel Medicine and Health*, 3rd edn. Eds. Robert Steffen, Herbert L. DuPont, and Annelies Wilder-Smith. Hamilton, ON: BC Decker, 2007.

Travel medicine training

The most comprehensive approach to training in the field of travel medicine is provided by ISTM, which has established a core curriculum termed the "Body of Knowledge." This outlines all the areas of study pertinent to achieving competence in the profession. ISTM also offers regular examination opportunities to sit for the Certificate in Travel Health. (http://www.istm.org/WebForms/Members/MemberResources/Cert_Travhlth/Default.aspx). In addition, ISTM provides an Online Learning Program (http://www.istm.org/WebForms/Activities/Online.aspx) with topics in a number of areas.

An Intensive Update Course in Clinical Tropical Medicine and Travelers' Health is offered a number of times a year by ASTMH. A Certificate of Knowledge in Clinical Tropical Medicine and Travelers' Health (http://www.astmh.org/Certification_Program/4978.htm) is awarded to those who successfully pass a biennial examination.

The Wilderness Medical Society (WMS) offers many courses relevant to travel medicine, and students can achieve the Diploma in Mountain Medicine (DiMM) (http://wms.org/education/dimm.asp).

There are various postgraduate educational opportunities offered by universities and colleges, and specific examples include:

- Diploma in Travel Medicine awarded by the Royal College of Physicians and Surgeons of Glasgow (http://www.rcpsg.ac.uk/travel-medicine/about-ftm/diploma-course.aspx)
- Graduate Certificate of Travel Medicine, James Cook University, Australia (http://www-public.jcu.edu.au/courses/course_info/index.htm?userText=73511-#.Unb4FFNMfTo)
- Postgraduate Certificate, Diploma and Masters in Travel Medicine (http://www.otago.ac.nz/wellington/departments/primaryhealthcaregeneralpractice/postgraduate/otago021119.html)
- Certificate of Competence in Travel Medicine, South African Society of Travel Medicine (http://www.sastm.org.za/students.php)
- Basic course in Travel Medicine, Royal College of Surgeons of Ireland (http://www.rcsi.ie/international_health_tropical_medicine_teaching).

There are also a number of well-known diploma and short courses in tropical medicine around the world. The Gorgas Memorial Institute of Tropical and Preventive Medicine (www.gorgas.org), based in Peru, in collaboration with the University of Alabama at Birmingham, provides clinical and academic training leading to a diploma in tropical medicine. Other tropical medicine courses (not an exhaustive list) are offered through Mahidol University, the Liverpool School of Tropical Medicine, Humboldt University, Bernhard Nocht Institute, James Cook University, University of Melbourne, the Royal College of Surgeons of Ireland, Tulane University, Prince Leopold Institute of Tropical Medicine, Baylor College, Uniformed Services University of the Health Sciences (USA), and the London School of Hygiene and Tropical Medicine.

Travel medicine practice guidelines

While the professional organizations, text books, journals, and courses mentioned above outline all the elements of travel medicine, the only guidance on clinical standards of care are laid out in "The Practice of Travel Medicine: Guidelines by the Infectious Diseases Society of America" (IDSA Practice Guidelines: http://www.idsociety.org/idsa_practice_guidelines/). Other guidance is also available from:

- *CDC Health Information for International Travel 2014: The Yellow Book.* Centers of Disease Control and Prevention, USA (http://www.cdc.gov/travel/yb/)
- *WHO International Travel and Health 2012* (http://www.who.int/ith/en/)
- *Immunisation Against Infectious Disease* (The Green Book). UK Department of Health, London (https://www.gov.uk/government/collections/immunisation-against-infectious-disease-the-green-book)
- *Health Information for Overseas Travel.* National Travel Health Network and Centre, London (http://www.nathnac.org/yellow_book/YBmainpage.htm)
- *The Australian Immunisation Handbook,* 10th edn., 2013 (http://www.health.gov.au/internet/immunise/publishing.nsf/Content/Handbook10-home)

International organizations

The World Health Organization (WHO) has a unit focused on international travel and health (www.who.int/ith/en). WHO regularly published a travel health guide called *International Travel and Health* (also known as The Green Book) (http://www.who.int/ith/chapters/en/index.html).

Governmental organizations

United States
The primary US federal agency focused on travelers' health is the Centers for Disease Control and Prevention (CDC). The CDC's Travelers' Health Branch maintains a website (www.cdc.gov/travel) with the latest updates, guidance for travelers and clinicians, and information on a variety of topics, including travel-related diseases, travel vaccines, and destinations. The Yellow Book (mentioned above) is produced by the Travelers' Health Branch and is also available on the website (www.cdc.gov/yellowbook).

Canada
Public Health Agency of Canada – Travel Health: http://www.phac-aspc.gc.ca/tmp -pmv/index-eng.php

United Kingdom

- The National Travel Health Network and Centre (NaTHNaC) promotes standards in travel medicine, providing travel health information for health professionals and the public (http://www.nathnac.org/)
- Public Health England: Travel Health (http://www.hpa.org.uk/Topics/Infectious Diseases/InfectionsAZ/TravelHealth/)
- Health Protection Scotland: Travel Health. (http://www.hps.scot.nhs.uk/travel/).

Australia
Smartraveller – The Australian Government's travel advisory and consular information service (http://www.smartraveller.gov.au/): Smartraveller provides travel advice for countries and events, guidance about travel insurance and staying safe and healthy, and getting help overseas.

Travel safety and security issues

United States
The US Department of State (DOS) maintains a website (www.travel.state.gov) focused on travel safety and security issues. The website provides country-specific

information, travel warnings, and travel alerts (http://travel.state.gov/travel/cis_pa
_tw/cis/cis_4965.html). DOS also provides the Smart Travelers Enrollment Program
(STEP), which allows US travelers to register their travel plans.

Canada
Country travel advice and advisories (http://travel.gc.ca/travelling/advisories): official information and advice from the Government of Canada on situations that may
affect safety and well-being abroad, and also other important travel issues such as
security, local laws and culture, entry and exit requirements, and health.

Australia
Travel Abroad (http://smartraveller.gov.au/).

United Kingdom
Foreign and Commonwealth Office Foreign Travel Advice (https://www.gov.uk/
foreign-travel-advice).

Surveillance, disease outbreaks, and epidemiologic bulletins

The WHO posts a Weekly Epidemiological Record (www.who.int/wer/) that contains
global epidemiologic information on cases and outbreaks of diseases. The alert,
response, and capacity building under the International Health Regulations (IHR)
website (www.who.int/ihr) encompasses an integrated system for epidemics and
other public health emergencies.

The CDC Travelers' Health website (http://wwwnc.cdc.gov/travel/notices) posts
travel health notices that are designed to inform travelers and clinicians about current health issues related to specific destinations. These issues may arise from disease
outbreaks, special events or gatherings, natural disasters, or other conditions that may
affect travelers' health.

The *Morbidity and Mortality Weekly Report* (MMWR) (www.cdc.gov/mmwr) series
is prepared by the CDC. Often called "the voice of CDC," the MMWR series is the
agency's primary vehicle for scientific publication of timely, reliable, authoritative,
accurate, objective, and useful public health information and recommendations.

The GeoSentinel Global Surveillance Network (www.geosentinel.org) of ISTM
and CDC is a worldwide communication and data collection network for the surveillance of travel-related morbidity. Aggregation of these data across a network of 57
globally dispersed medicine clinics on all continents allows linking of final diagnoses
in migrating populations with similar geographic exposures.

The European Centre for Disease Prevention and Control (ECDC) publishes a
weekly Communicable Disease Threat Report (http://ecdc.europa.eu/en/publications
/surveillance_reports/Communicable-Disease-Threats-Report/Pages/Communicable
-Disease-Threats-Report.aspx).

Additionally, a number of non-government organizations monitor situations that may impact the health of travelers:
- Eurosurveillance (www.eurosurveillance.org)
- ProMED (www.promedmail.org)
- WHO Global Response and Alert (http://www.who.int/csr/en/)
- WHO The Weekly Epidemiological Record (WER) (http://www.who.int/wer/en/)
- HealthMap (www.healthmap.org/en).

Vaccine resources

The CDC provides a number of vaccine resources:
- The Pink Book outlines the epidemiology and prevention of vaccine-preventable diseases (www.cdc.gov/vaccines/pubs/pinkbook/index.html).
- The US Advisory Committee on Immunization Practices (ACIP) provides the official US recommendations for vaccination use (www.cdc.gov/vaccines/pubs/ACIP -list.htm).
- Vaccine information statements (VIS) can be found at http://www.cdc.gov/vaccines /pubs/vis/default.htm.

The WHO also publishes a series of regularly updated position papers on vaccines that summarize essential information on diseases and vaccines and provide the current WHO position on the use of vaccines worldwide vaccine use (http://www.who.int/immunization/position_papers/en/) and presents country-specific routine immunization schedules (http://apps.who.int/immunization _monitoring/en/globalsummary/ScheduleSelect.cfm).

A comprehensive list of health topics including those related to travel medicine can be found at WHO Health Topics: A–Z List (http://www.euro.who.int/en/health-topics/View-A-Z-list).

Canada: *Canadian Immunization Guide* (http://www.phac-aspc.gc.ca/publicat/cig -gci/index-eng.php).

United Kingdom: *Immunization Against Infectious Disease*. The Green Book, published by Public Health England and the UK Department of Health, has the latest information on vaccines and vaccination procedures for all vaccine-preventable infectious diseases (https://www.gov.uk/government/collections/immunisation-against-infectious-disease-the-green-book).

Australia: *The Australian Immunisation Handbook*, 10th edn., 2013, provides clinical advice for health professionals on the safest and most effective use of vaccines in their practice (http://www.health.gov.au/internet/immunise/publishing.nsf/Content/ Handbook10-home).

Overseas medical assistance

The US Department of State provides information for travelers seeking medical assistance while abroad (http://travel.state.gov/travel/tips/brochures/brochures _1215.html).

A further resource is the US Overseas Security Advisory Council (OSAC) (www.osac.gov).

A number of professional and commercial organizations offer similar resources:

- International Association for Medical Assistance to Travelers (www.iamat.org)
- International SOS (www.internationalsos.com)
- MEDEX (www.medexassist.com)
- Divers Alert Network (DAN) (http://www.diversalertnetwork.org/).

Disease information

The CDC provides a complete list of diseases and conditions on its website (www.cdc.gov/DiseasesConditions), and the Yellow Book (www.cdc.gov/yellowbook) has a chapter devoted to travel-related diseases.

The WHO has a similar description of health topics (www.who.int/topics/en) and also specific sites for rabies (www.who-rabies-bulletin.org), polio (www.polioeradication.org), schistosomiasis (www.who.int/schistosomiasis), and water and sanitation issues (www.who.int/water_sanitation_health).

Some other national sites with similar information include (not exhaustive):

- National Travel Health Network and Centre (NaTHNaC) (www.nathnac.org)
- Public Health Agency of Canada, Travel Health (http://www.phac-aspc.gc.ca/tmp -pmv/)
- Fitfortravel, Health Protection Scotland (http://www.fitfortravel.nhs.uk/home .aspx)
- Travax; Health Protection Scotland (http://www.travax.nhs.uk/)
- Public Health England (https://www.gov.uk/government/organisations/public-health-england).

Electronic discussion forums/listservs

An electronic discussion forum is an online discussion site where people subscribe to the list, post messages, and establish a "thread" on a topic. Forums specific to travel medicine include the following:

- GovDelivery (CDC) (www.cdc.gov/emailupdates/index.html)
- TravelMed (ISTM) (www.istm.org/WebForms/Members/MemberActivities/listserve.aspx).

RSS feeds

RSS stands for Really Simple Syndication, which uses a web feed format so that people can publish frequently updated information, and includes full or summarized text. The material is then made available automatically to multiple other sites and is therefore accessible to many people as timely updates. RSS feeds specific to travel medicine include the following:

- CDC Travelers' Health (www.cdc.gov/travel)
- CDC (www.cdc.gov/podcasts/rss.asp)
- US Department of State (www.state.gov/misc/echannels/66791.htm)
- World Health Organization (www.who.int/about/licensing/rss/en)
- Pan American Health Organization (www.paho.org/english/dd/pin/rssfeed.htm)
- CDC MMWR (www.cdc.gov/mmwr/rss/rss.html)
- ProMED-mail (http://ww2.isid.org/rss/)
- Eurosurveillance (www.eurosurveillance.org/Public/RSSFeed/RSSFeed.aspx)
- US Central Intelligence Agency (CIA): The World Factbook (https://www.cia.gov/news-information/your-news/index.html)
- ReliefWeb (http://reliefweb.int/rss)
- Divers Alert Network (www.diversalertnetwork.org/rss/index.asp)
- International Association for Medical Assistance to Travelers (www.iamat.org/blog/rss.cfm).

Applications for smart phones and devices

There has been a rapid rise in the use of Smart Phones and Devices and as a consequence there has been the development of a range of applications or "Apps," which are basically programs that run on the operating systems of these devices. Some of those relevant to travel medicine include the following:

- Travel Health Guide, WaKi Apps Limited (https://itunes.apple.com/au/app/travel-health-guide/id355832434?mt=8)
- Travel Med, USBMIS (https://itunes.apple.com/en/app/travel-med/id411753521?mt=8)
- Travel iClinic, Dr iSeb Limited (https://itunes.apple.com/cy/app/dr.-iseb/id406154001?mt=8)
- Fit2travel, GlaxoSmithKline Australia (https://itunes.apple.com/au/app/fit2travel/id428933753?mt=8)
- The CDC has two mobile apps available; "Can I eat this?" and TravWell (http://wwwnc.cdc.gov/travel/page/apps-about)

Travel-related infectious diseases

CHAPTER 6

Travelers' diarrhea

Charles D. Ericsson
University of Texas Medical School at Houston, Houston, TX, USA

The syndrome: clinical definitions, epidemiology, and microbiology

Whereas complex definitions of diarrhea include features such as volume of stool passed, for the purpose of advising travelers, travelers' diarrhea refers to the abrupt onset of passage of unformed (soft – takes the shape of the container; or watery – can be poured) stools, accompanied by nausea, vomiting, abdominal cramps, or low-grade fever. Tenesmus and passage of bloody stools are uncommon but as a rule predict an invasive pathogen such as *Shigella*. The problem in trying to differentiate between invasive and secretory diarrhea in the differential use of antimicrobial agents in clinical management is overlap of clinical syndromes [1]. Antibiotics cannot logically be limited to invasive pathogens, for instance, because even the archetypical pathogen *Shigella* often presents with watery diarrhea and not the more typical dysenteric picture that might follow. Diarrhea caused by enterotoxigenic *Escherichia coli*, a secretory pathogen and the most common cause of travelers' diarrhea in many parts of the world, also responds better to antibiotic-containing regimens rather than antisecretory agents alone [2,3].

The world can be divided into areas with high, intermediate, and low rates; however, the only clinically helpful designation is low rate, because rates in both intermediate- and high-risk areas arguably require the same approach to preparing the traveler to prevent and/or self-treat the syndrome [4]. Basically, low rates are only found in developed countries. High rates of diarrhea for persons traveling from industrialized countries to developing regions are in the order of 40–60% over a 2–3-week vacation. Although most travelers' diarrhea is self-limiting within 3–5 days, a substantial percentage of travelers will change their activities (25%), and some will be confined to bed (15%), which has been a major reason for considering arming the traveler with drugs for self-treatment. Mounting evidence indicates up to a 10% prevalence of irritable bowel syndrome (IBS) that persists for 6 months after a bout of travelers' diarrhea, despite treatment of the initial bout of diarrhea with antimicrobial agents. This, coupled with the largely disappointing status of vaccine prevention of enteric pathogens, has prompted renewed interest in the prevention of the syndrome through education and possibly chemoprophylaxis.

Essential Travel Medicine, First Edition.
Edited by Jane N. Zuckerman, Gary W. Brunette and Peter A. Leggat.
© 2015 John Wiley & Sons, Ltd. Published 2015 by John Wiley & Sons, Ltd.

Diarrhea associated with travel can result from multiple causes, including a change in the normal diet, food poisoning (toxins), and infection with viruses (*Rotavirus* and *Norovirus*) and parasites (*Giardia lamblia, Entamoeba histolytica,* and *Cryptosporidium*). However, bacteria (enterotoxigenic, enteroaggregative, and enteroinvasive *E. coli, Shigella, Campylobacter jejuni,* and *Aeromonas, Salmonella, Vibrio,* and *Plesiomonas* spp., among others) account for the majority of causes. The major causal role of bacteria explains the benefits of antimicrobial agents in the treatment and prevention of the syndrome.

The risk of traveler's diarrhea is highest wherever sanitation, food storage practices, and fuel for cooking are inadequate [5]. Contaminated water appears to be a risk factor for some viruses and parasites, but contaminated food is the most common risk factor among most travelers to the developing world. Inadequate public health practices appear to be a more important risk than contamination of specific food items. As such, the risk of ingesting contaminated food is ubiquitous and travelers find it difficult to prevent diarrhea only by exercising safe beverage and food choices. Nevertheless, travelers should seek locations of food consumption that have an excellent reputation for safety. Clean bottled water is generally readily available in developing countries. Carbonated beverages are inherently safe. Being prepared to use filters, boil water, or disinfect water with iodine is generally not necessary for the average traveler. Piping hot, thoroughly cooked food, dry food, and fruits and vegetables peeled by the traveler are considered generally safe. Tap water, ice cubes, unpasteurized fruit juices or dairy products, fresh salads, cold sauces and toppings, some desserts, open buffets, and undercooked or incompletely reheated foods should be avoided. Most travel medicine experts feel that travelers simply cannot abide by these recommendations and that travelers should be prepared to self-treat. Some experts consider that fluid replacement alone suffices; however, far more experts consider that symptomatic relief afforded by self-treatment with antidiarrheal agents outweighs concerns about side-effects or the theoretical fostering of antimicrobial resistance. The use of antimicrobial prophylaxis, on the other hand, remains a very controversial approach, particularly among European, as compared with North American, travelers [6].

Chemoprophylaxis of travelers' diarrhea

Chemoprophylaxis might be a reasonable strategy for a traveler who is taking a brief trip to a high-risk area and cannot afford to be ill for even a single day [7]. Traditionally, the benefits and safety of chemoprophylaxis with antimicrobials were weighed against obtaining prompt relief of diarrhea by the use of the antisecretory/antimotility agent loperamide, plus an antimicrobial agent. Travelers who might have been offered chemoprophylaxis included competitive athletes, politicians, business travelers, and people going to special events. The confirmation that up to 10% of those developing travelers' diarrhea have symptoms of IBS up to 6 months later and the availability of a safe, minimally absorbed antimicrobial agent, rifaximin, have rekindled interest in the chemoprophylaxis of travelers' diarrhea.

Lactobacillus rhamnosus GG is a safe agent for the prevention of travelers' diarrhea. However, it achieved only modest efficacy in one study and was less effective in others. Likewise, other probiotics have demonstrated geographically patchy and inconsistent efficacy. Probiotics cannot be recommended for routine prophylaxis of travelers' diarrhea. Probiotics are safe, however, and popular among some travelers, so probably need not be discouraged provided that the traveler understands that predictably more effective regimens for prevention are available.

Bismuth subsalicylate-containing compounds and antimicrobial agents are efficacious in the prevention of travelers' diarrhea. Bismuth subsalicylate, which is active in large part because it is an antimicrobial agent, can successfully prevent approximately 65% of travelers' diarrhea. Disadvantages of this regimen include cost, the bulk of the liquid product in luggage, the potential risks of the absorbed salicylate, and the development of a black tongue and stools. Although the black discoloration is trivial, related to precipitates of bismuth salts, travelers are disconcerted by an unsightly black tongue and sometimes alarmed that they might have melena. Also, bismuth subsalicylate-containing products are not readily available in many parts of the world.

Trimethoprim–sulfamethoxazole can no longer be advocated for the prevention of travelers' diarrhea owing to developing resistance worldwide. Fluoroquinolones successfully prevent up to 80% of travelers' diarrhea, but a cogent argument can be made for reserving this class of agents for the treatment of numerous medical conditions and not risk the development of fluoroquinolone resistance through their use in prevention of travelers' diarrhea. Rifaximin is a non-absorbed (<0.4%) antimicrobial agent with an excellent safety profile and proven usefulness in the management of certain enteric diseases and long term prevention of hepatic encephalopathy. A daily dose of rifaximin prevents illness about as effectively as bismuth subsalicylate [8]. Emergence of resistance has not been a clinical problem.

Although some experts still question the wisdom of routine chemoprophylaxis of travelers' diarrhea and routinely favor self-treatment instead, the concept of preventing IBS by preventing travelers' diarrhea in the first place, has caused others to reconsider the use of chemoprophylaxis of travelers' diarrhea in most if not all short-term travelers. Agents useful in the prevention of travelers' diarrhea are listed in Table 6.1.

Symptomatic treatment of travelers' diarrhea

Fluid replacement has long been the cornerstone of therapy for travelers' diarrhea. Arguably, dehydration from loss of fluids and decreased oral intake is the greatest risk to health in young children and debilitated or older people. However, when loperamide was used to treat the syndrome, additional use of oral rehydration solution did not add to the clinical benefit of loperamide alone [9]. Generally, fruit juices or flavored mineral water suffice for oral rehydration during most episodes of travelers' diarrhea. Packets of oral rehydration salts, which can be reconstituted with clean water to make oral rehydration solution, are increasingly available in pharmacies throughout the world. Treatment with oral rehydration solution is a wise

Table 6.1 Recommended agents for travelers' diarrhea chemoprophylaxis.

Agent	Dosage	Comments
Bismuth subsalicylate (Pepto Bismol®)	Two tablets chewed four times per day	Avoid in persons who should not take aspirin or who are on anticoagulants. Black stool and tongue may occur
Fluoroquinolones[a]		
Norfloxacin	400 mg PO daily	Occasional gastrointestinal upset, rash, and allergic reactions
Ciprofloxacin	500 mg PO daily	
Rifaximin	200–400 mg PO daily	Well tolerated since rifaximin is not absorbed (<0.4%). Dose for South-East Asia has not been studied, but since *Campylobacter* minimal inhibitory concentrations are higher than for other enteric pathogens, 400 mg per day is recommended

[a]Other fluoroquinolones can be predicted to be effective but they have not been studied in prophylaxis.

consideration for diarrhea in children, elderly adults, and those who might develop diarrhea a long distance from medical attention. In adults, a diet restricted to liquids and bland foods may not offer additional treatment benefit when diarrhea is also being treated with antibiotics [10].

Medications and their doses for symptomatic relief of travelers' diarrhea are listed in Table 6.2 [11]. Agents that offer no or insufficient relief include anticholinergics, adsorbents such as kaolin–pectin preparations, and probiotics such as *Lactobacillus*. Owing to insufficient information or lack of availability, calmodulin and enkephalinase inhibitors cannot be recommended.

Bismuth subsalicylate reduces the number of stools passed in travelers' diarrhea by approximately 16–18%. Although it can be recommended in mild diarrhea, for

Table 6.2 Recommended agents for symptomatic treatment of travelers' diarrhea.

Agent	Dosage	Comments
Bismuth subsalicylate (Pepto Bismol)	1 oz PO every 30 minutes for 8 doses	Delayed onset of action. Avoid in persons who should not take aspirin or who are on anticoagulants. May interfere with absorption of other antimicrobials, notably fluoroquinolones and doxycycline. Black stools and tongue may occur
Loperamide (Imodium)	4 mg PO then 2 mg after each loose stool, not to exceed 8 mg daily	Rapid onset of action. Best results occur with loperamide plus an antimicrobial agent. Very well tolerated

moderate to severe disease loperamide works better and with a faster onset of action. Opiates and diphenoxylate are effective, but central nervous system and other side-effects, plus poor tolerance among the elderly, limit their usefulness. Because it is safe and efficacious, loperamide has become the symptomatic treatment agent of choice. Concerns over side-effects or complications due to the use of an antimotility agent such as loperamide generally have arisen from case reports involving subjects who took the drug for far longer than advised or during episodes of bloody diarrhea when an antimicrobial agent was not given concurrently.

The combination of loperamide and an antimicrobial agent (e.g., a fluoro-quinolone or azithromycin) is especially efficacious in the treatment of travelers' diarrhea [12]. Loperamide appears to be safe, even in children, provided that doses are kept in the recommended range and the drug is stopped if diarrhea persists despite several days of treatment. Most experts prefer, however, to avoid using loperamide in children. Although the combination of loperamide and an antibiotic was more efficacious than antibiotic alone in the treatment of *Shigella* dysentery [13], most experts prefer not to use loperamide when the patient has high fever and passage of grossly bloody stools.

Antibiotic treatment of travelers' diarrhea

Travelers' diarrhea can be relieved in a little over 1 day after empirical antibiotic therapy is instituted [11]. With the concurrent use of loperamide, relief (defined as passage of no additional unformed stools) is realized in a matter of hours [12]. In the face of increasing resistance among enteric enteropathogens worldwide, trimethoprim–sulfamethoxazole can no longer be recommended. Until recently, a fluoroquinolone had been the drug of choice for empirical treatment of travelers' diarrhea. With recognition that *Campylobacter jejuni* is a common cause of travelers' diarrhea in South-East Asia and resistance to fluoroquinolones among *Campylobacter* in this region is up to 90%, the preferred agent for the empiric treatment of travelers' diarrhea has become azithromycin [12]. Rifaximin, with broad activity against enteric pathogens, is effective in the treatment of travelers' diarrhea in regions of the world where enterotoxigenic *E. coli* is the predominate pathogen. However, it is not recommended for the treatment of bloody diarrhea or when invasive pathogens are suspected, limiting its usefulness as a therapeutic agent in regions such as South-East Asia [14]. The most appropriate use of rifaximin is arguably as a chemoprophylactic agent since it can prevent (but not treat) diarrhea caused by invasive pathogens. Either a fluoroquinolone or azithromycin can be used for the treatment of any illness that occurs despite prophylaxis, except azithromycin is preferred in South-East Asia. Recommended dosages of antimicrobial agents are given in Table 6.3. Often a single dose suffices [15]. For "savvy" travelers, instructions can be to take a single dose of antibiotic and 24 hours later re-evaluate themselves. If they are well, no further antibiotic is necessary. Prescribing a 3-day supply of antibiotic is aimed at the few travelers who might have exceptionally severe diarrhea. Travelers who do not respond to empirical antibiotic treatment or who have persistent diarrhea of more than 1 week's duration should seek medical attention.

Table 6.3 Recommended antimicrobial agents for the treatment of travelers' diarrhea.

Agent	Dosage	Comments
Fluoroquinolones[a]		
Ciprofloxacin	500 mg PO BID for 3 days OR 750 mg PO once	Occasional gastrointestinal upset, rash, and allergic reactions. After 24 hours, patients can re-evaluate themselves before taking the next dose. If diarrhea persists, or if fever or passage of bloody stools was present, finish 3 days of therapy
Levofloxacin	500 mg PO QD for 3 days OR 500–750 mg PO once	
Azithromycin	1000 mg PO once OR 500 mg daily for 2–3 days	Agent of choice for diarrhea occurring in South-East Asia. A single 500 mg dose suffices when *E. coli* is the predominant enteropathogen. A 500 mg dose regimen is preferred for small adults in the hope of minimizing gastrointestinal upset
Rifaximin	200 mg PO TID for 3 days[b]	Should not be used to treat persons in whom an invasive enteropathogen is suspected, or in those with fever or grossly bloody stools

[a]Single doses of levofloxacin have been studied and appear equivalent to 3-day regimens. Likely single doses of any fluoroquinolone will suffice.
[b]400 mg PO BID for 3 days is also efficacious.

References

1 Mattila L. Clinical features and duration of travelers' diarrhoea in relation to its etiology. *Clin Infect Dis* 1994; **19**: 728–734.
2 DuPont HL, Ericsson CD. Prevention and treatment of travelers' diarrhoea. *N Engl J Med* 1993; **328**: 1821–1827.
3 Ericsson CD, DuPont HL. Travellers' diarrhoea: approaches to prevention and treatment. *Clin Infect Dis* 1993; **16**: 616–624.
4 Shah N, DuPont HL, Ramsey DJ. Global etiology of travelers' diarrhoea: systematic review from 1973 to the present. *Am J Trop Med Hyg* 2009; **80**: 609–614.
5 Castelli F, Black RE. Epidemiology of travelers' diarrhoea. In: Ericsson CD, DuPont HL, Steffen R (eds.) *Travelers' Diarrhoea*, 2nd edn. Hamilton, ON: BC Decker, 2008, pp. 92–104.
6 Ericsson CD, Melgarejo NA, Jelinek T, et al. Travelers' preferences for the treatment and prevention of acute diarrhea. *J Travel Med* 2009; **16**: 172–178.
7 DuPont HL, Ericsson CD, Farthing MJG, et al. Expert review of the evidence base for prevention of travelers' diarrhea. *J Travel Med* 2009; **16**: 149–160.
8 Martinez-Sandoval F, Ericsson CD, Jiang, Z-D, et al. Prevention of travelers' diarrhea with rifaximin in US travellers to Mexico. *J Travel Med* 2010; **17**: 111–117.
9 Caeiro JP, DuPont HL, Albrecht, H, et al. Oral rehydration therapy plus loperamide versus loperamide alone in the treatment of travelers' diarrhea. *Clin Infect Dis* 1999; **28**: 1286–1289.

10 Huang DB, Awasthi M, Le J, et al. The role of diet in the treatment of travelers' diarrhea: a pilot study. *Clin Infect Dis* 2004; **39**: 468–471.

11 DuPont HL, Ericsson CD, Farthing MJG, et al. Expert review of the evidence base for self-therapy of travelers' diarrhea. *J Travel Med* 2009; **16**, 161–171.

12 Ericsson CD, DuPont HL, Okhuysen PC, et al. Loperamide plus azithromycin more effectively treats travelers' diarrhea in Mexico than azithromycin alone. *J Travel Med* 2007; **14**: 312–319.

13 Murphy GS, Bodhidatta L, Echeverria P, et al. Ciprofloxacin and loperamide in the treatment of bacillary dysentery. *Ann Intern Med* 1993; **118**: 582–586.

14 Taylor DN, Bourgeois AL, Ericsson CD, et al. A randomized, double-blind, multicenter study of rifaximin compared with placebo and with ciprofloxacin in the treatment of travelers' diarrhea. *Am J Trop Med Hyg* 2006; **74**: 1060–1066.

15 Ericsson CD, DuPont HL, Mathewson IJ. Single dose ofloxacin plus loperamide compared with single dose or three days of ofloxacin in the treatment of travelers' diarrhea. *J Travel Med* 1997; **4**: 3–7.

CHAPTER 7

Vector-borne diseases

Annelies Wilder-Smith

Nanyang Technological University, Singapore

Epidemiology

Dengue

Dengue virus is transmitted to humans primarily through the bite of an infected *Aedes* sp. mosquito. Dengue is now the most common arboviral disease in the tropics and subtropics [1]. The main vector is *Aedes aegypti*, which is an effective vector because of its day-biting habits, its imperceptible bite, and its peridomestic breeding behavior. *Aedes albopictus* is the secondary vector, less efficient, but with a more expanded geographic distribution, including large parts of the United States and southern Europe. The dengue virus (DENV) has four serotypes. Increasingly, all four serotypes co-circulate the tropics and subtropics, contributing to enhanced epidemics of more severe disease.

The World Health Organization (WHO) estimates that 100,000 cases of dengue, including 20,000 deaths, occur annually worldwide [1]. Recent modeling and consensus estimates that also include asymptomatic disease indicate as many as 400 million cases annually [2]. South-East Asia, South Asia, Central and South America, parts of the Caribbean, and the western Pacific region all experience epidemic or endemic dengue. Reports of indigenous transmission are now also increasing from Africa and the Middle East [3,4]. The threat of dengue to more temperate regions is also increasing, with frequently reported small outbreaks in Florida and Texas, USA, occasional cases in Hawaii, a major outbreak in Madeira, and reports of less than a handful of cases in southern Europe (southern France and Croatia) [5]. Dengue has seen a 30-fold increase over the past decades, and is likely to increase further both in incidence and in further geographic spread into currently non-endemic areas, including temperate climates. This is due to various factors, including increasing international travel and population mobility, the expansion of the dengue vector habitats, continued human population growth, increasing urbanization, and the inability to sustain vector control effectively [6].

Novel vector control strategies that involve releasing *Wolbachia*-infected mosquitoes or genetically engineered mosquitoes appear promising, but their deployment may be controversial and not thought likely to occur on a large scale in the near future. A vaccine against dengue is urgently needed.

Essential Travel Medicine, First Edition.
Edited by Jane N. Zuckerman, Gary W. Brunette and Peter A. Leggat.
© 2015 John Wiley & Sons, Ltd. Published 2015 by John Wiley & Sons, Ltd.

Chikungunya

Chikungunya is a viral disease (genus *Alphavirus*) that is transmitted to humans by the same mosquitoes as for dengue, namely *Aedes aegypti* and *Aedes albopictus* [7]. The name chikungunya originates from a verb in the Kimakonde language, meaning "to become contorted." Chikungunya was first identified in Tanzania in the early 1950s and has caused periodic outbreaks in Asia and Africa, with outbreaks usually separated by periods of more than 10 years. Chikungunya virus (CHIKV) emerged in Indian Ocean islands in 2005 and caused a major outbreak that involved >260,000 patients (about one-third of the population!), including travelers returning home from these islands [8]. The complete genomic sequence identified a new CHIKV variant emerging from the East/Central African evolutionary lineage, which may have contributed to the extent of the outbreak. In 2006, a major outbreak of CHIK occurred in India, with more than 1.5 million cases, with *Aedes aegypti* as vector. *Aedes albopictus*, the implicated vector of CHIKV in Indian Ocean islands, has dispersed worldwide in recent decades, which may explain the first outbreak of CHIK in Europe when an Indian traveled to Northern Italy in 2007 [9], triggering an outbreak of 197 CHIK cases in Italy.

Japanese encephalitis

Japanese encephalitis virus (JEV), a mosquito-borne flaviviral zoonotic infection, is the most common vaccine-preventable cause of encephalitis in Asia. JEV is transmitted in an enzootic cycle between species of *Culex* mosquitoes and vertebrates, primarily birds, with pigs serving as amplifying hosts. Nearly half the human population, 3 billion people, currently lives in countries where JE occurs [10]. JE is concentrated in China, India, and South-East Asia, where it is the leading cause of viral neurologic disability, with incidence exceeding that of herpes simplex virus encephalitis [11]. It has emerged in northern Australia, especially the islands of the Torres Strait [12,13]. In highly endemic areas, incidence rates of the disease may be 10 per 100,000 population [14]. In the past decade, 30,000–50,000 cases of JE have been notified to the WHO from Asia and Australia, resulting in about 10,000 deaths and an estimated 15,000 cases with long-term neurologic and/or psychiatric sequelae [15]. Proximity to rice fields breeding *Culex tritaeniorhynchus* or *Culex vishnui* species and pig farms have been identified as risk factors for JE [16]. Surveillance generally underestimates the true burden of infection, as a majority of infections are asymptomatic, resulting in a case-to-infection ratio of approximately 1 in 250 [17]. Major JE outbreaks have occurred over the past two decades in Uttar Pradesh, India, and in Nepal [18,19], possibly related to the increased acreage allocated to cultivating wet rice. Transmission may be increasing in Bangladesh, Cambodia, Indonesia, Laos, Myanmar, and Pakistan, due to in part to growing human populations and in some cases to the introduction of large-scale pig rearing [20,21]. Enhanced agricultural cultivation such as rice crops gives rise to growing habitats for the mosquitoes.

Clinical manifestations

Dengue

The clinical manifestation of dengue ranges from asymptomatic to severe life-threatening disease. Most people, in particular children, infected with DENV are asymptomatic. Classical dengue fever is characterized by high fever, headache, rash, eye pain, muscle aches, joint pain, and severe fatigue. The more severe forms, dengue hemorrhagic fever (DHF) and dengue shock syndrome (DSS), include a plasma leakage syndrome characterized by petechiae, hemoconcentration, and pleural and/or peritoneal effusions that can lead to a fulminant course with shock and death if not treated appropriately. Most of the more severe cases occur following secondary infection. The most prominent hypothesis to explain this observation is the antibody-dependent enhancement (ADE) theory, proposed by Scott Halstead. ADE proposes that non-neutralizing cross-reactive antibodies bind to non-homologous virus and facilitate uptake into Fc receptor-bearing cells that in turn results in greater virus loads and cytokine storm. Other explanatory possibilities include the theory of "antigenic sin." In view of the fact that severe disease is a relatively rare event compared with the number of individuals with secondary infection, it is assumed that DHF only results under specific circumstances where additional factors are needed, in particular host factors. Differences in viral strains, including viral genotypes, and the sequence of infection in addition to genetic factors play a role.

The hallmark of DHF and DSS is a capillary leakage syndrome, accompanied by hemorrhagic manifestations. Despite the name, hemorrhagic manifestations are usually mild and include epistaxis, gingival bleeding, and petechiae. Major hemorrhagic manifestations such as massive intestinal bleeding or severe hypermenorrhagia occur only rarely, and usually more in adults than in children. Patients with DHF or DSS present in the first days similarly to those with classical dengue fever, but then plasma leakage develops at the time of defervescence around 5–7 days after onset of symptoms. Abdominal pain and vomiting, restlessness, change in level of consciousness, and a sudden change from fever to hypothermia may be the first clinical warning signs, associated with a significant decrease in platelets [22]. Mortality of DHF can be up to 20%, but in experienced dengue management hospitals, the case fatality rate is far below 1%. Rare severe manifestations or complications beyond DHF and DSS include fulminant hepatitis, myocarditis, encephalitis, blindness due to retinal bleeding, and hemophagocytic syndrome.

The WHO has published a new dengue case classification with a binary classification into "dengue" and "severe dengue" [23]. A WHO subclassification with dengue presenting with warning signs will aid clinicians in identifying those patients who will need immediate hospitalization versus further daily monitoring as an outpatient. The revised dengue classification has a high potential for facilitating dengue case management and surveillance [24], and further refinement of the warning signs is currently ongoing in a multi-country study [25].

Chikungunya

Similarly to dengue, a large proportion of patients remain asymptomatic, and the incubation time is around 3–7 days. Disease is most often characterized by a sudden onset of high fever and severe joint pain (arthralgia) and myalgia, with or without rash, headache, fatigue, nausea, and vomiting. Fevers typically last from several days up to 1 week. Rare but serious complications of the disease can occur, including myocarditis, ocular disease (uveitis, retinitis), hepatitis, acute renal disease, bulbous skin lesions, and meningoencephalitis, Guillain–Barré syndrome, paresis, or palsies. Although the case fatality rate is extremely low for CHIK, incapacitating joint pain, stiffness, or tenosynovitis may last for weeks or months.

Japanese encephalitis

As with all other flaviviral infections, the asymptomatic-to-symptomatic ratio is high. The case fatality rate increases with age [20]. In persons who develop symptoms, the incubation period (time from infection until illness) is typically 5–15 days, and initial symptoms often include fever, headache, and vomiting. Mental status changes, neurologic symptoms, weakness, and movement disorders might develop over the next few days. Seizures are common, especially among children. Clinical JE is a severe disease with a high case fatality rate (30%) [26]. About 25–50% of persons who survive encephalitis suffer from long-term or permanent disabilities such as physical and mental impairments [27].

Diagnosis

Dengue

Non-specific fever with or without a rash, in particular if associated with thrombocytopenia and leukopenia, should alert the clinician to the diagnosis of dengue fever and should initiate laboratory confirmation. The appropriate tests depend on the day of illness, with virus-based investigations carried out in the first 4–5 days of illness, and serological assays from day 4–5 of illness. Probable diagnosis of dengue infection is made based on a positive dengue immunoglobulin M (IgM) test, the most common assay in most countries, or a titer of greater than 1:1280 with the hemagglutination inhibition test. Confirmed diagnosis of dengue requires at least one of the following: fourfold or greater rise in serum IgG titers specific to dengue virus between acute and convalescent serum; detection of dengue virus in serum tissue, or autopsy samples; and a positive dengue-specific polymerase chin reaction (PCR). Lateral flow tests for NS1 detection are the most feasible methods for early diagnosis of dengue [28], as they have about the same sensitivity as PCR, are less expensive, and require less expertise.

Chikungunya

Abnormal laboratory findings can include thrombocytopenia, lymphopenia, and elevated creatinine and liver function tests, hence based on those findings it is impossible to differentiate from dengue. CHIK can be confirmed with PCR or viral culture in the first week of illness. Numerous quantitative reverse transcription polymerase chain reactions (RT-PCRs) have been developed. CHIKV-specific IgM-neutralizing antibodies normally develop towards the end of the first week of illness and a few days later CHIKV-specific IgG. Convalescent-phase samples should be obtained from patients whose acute-phase samples test negative.

Japanese encephalitis

The cerebrospinal fluid (CSF) opening pressure is elevated in about 50% of patients. CSF findings are typically a mild to moderate pleocytosis of 10 to several hundred white blood cells/mm^3 with lymphocytic predominance, slightly elevated protein, and normal CSF-to-plasma glucose ratio. Magnetic resonance imaging is more sensitive than computed tomography scanning for detecting JEV-associated abnormalities such as changes in the thalamus, basal ganglia, midbrain, pons, and medulla. Thalamic lesions are the most commonly described abnormality. EEG abnormalities may include theta and delta coma, burst suppression, epileptiform activity, and occasionally alpha coma. JE is diagnosed serologically by detection of JEV-specific IgM antibodies in CSF or serum by an enzyme-linked immunosorbent assay (ELISA). The presence of JEV-specific IgM antibodies in CSF confirms recent central nervous system infection. IgM antibody in serum, detectable about 5–8 days after symptom onset, is suggestive of JE but could indicate asymptomatic infection, or infection in the recent past, or recent JEV vaccination. If JE is suspected and acute samples are negative, a convalescent serum sample should be collected. As serodiagnosis of flaviviral infections is not straightforward and cross-reactivity is common, samples positive by ELISA should be referred to a reference laboratory for confirmatory plaque reduction neutralization testing (PRNT).

Virus isolation or detection of viral RNA with a nucleic acid amplification test (NAAT) can provide a definitive diagnosis, but positive results from CSF or blood are rare because of low levels of transient viremia and high levels of neutralizing antibodies by the time distinctive clinical symptoms are recognized. Hence virus isolation and NAATs are insensitive for the detection of JEV or JE viral RNA in blood or CSF. In fatal cases, nucleic acid amplification, histopathology with immunohistochemistry, and virus culture of autopsy tissues can be useful.

Clinical management

Dengue

There is no specific antiviral treatment against dengue. Clinical management is therefore symptomatic and supportive, with the primary aim being to prevent mortality from severe leakage syndrome [29]. Classic dengue is treated with antipyretics, such as paracetamol, bed rest, and oral (rarely parenteral) fluid replacement, and most cases can be managed on an outpatient basis, provided that platelet and hematocrit counts can be carried out on a regular basis. The critical period is usually around days 4–7 of the illness. Prompt institution of intravenous fluid replacement is indicated, with either normal saline or Ringer's solution, if clinical symptoms and signs of leakage occur, which include narrowing of the pulse pressure, rise in hematocrit, and other warning signs. The WHO publishes a treatment algorithm for rehydration therapy and the indication for blood transfusions or fresh frozen plasma/platelets [30].

Chikungunya and Japanese encephalitis

Similarly to dengue, there is no specific antiviral therapy. Care is based on symptoms and relief of joint pains for chikungunya, and for Japanese encephalitis on management of encephalitis and seizures.

Risk for international travelers

Dengue
The risk of dengue for travelers to dengue-endemic countries depends on the travel destination, duration of travel, activities during travel, and the season of travel [31]. The GeoSentinel network of travel medicine providers report an increasing trend of dengue in travelers associated with a cyclic pattern [32]. Dengue is now the second most common cause of fever in returning travelers [31]. The main risk destinations are South-East Asia, followed by Latin America and the Caribbean. Despite the fact that dengue is frequently reported in travelers, death remains a rare event [33]. Nevertheless, dengue is often not a mild disease and leads to disruption of travel plans, and even to evacuations in 30% in some case series [31].

Chikungunya
The risk for travelers is highest with travel to areas experiencing ongoing epidemics of the disease. The risk was highest in the period 2006–2009, but with abating epidemics the risk has declined again. Given the high level of viremia in humans, and the worldwide distribution of *Ae. aegypti* and *Ae. albopictus*, there is a risk of importation of chikungunya virus into new areas by infected travelers. For example, in 2006 the migration of infected people introduced the infection to many temperate countries, with a dominance in France. Migration also triggered the 2007 CHIK outbreak in a coastal village in Northern Italy via a traveler from India [34].

Japanese encephalitis
JE is a rare problem for travelers, but when it occurs, it is a devastating disease. The risk of JE in travelers to South-East Asia may be of the order of 1 per million travelers [20]. Before 1973, more than 300 cases of JE occurred among US military personnel [35]. The risk to the traveler visiting rural endemic areas in the peak transmission season has been estimated to be as high as one in 5000 for a 4-week stay or one in 20,000 for a 1-week stay [36]. During 1973–2008, a total of 55 cases of travel-associated JE were reported [35]. The countries where infection was most commonly acquired were Thailand, followed by Indonesia, China, the Philippines, Japan, and Vietnam [35]. Duration of travel, when known, ranged from 10 days to 34 years, but was shorter than 1 month for 65% of travelers. Several dozen sporadic cases of JE among travelers, many on seemingly benign and short itineraries, have been reported in the past 30 years [37,38], underscoring the difficulty of providing prescriptive guidance for preventing a disease that occurs infrequently but, if acquired, has serious consequences.

Prevention and control

Prevention of dengue and chikungunya
Aedes mosquito control follows three main strategies: source reduction, use of larvicides, and use of ultralow-volume aerosolized adulticides. Biological control

of larvae in the form of larvivorous fish or predatory copepods has shown some efficacy in small-scale studies. A novel promising approach is the use of *Wolbachia* as a biologic control agent. *Wolbachia* introduced into *Aedes* mosquitoes reduce the lifespan of the mosquito, affect reproduction, and inhibit viral replication [39]. An approach based on mosquitoes carrying a conditional dominant lethal gene (release of insects carrying a dominant lethal, RIDL) is being developed to control the transmission of dengue viruses by vector population suppression [40]. Personal protection against *Aedes* mosquitoes is difficult to sustain on a long-term basis as it requires daily protective measures with insect repellent, applied throughout the day as *Aedes* mosquitoes are day-biting mosquitoes. Bed nets are therefore limited in their efficiency for dengue or CHIK prevention, in contrast to malaria. A dengue vaccine for the endemic population is urgently needed, and in advanced development. More information can be found in a recent excellent review by Thomas and Endy [41]. The increasing incidence of dengue in travelers also warrants a dengue vaccine for travelers [42]. Development of a vaccine against chikungunya is also ongoing.

Prevention of Japanese encephalitis

Vaccination against JE is part of many national immunization programs in JE-endemic countries, and as a result the incidence of JE in humans has declined in those countries, although JE virus continues to circulate. All travelers to JE-endemic areas should take precautions to avoid mosquito bites, which include using insect repellents, permethrin-impregnated clothing, and bed nets, and staying in accommodation with screened or air-conditioned rooms [20]. JE vaccination is recommended for travelers at risk [43].

Vaccines against Japanese encephalitis

The inactivated mouse brain-derived vaccine is now obsolete owing to safety concerns, and is commonly replaced by cell culture-based vaccines. For international travelers, a Vero cell-derived, inactivated and alum-adjuvanted JE based on the SA 14-14-2 strain is available in North America, Australia, and various European countries (IXIARO, referred to as IC51; Intercell, Vienna, Austria). The primary two doses are administered 4 weeks apart. A booster dose is recommended 1–2 years after the primary immunization. In most countries, the lower age limit is 2 years, although in some countries the vaccine remains licensed only for use in individuals 18 years and older. Another Vero cell-derived inactivated JE vaccine was licensed by the Japanese authorities in February 2009 and a similar Japanese vaccine was licensed in 2011. These two vaccines use the same strain of JE virus (Beijing-1) as the mouse-brain-derived vaccine. Clinical trials have shown that all these Vero cell-based inactivated JE vaccines are safe and immunogenic, with seroconversion rates exceeding 95% [44].

A live attenuated vaccine based on the SA 14-14-2 strain of the JE virus is widely used in China and in an increasing number of countries within the Asian region, including India, the Republic of Korea, Sri Lanka, and Thailand [43], given either as a single dose or as two doses usually 1 year apart. In addition, a live-attenuated yellow fever–Japanese encephalitis chimeric vaccine (IMOJEV, referred to as Japanese encephalitis-CV; Sanofi Pasteur, Lyon, France) was licensed in Australia and Thailand and is under review in other Asian countries. The advantage of this vaccine is its single dose and the duration of protection is thought to be long, although the need for and timing of a booster dose are still unknown.

References

1 Murray NE, Quam MB, Wilder-Smith A. Epidemiology of dengue: past, present and future prospects. *Clin Epidemiol* 2013; **5**: 299–309.

2 Bhatt S, Gething PW, Brady OJ, et al. The global distribution and burden of dengue. *Nature* 2013; **496**: 504–507.

3 Sessions OM, Khan K, Hou Y, et al. Exploring the origin and potential for spread of the 2013 dengue outbreak in Luanda, Angola. *Glob Health Action* 2013; **6**: 21822.

4 Amarasinghe A, Kuritsk JN, Letson GW, Margolis HS. Dengue virus infection in Africa. *Emerg Infect Dis* 2011; **17**: 1349–1354.

5 Tomasello D, Schlagenhauf P. Chikungunya and dengue autochthonous cases in Europe, 2007–2012. *Travel Med Infect Dis* 2013; **11**: 274–284.

6 Wilder-Smith A, Gubler DJ. Geographic expansion of dengue: the impact of international travel. *Med Clin North Am* 2008; **92**: 1377–1390, x.

7 Chen LH, Wilson ME. Dengue and chikungunya in travelers: recent updates. *Curr Opin Infect Dis* 2012; **25**: 523–529.

8 Parola P, de Lamballerie X, Jourdan J, et al. Novel chikungunya virus variant in travelers returning from Indian Ocean islands. *Emerg Infect Dis* 2006; **12**: 1493–1499.

9 Rezza G, Nicoletti L, Angelini R, et al. Infection with chikungunya virus in Italy: an outbreak in a temperate region. *Lancet* 2007; **370**: 1840–1846.

10 Halstead SB, Jacobson J, Dubischar-Kastner, K. Japanese encephalitis vaccines. In: Plotkin SA, Orenstein WA, Offit PA (eds.) Vaccines, 6th edn. Philadelphia, PA: Saunders Elsevier, 2013, pp. 312–351.

11 Wilder-Smith A, Freedman DO. Japanese encephalitis: is there a need for a novel vaccine? *Expert Rev Vaccines* 2009; **8**: 969–972.

12 Hanna JN, Ritchie SA, Phillips DA, et al. Japanese encephalitis in north Queensland, Australia, 1998. *Med J Aust* 1999; **170**: 533–536.

13 Hanna JN, Ritchie SA, Phillips DA, et al. An outbreak of Japanese encephalitis in the Torres Strait, Australia, 1995. *Med J Aust* 1996; **165**: 256–260.

14 Koff WC, Elm JL, Jr.,, Halstead SB. Suppression of dengue virus replication in vitro by rimantadine hydrochloride. *Am J Trop Med Hyg* 1981; **30**: 184–189.

15 WHO. Japanese encephalitis vaccines: WHO position paper. *Wkly Epidemiol Rec* 2006; **81**: 331–340.

16 Liu W, Gibbons RV, Kari K, et al. Risk factors for Japanese encephalitis: a case–control study. *Epidemiol Infect* 2010; **138**: 1292–1297.

17 Konishi E, Suzuki T. Ratios of subclinical to clinical Japanese encephalitis (JE) virus infections in vaccinated populations: evaluation of an inactivated JE vaccine by comparing the ratios with those in unvaccinated populations. *Vaccine* 2002; **21**: 98–107.

18 Arunachalam N, Samuel PP, Paramasivan R, et al. Japanese encephalitis in Gorakhpur Division, Uttar Pradesh. *Indian J Med Res* 2008; **128**: 775–777.

19 Bista MB, Shrestha JM. Epidemiological situation of Japanese encephalitis in Nepal. *JNMA J Nepal Med Assoc* 2005; **44**: 51–56.

20 Burchard GD, Caumes E, Connor BA, et al. Expert opinion on vaccination of travelers against Japanese encephalitis. *J Travel Med* 2009; **16**: 204–216.

21 Gingrich JB, Nisalak A, Latendresse JR, et al. A longitudinal study of Japanese encephalitis in suburban Bangkok, Thailand. *Southeast Asian J Trop Med Public Health* 1987; **18**: 558–566.

22 Gibbons RV, Vaughn DW. Dengue: an escalating problem. *BMJ* 2002; **324**: 1563–1566.

23 Farrar JJ, Hien TT, Horstick O, et al. Dogma in classifying dengue disease. *Am J Trop Med Hyg* 2013; **89**: 198–201.

24 Barniol J, Gaczkowski R, Barbato EV, et al. Usefulness and applicability of the revised dengue case classification by disease: multi-centre study in 18 countries. *BMC Infect Dis* 2011; **11**: 106.

25 Jaenisch T, IDAMS, Sakuntabhai A, et al. Dengue research funded by the European Commission – scientific strategies of three European dengue research consortia. *PLoS Negl Trop Dis* 2013; **7**(12): e2320.

26 Burchard GD, Caumes E, Connor BA, et al. Expert opinion on vaccination of travelers against Japanese encephalitis. *J Travel Med* 2009; **16**: 204–216.

27 Gould EA, Solomon T. Pathogenic flaviviruses. *Lancet* 2008; **371**: 500–509.

28 Ferraz FO, Bomfim MR, Totola AH, et al. Evaluation of laboratory tests for dengue diagnosis in clinical specimens from consecutive patients with suspected dengue in Belo Horizonte, Brazil. *J Clin Virol* 2013; **58**: 41–46.

29 Wilder-Smith A, Ooi EE, Vasudevan SG, Gubler DJ. Update on dengue: epidemiology, virus evolution, antiviral drugs, and vaccine development. *Curr Infect Dis Rep* 2010; **12**: 157–164.

30 WHO. *Dengue: Guidelines for Diagnosis, Treatment, Prevention and Control*. Geneva: World Health Organization, 2009.

31 Wilder-Smith A, Schwartz E. Dengue in travelers. *N Engl J Med* 2005; **353**: 924–932.

32 Leder K, Torresi J, Brownstein JS, et al. Travel-associated illness trends and clusters, 2000–2010. *Emerg Infect Dis* 2013; **19**: 1049–1073.

33 Wilder-Smith A, Tambyah PA. Severe dengue virus infection in travelers. *J Infect Dis* 2007; **195**: 1081–1083.

34 Chen LH, Wilson ME. Travel-associated dengue infections in the United States, 1996 to 2005. Letter 1. *J Travel Med* 2010; **17**: 285; author reply, 286.

35 CDC. Japanese encephalitis vaccines. Recommendations of the Advisory Commitee on Immunization Practices (ACIP). *MMWR Morb Mortal Wkly Rep* 2010; **59**: 1–21.

36 CDC. Inactivated Japanese encephalitis vaccine. Recommendations of the Advisory Committee on Immunization Practices (ACIP). *MMWR Morb Mortal Wkly Rep* 1993; **42**: 1–15.

37 Wittesjo B, Eitrem R, Niklasson B, et al. Japanese encephalitis after a 10-day holiday in Bali. *Lancet* 1995; **345**: 856–857.

38 Buhl MR, Black FT, Andersen PL, Laursen A. Fatal Japanese encephalitis in a Danish tourist visiting Bali for 12 days. *Scand J Infect Dis* 1996; **28**: 189.

39 Hoffmann AA, Montgomery BL, Popovici J, et al. Successful establishment of *Wolbachia* in *Aedes* populations to suppress dengue transmission. *Nature* 2011; **476**: 454–457.

40 Wise de Valdez MR, Nimmo D, Betz J, et al. Genetic elimination of dengue vector mosquitoes. *Proc Natl Acad Sci U S A* 2011; **108**: 4772–4775.

41 Thomas SJ, Endy TP. Current issues in dengue vaccination. *Curr Opin Infect Dis* 2013; **26**: 429–434.

42 Wilder-Smith A, Deen JL. Dengue vaccines for travelers. *Expert Rev Vaccines* 2008; **7**: 569–578.

43 Wilder-Smith A, Halstead SB. Japanese encephalitis: update on vaccines and vaccine recommendations. *Curr Opin Infect Dis* 2010; **23**: 426–431.

44 Halstead SB, Thomas SJ. Japanese encephalitis: new options for active immunization. *Clin Infect Dis* 2010; **50**: 1155–1164.

CHAPTER 8

Yellow fever

Mark D. Gershman[1] & J. Erin Staples[2]

[1] *Centers for Disease Control and Prevention, Atlanta, GA, USA*
[2] *Centers for Disease Control and Prevention, Fort Collins, CO, USA*

Epidemiology

Yellow fever (YF) virus is transmitted to humans primarily through the bite of an infected *Aedes* or *Haemagogus* sp. mosquito. The virus is present in sub-Saharan Africa and tropical South America, where it is endemic and intermittently epidemic [1]. The World Health Organization (WHO) estimates that 200,000 cases of YF, including 30,000 deaths, occur annually worldwide.

YF virus has three transmission cycles: sylvatic (jungle), intermediate (savannah), and urban [2]. Most YF disease in humans is due to sylvatic or intermediate transmission cycles. However, urban YF occurs periodically in Africa and sporadically in the Americas.

In Africa, most outbreaks have been reported from West Africa, with fewer outbreaks being reported from Central and East Africa [2]. YF virus transmission in rural West Africa is seasonal, with an elevated risk during the end of the rainy season and the beginning of the dry season (usually July–October) [3]. However, YF virus may be episodically transmitted by *Ae. aegypti* even during the dry season in both rural and densely settled urban areas [2].

In South America, transmission of YF virus occurs predominantly in sparsely-populated forested areas. Consequently, YF occurs most frequently in unimmunized young men who are exposed to mosquitoes through work in forested areas [2]. The risk for infection in South America is highest during the rainy season (January–May) [3].

Clinical manifestation, diagnosis, and treatment

Most people infected with YF virus are asymptomatic. For symptomatic illness, the incubation period is typically 3–6 days. The initial illness presents as a non-specific febrile illness with sudden onset of fever, headache, myalgias, nausea, and vomiting [2]. Most patients improve after the initial presentation; however, approximately 15% of patients progress, after a brief remission of hours to 1 day, to more severe

Essential Travel Medicine, First Edition.
Edited by Jane N. Zuckerman, Gary W. Brunette and Peter A. Leggat.
© 2015 John Wiley & Sons, Ltd. Published 2015 by John Wiley & Sons, Ltd.

disease with jaundice, hemorrhagic symptoms, and multisystem organ failure. The case–fatality ratio for patients with hepatorenal dysfunction is 20–50% [2].

The preliminary diagnosis is based on the patient's clinical features and travel details. Laboratory diagnosis is typically made by detecting virus-specific immunoglobulin M (IgM) antibodies, followed by confirmation by more specific antibody testing, such as a plaque reduction neutralization test. Samples collected in the first few days of the illness may be positive by YF virus isolation or nucleic acid amplification tests.

No specific medications are available to treat YF virus infections; treatment is supportive (e.g., rest, fluids, analgesics, and antipyretics).

Yellow fever among travelers

A traveler's risk for acquiring YF is determined by various factors, including immunization status, travel details, and local rate of virus transmission at the destination during the time of travel [4]. Although reported cases of human disease are the principal indicator of disease risk, case reports may be absent because of a low level of transmission, a high level of immunity in the population (e.g., because of vaccination), or insensitive surveillance. This "epidemiologic silence" does not equate to absence of risk and should not lead to travel without protective measures.

From 1970 through 2012, nine YF cases were reported in unvaccinated travelers from the United States and Europe and one in a vaccinated traveler [2]. Eight of the nine unvaccinated travelers died and the vaccinated traveler survived.

For a 2-week stay, the estimated risks for illness and death attributable to YF for an unvaccinated traveler visiting an endemic area of West Africa are 50 and 10 cases per 100,000, respectively; for South America, the risks for illness and death are 5 and 1 case per 100,000, respectively [3].

Prevention

All travelers to YF-endemic countries should be advised of the disease risk and prevention methods, including personal protective measures and vaccine.

Personal protection measures

All travelers should take precautions to avoid mosquito bites, including using insect repellent, wearing permethrin-impregnated clothing, and staying in accommodations with screened or air-conditioned rooms [5].

Vaccines

All YF vaccines currently manufactured are live-attenuated viral vaccines. YF vaccine is recommended for people aged 9 months or more who are traveling to or living in areas with risk for YF virus transmission in South America and Africa [6,7]. In addition, some countries require proof of YF vaccination for entry. To minimize the risk of serious adverse events, clinicians should observe the contraindications to and precautions for vaccination and vaccinate only persons who are at risk for exposure or are visiting a country that requires proof of vaccination for entry [6].

Vaccine administration

For persons of all ages for whom vaccination is indicated, a single subcutaneous injection of reconstituted vaccine should be administered. In 2013, the World Health Organization (WHO) stated that a single dose of YF vaccine is sufficient to confer life-long protective immunity against YF disease, and a booster dose is not necessary [6]. However, the International Health Regulations (IHR) continue to require revaccination at 10-year intervals. Therefore, clinicians and travelers should review country entry requirements, including for booster doses, prior to traveling [7].

Vaccine safety and adverse reactions

Reactions to YF vaccine are generally mild; 10–30% of vaccinees report mild systemic adverse events, including low-grade fever, headache, and myalgias [2].

Three well-characterized serious adverse events occur following YF vaccine administration: immediate hypersensitivity or anaphylactic reactions, YF vaccine-associated neurologic disease (YEL-AND), and YF vaccine-associated viscerotropic disease (YEL-AVD) [4].

- Immediate hypersensitivity reactions are characterized by rash, urticaria, and/or bronchospasm. Anaphylaxis after YF vaccine is reported to occur at a rate of 0.8–1.8 cases per 100,000 doses distributed.
- YEL-AND manifests as distinct clinical syndromes, including meningoencephalitis, Guillain–Barré syndrome, and acute disseminated encephalomyelitis. Illness onset is 3–28 days after vaccination, and almost all cases have been reported in first-time vaccinees [4]. YEL-AND is rarely fatal. The incidence of YEL-AND among US travelers is reported to be 0.4–0.8 per 100,000 doses distributed [4].
- YEL-AVD is similar to wild-type disease, with widespread vaccine virus dissemination, and often multisystem organ failure and death [4]. More than 60 cases have been reported worldwide. Symptom onset is 0–8 days after vaccination, and all cases have been reported in first-time vaccinees. The case–fatality ratio is 63% [2]. The incidence of YEL-AVD among US travelers is 0.3–0.4 cases per 100,000 doses of vaccine distributed [4].

Contraindications

Persons who have a contraindication to YF vaccination should be not vaccinated and should avoid travel to YF-endemic areas. If travel to endemic areas is unavoidable, the clinician should provide a medical waiver and inform the traveler of increased risk for YF associated with lack of vaccination, and also protective measures.

Infants younger than 6 months

YF vaccine is contraindicated for infants aged <6 months because of a relatively high rate of YEL-AND documented in vaccinated young infants [2].

Hypersensitivity

YF vaccine is contraindicated for people with a history of hypersensitivity to any of the vaccine components, including eggs, egg products, chicken proteins, and gelatin. Skin testing and desensitization can be performed (see the vaccine package insert) in persons needing vaccination but for whom there is a concern about hypersensitivity reaction to the vaccine.

Altered immune status

YF vaccine is contraindicated for people with altered immune status caused by any of the following conditions [4,6]:

- Thymus disorder associated with abnormal immune cell function, such as thymoma or myasthenia gravis.
- AIDS or other clinical manifestations of HIV, including people with CD4 T-lymphocyte values <200/mm^3 or <15% of total lymphocytes for children aged <6 years.
- Primary immunodeficiencies, malignant neoplasms, and transplantation.
- People whose immunologic response is either suppressed or modulated by current or recent radiation therapies or drugs. Drugs with known immunosuppressive or immunomodulatory properties include, but are not limited to, high-dose systemic corticosteroids, alkylating drugs, antimetabolites, tumor necrosis factor-α inhibitors, interleukin blocking agents, and other monoclonal antibodies targeting immune cells [5]. If these therapies are discontinued, YF vaccine should be deferred until immune function has improved.

Family members of people with altered immune status, who themselves have no contraindications, can receive YF vaccine.

Precautions

If a person who has a condition that is considered a precaution to YF vaccination cannot postpone or avoid travel to YF-endemic countries, vaccination can be considered based on weighing risk versus benefits. If international travel requirements, not risk of YF, are the only reason for vaccination, the person should be excused from YF immunization and issued a waiver.

Infants aged 6–8 months

Age 6–8 months is a precaution for YF vaccination. Two cases of YEL-AND have been reported among infants aged 6–8 months [4].

Adults 60 years of age or older

Age 60 years or more is a precaution for YF vaccination because the reporting rate for YEL-AND and YEL-AVD is increased among people aged 60 years or more [4]. Given that YEL-AND and YEL-AVD are seen almost exclusively in primary vaccinees, caution should be exercised with older travelers who are receiving their first YF vaccination.

Asymptomatic HIV infection with moderate immune suppression

Asymptomatic HIV infection with CD4 T-lymphocyte values 200–499/mm^3 or 15–24% of total lymphocytes for children aged <6 years is associated with moderate immune suppression and hence is a precaution for YF vaccination. The relatively few observational studies performed have reported no serious adverse events following YF vaccination among patients considered moderately immunosuppressed based on their CD4 counts.

Note. If an asymptomatic HIV-infected person has no evidence of immune suppression based on CD4 counts (CD4 T-lymphocyte values $\geq 500/mm^3$ or $\geq 25\%$ of total lymphocytes for children aged <6 years), YF vaccine can be administered if recommended.

Pregnancy

Pregnancy is a precaution for YF vaccine administration. The safety of YF vaccination during pregnancy has not been studied in a large prospective trial. However, among pregnant women who received YF vaccination, limited studies have found no major malformations in their infants, and results are conflicting regarding an association with spontaneous abortions. The seroconversion rate among women vaccinated during pregnancy is variable and might depend on the trimester of vaccination. Although there are no specific data, women should be advised to wait 4 weeks after YF vaccination before conceiving.

Breastfeeding

Breastfeeding is a precaution for YF vaccine administration. Three YEL-AND cases have been reported in exclusively breastfed infants, aged <1 month, whose mothers were vaccinated with YF vaccine [2].

Simultaneous administration of other vaccines

Because no evidence exists that inactivated vaccines interfere with the immune response to YF vaccine, they can be administered either simultaneously or at any time before or after YF vaccination. YF vaccine should be given simultaneously or 30 days apart from other live-virus vaccines because the immune response to one live-virus vaccine might be impaired if administered within 30 days of another live-virus vaccine [6]. However, oral typhoid vaccine can be administered simultaneously or at any interval before or after YF vaccine.

International certificate of vaccination or prophylaxis (ICVP)

The IHR allow countries to require proof of YF vaccination from travelers, even if only in transit, arriving from a country with risk of YF virus transmission, to prevent importation and indigenous spread of YF virus [7]. Some countries require evidence of vaccination from all entering travelers [5]. Travelers without proof of YF vaccination who arrive in a country with a YF vaccination entry requirement may be quarantined for up to 6 days, refused entry, or vaccinated on-site.

As proof of YF vaccination, all vaccinees should possess a completed International Certificate of Vaccination or Prophylaxis (ICVP) validated with the provider's signature and the YF vaccination stamp of the administering YF vaccination center [5].

The ICVP must be signed by a medical provider supervising the administration of the vaccine, who may be a licensed physician or a healthcare worker designated by the physician.

An incomplete ICVP is not considered valid, and the traveler could be treated the same as a person without proof of vaccination at the port of entry. The ICVP is valid for 10 years, beginning 10 days after the date of vaccination. When a booster dose of the vaccine is given within this 10-year period, the certificate is considered valid from the date of revaccination.

Medical waivers (exemptions)

A traveler who has a specific contraindication to YF vaccine and who cannot avoid travel to a country requiring vaccination should be issued a waiver before departure. The clinician issuing a waiver should fill out and sign the Medical Contraindications to Vaccination section of the ICVP and give the traveler a signed and dated exemption letter on letterhead stationery. The letter should clearly state the contraindications to vaccination and bear the stamp of the YF vaccination center. The clinician should also inform the traveler of the increased risk for YF associated with lack of vaccination and how to minimize this risk by avoiding mosquito bites. Reasons other than medical contraindications or precautions are not acceptable for exemption from vaccination. The traveler should be advised that issuance of a waiver does not guarantee its acceptance by the destination country.

Requirements versus recommendations

Country entry requirements for proof of YF vaccination under the IHR differ from YF vaccination recommendations, such as those published by the WHO [5,7]. YF vaccine entry requirements are established by countries to prevent the importation and transmission of YF virus. Travelers must comply with these to enter the country, unless they have been issued a medical waiver. Country requirements are subject to change at any time; therefore, travelers are encouraged to check with the relevant embassy or consulate before departure.

YF vaccine recommendations are advice given by public health authorities to prevent YF virus infections among travelers. Recommendations are subject to change at any time because of changes in YF virus circulation, and travelers should check relevant websites for updates.

YF risk classification for travelers

The four categories of risk for YF virus transmission apply to all geographic areas: endemic, transitional, low potential for exposure, and no risk [1]. YF vaccination is recommended for travel to endemic and transitional areas. Although vaccination is generally not recommended for travel to areas with low potential for exposure, it

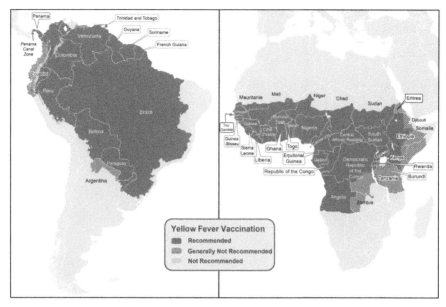

Figure 8.1 Yellow fever vaccine recommendations. Source: Adapted from Centers for Disease Control and Prevention 2014 [5].

might be considered for a small subset of travelers who may be at increased risk for exposure to YF virus because of prolonged travel, heavy exposure to mosquitoes, or inability to avoid mosquito bites.

References

1 Jentes ES, Poumerol G, Gershman MD, et al. The revised global yellow fever risk map and recommendations for vaccination, 2010: consensus of the Informal WHO Working Group on Geographic Risk for Yellow Fever. *Lancet Infect Dis* 2011; **11**: 622–632.

2 Monath TP, Gershman M, Staples JE, Barrett ADT. Yellow fever vaccine. In: Plotkin SA, Orenstein WA, Offit PA (eds.) *Vaccines*, 6th edn. Philadelphia, PA: Saunders Elsevier, 2013, pp. 870–968.

3 Monath TP, Cetron MS. Prevention of yellow fever in persons traveling to the tropics. *Clin Infect Dis* 2002; **34**: 1369–1378.

4 Staples JE, Gershman MD, Fischer M. Recommendations of the Advisory Committee on Immunization Practices (ACIP): yellow fever vaccine. *MMWR Morb Mortal Wkly Rep* 2010; **59**(RR-7): 1–27.

5 Centers for Disease Control and Prevention. *CDC Health Information for International Travel 2014*. New York: Oxford University Press, 2014.

6 WHO. Vaccines and vaccination against yellow fever: WHO position paper – June 2013. *Wkly Epidemiol Rec* 2013; **88**: 269–284.

7 WHO. *International Travel and Health* 2012. Geneva: *World Health Organization*, 2012.

CHAPTER 9

Malaria

Tomas Jelinek

Berlin Center for Travel and Tropical Medicine, Berlin, Germany

The disease and its lifecycle

Epidemiology

At least 2 billion people live in malarious areas [1]. Consequently, malaria remains one of the most important global public health challenges. It caused an estimated 225 million clinical cases and more than 655,000 deaths in 2011, mainly in children aged less than 5 years old living in sub-Saharan Africa [1–3]. The disease primarily affects poor populations in tropical and subtropical areas, where the temperature and rainfall are most suitable for the development of the malaria-causing *Plasmodium* parasites in *Anopheles* mosquitoes. Malaria also represents a serious health hazard to travelers to endemic areas. According to the World Tourism Organization, there were approximately 940 million travel-related arrivals worldwide in 2010, of which approximately 180 million were arrivals in malarious areas [4]. Imported malaria is seen in travelers returning from endemic countries or in migrants. A large proportion of the latter group consists of migrants living in Europe and returning from visiting friends and relatives (VFR) in a malarious area. VFRs traveling to sub-Saharan Africa have more than eight times the risk than tourists of being diagnosed with malaria, and more than twice the odds of being diagnosed with malaria after travel to Asia [5]. As international air travel to tropical destinations has become more and more popular, recent decades have brought a steady increase in imported cases in non-endemic countries [6–9]. After some years of declining numbers, the latest data from Europe [3,10] show increasing trends in imported malaria and US statistics show a 40-year high in imported malaria for 2011 [11]. One study found that the crude risk of malaria infection for travelers varied from one per 100,000 travelers to Central America and the Caribbean to 357 per 100,000 in Central Africa [12]

The parasite and its life cycle

Malaria arises from the infection of red blood cells with plasmodia. Species that infect humans are *Plasmodium falciparum, P. vivax, P. ovale, P. malariae*, and the recently detected *P. knowlesi* in South-East Asia. Severe manifestations are mainly due to *P. falciparum*, but *P. knowlesi* and in exceptional circumstances *P. vivax* are also capable of causing lethal disease. *P. falciparum* is the most virulent among the five *Plasmodium*

Essential Travel Medicine, First Edition.
Edited by Jane N. Zuckerman, Gary W. Brunette and Peter A. Leggat.
© 2015 John Wiley & Sons, Ltd. Published 2015 by John Wiley & Sons, Ltd.

species that cause malaria in humans. It is also distinguished by its particular pathophysiology, in particular through its ability to bind to endothelium during the blood stage of the infection and to sequester in organs, including the brain. This is the cause of most of the deaths from malaria. *P. vivax* is a far less deadly parasite but highly disabling; it is common in tropical areas outside Africa. The ability of *P. vivax* and also the very similar *P. ovale* to remain dormant for months as hypnozoites in the liver makes infection with these parasites difficult to eradicate. *P. malariae* does not form hypnozoites, but it can persist for decades as an asymptomatic blood stage infection. Originally a parasite causing infection in monkeys in South-East Asia, *P. knowlesi* has only recently been acknowledged as pathogenic for humans. It has spread locally and has a tendency to multiply rapidly inside erythrocytes, thus causing rapid and potentially lethal disease. However, unlike *P. falciparum*, it does not cause sequestration.

The *Plasmodium* life cycle leads to numerous transitions and stages of the parasite, all necessitating a specific immune response during this particular part of the cycle (Figure 9.1). Following inoculation by an *Anopheles* mosquito into the human dermis, motile sporozoites access blood vessels in the skin, are transported to the liver, and then transit through macrophages and hepatocytes to initiate liver stage infection. Subsequently, each sporozoite yields tens of thousands of merozoites. After an incubation period of 1–4 weeks, infected hepatocytes rupture and release merozoites, and the clinical disease begins. The merozoites invade erythrocytes, then further develop and multiply within these cells while digesting the hemoglobin. Asexual blood stage parasites produce 8–20 new merozoites every 36–48 hours (or 72 hours for *P. malariae*), causing parasite numbers to rise rapidly to levels as high as 10^{13} per host (Table 9.1). The asexual stages are pathogenic, and infected individuals can present with diverse sequelae affecting different organ systems. The blood stages of infection also include gametocytes (male and female sexual forms), that

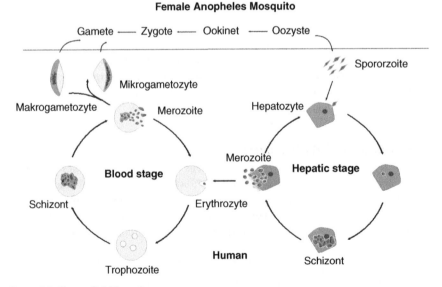

Figure 9.1 Plasmodial life cycle.

Table 9.1 Human malaria – essentials.

Parasite	*P. falciparum*	*P. vivax*	*P. ovale*	*P. malariae*	*P. knowlesi*
Disease	Falciparum malaria	Tertian (vivax) malaria	Tertian (ovale) malaria	Quartan malaria	Knowlesi malaria
No. of merozoites during hepatic stage	40,000	10,000	15,000	15,000	?
No. of merozoites in erythrocyte	8–12	16–24	10–12	8–12	8–12
Incubation period	7–28 days	12 days–1 year	12 days–1 year	20–50 days	7 days–months?
Longest reported incubation period (months)	>2	12	12	18	?
Max. duration of untreated infection (years)	1–2	1–5	1–5	3–50	1–2
Max. parasitemia (%)	Unlimited	1–2	1–2	1–2	Unlimited

await ingestion by mosquitoes before developing further. Sexual stage parasites are non-pathogenic but are transmissible to the *Anopheles* vector, where they recombine and generate genetically distinct sporozoites. The mosquito becomes infectious to its next blood meal donor 1–2 weeks after ingesting gametocytes, a time frame that is influenced by the external temperature. Development of *P. vivax* within the mosquito can occur at a lower environmental temperature than that required for the development of *P. falciparum*, explaining the preponderance of *P. vivax* infections outside tropical and subtropical regions.

Clinical presentation of malaria in travelers

Health practitioners face a broad spectrum of patient characteristics when encountering malaria, from the moderately compromised individual with few symptoms to the critically ill patient with organ failure. The majority of imported cases remain uncomplicated [5,6]. The mortality of imported *P. falciparum* malaria cases varies from 0.4% in a large cohort from France to 5% in a recent cluster of cases imported from the Gambia [13,14]. Most patients with *P. falciparum* infections become symptomatic within 30 days after return from the malaria-endemic area. Longer incubation periods are seen with the other *Plasmodium* species and are prolonged by incomplete malaria chemoprophylaxis, which may reduce parasitemia without achieving full protection. Prodromal symptoms, which may precede the fever for up to 2 days, are fatigue, loss of appetite, headache, and body pains. In non-immune patients, malaria usually starts suddenly with a severe feeling of sickness and fever, often reaching 39 °C and higher [15]. Not all patients show typical fever paroxysms and absence of fever does not remove the suspicion of malaria in an ill patient. If present, the frequency of the febrile episodes depends on the parasite species, occurring every 48 hours (tertian) for *P. vivax* and *P. ovale*, every 72 hours (quartan) for *P. malariae*, and every 24 hours (quotidian) for *P. knowlesi*. In *P. falciparum* malaria, the fever usually lacks a regular pattern. Common symptoms are headache and myalgia; nausea is frequent. Other symptoms may include vomiting, dry cough, icterus, confusion, and respiratory distress. Compromised circulation leads to renal failure and impaired tissue perfusion, resulting in acidosis. Gastrointestinal complaints unrelated to treatment, including vomiting and diarrhea, are less frequent. Clinical examination is non-specific since it often takes some time before anemia or hepatosplenomegaly develop.

As an effect of previously acquired semi-immunity, malaria in adult migrants is characterized by a milder clinical presentation, lower levels of parasitemia, shorter parasite clearance time after treatment, and shorter fever duration compared with malaria in non-immune travelers [16–18]. A high proportion of migrants have few symptoms and present long after arrival in the host country [19], with periods of months up to several years recorded [19–23]. If semi-immunity is lost after living 2 years or longer in non-endemic areas, traveling migrants have a risk of clinical malaria approaching that of non-immune travelers [24,25].

Malaria diagnosis

Early and fast diagnosis is crucial to prevent uncomplicated malaria progressing to complicated disease. Microscopic examination of Giemsa-stained thin and thick blood films remains the gold standard. In expert hands, the method is simple, rapid, and sensitive [26], with a sensitivity reaching five parasites per microliter [27]. More sensitive thick blood films are combined with thin blood films for determination of parasitemia and species identification. However, expert microscopy is frequently not available when patients need to be diagnosed quickly, thus reducing the use of this method significantly. Even after the start of specific treatment, there is a lag-phase before the parasite density begins to decline [28], and there may even be an increase in parasitemia in the first 24 hours after onset of therapy. Rapid diagnostic tests (RDTs) based on the detection of parasite-specific antigens by monoclonal antibodies have been developed to make the first assessment of a potential malaria patient simpler and potentially more reliable. Antigens commonly used are histidine-rich protein 2 (HRP2), pan-plasmodial aldolase, and parasite-specific lactate dehydrogenase (LDH). Assays are available that detect all species, i.e. *P. falciparum*, *P. vivax*, *P. ovale*, and *P. malariae* [29]. *P. knowlesi* infections may be detected by rapid tests that include the pan-plasmodial aldolase or LDH antigens, but sensitivity appears to be limited [30]. For falciparum malaria, many RDTs show a 100% parasite detection score down to a parasite density level of 200 parasites per microliter, equivalent to a parasitemia of approximately 0.004% [31]. However, there are limitations. Rapid tests cannot determine the parasite density. False-negative RDTs in patients with very high parasite densities have been described, probably due to the so-called "pro-zone" effect [32,33]. Mutations in the HRP2 gene may also result in false-negative tests [34,35] and rheumatoid factor may lead to false positives [36]. Results of a WHO multicenter evaluation of different rapid diagnostic tests showed that the best performance was found with tests based on a combination of the HRP2 and pan-plasmodial proteins [31]. Clinicians using rapid tests need to be aware that no RDT test so far is 100% reliable and that they should be used in parallel with and not instead of blood film examination. RDTs also are a potential option for travelers without access to qualified medical care. However, rapid tests may be difficult to perform and interpret by untrained persons, particularly those in distress [37,38] Emphasis should be placed on proper instructions and training if tests are recommended to travelers [39].

Methods of prevention including prophylaxis and emergency stand-by treatment

Exposure prophylaxis

Avoiding mosquito bites is a crucial step towards avoiding malaria, hence counseling on effective exposure prophylaxis is a main pillar of counseling for travel to malarious areas. Anopheles mosquitoes are active from sunset to dawn, often in the vicinity of their breeding areas (lakes, rivers, ponds). Travelers need to be aware of potential sources of mosquito bites and should protect themselves accordingly. This includes sleeping in air-conditioned rooms or the use of permethrine-impregnated bed nets, the treatment of clothes with permethrine, and the application of repellents to the unprotected skin. The most effective repellent is diethyltoluamide (DEET), a chemical that effectively confuses the sensory functions of mosquitoes and renders them less capable of smelling humans. The most effective concentrations are 30–50%.

Chemoprophylaxis

Drug details can be found in Table 9.2. Recommendations for malaria chemoprophylaxis vary according to destination, season, and individual specifics of travelers [40]. Time, destination, and duration of travel and also the specifics of the traveler need to be taken into account when counseling on malaria prophylaxis. Adherence to recommendations is a crucial issue. Since effective vaccines are not available, chemoprophylaxis is recommended for destinations with a high risk of malaria. Although this strategy cannot prevent infection, it will usually prevent manifestation of disease. Effective antimalarials for this strategy include atovaquone–proguanil, doxycycline, mefloquine, and chloroquine in areas without resistance (Table 9.2). The risk of severe adverse events due to chemoprophylaxis has to be calculated against the risk of potentially life-threatening malaria. It has been shown that adherence to recommended prophylaxis protocols is severely diminished by the occurrence of side-effects [40–42].

The efficacy of chloroquine as a chemoprophylactic drug is severely diminished by the resistance of *P. falciparum* to this compound. Hence it is only rarely indicated, exceptions being destinations in Central America and the Caribbean.

The chloroquine–proguanil combination has been used for several years in order to override widespread resistance against one or both of the drugs. Since particularly *P. falciparum* has become resistant against the combination and since both drugs frequently produce unpleasant side-effects, their use is no longer recommended.

Mefloquine has been used for decades as a chemoprophylactic drug and its efficacy and side-effects are well documented. It can still be used in many parts of the world since resistance has been slow to develop. It also is the only widely effective

Table 9.2 Antimalarials for treatment and prophylaxis.

Substance or combination	Therapy/SBET		Prophylaxis	
	Adults	**Children**	**Adults**	**Children**
Chloroquine (only if no resistance)	1 tab. = 150 mg base (~500 mg salt): initially 1 × 4 tab., 6 h later 2 tab., 24 h later 2 tab., 48 h later 2 tab.	Initially 10 mg base/kg (~8.3 mg salt/kg), 6 h later 5 mg base/kg, 24 h later 5 mg base/kg, 48 h later 5 mg base/kg	1 tab. = 150 mg base (~500 mg salt); 1 × 2 tab./week, >75 kg: 1 × 3 tab./week., start 1 week before travel, stop 4 weeks after travel	5 mg/kg (~8.3 mg salt/kg) once per week., max. Adult dose, start 1 week before travel, stop 4 weeks after travel
Proguanil (in combination with chloroquine; only if no resistance)	Not effective	Not effective	1 × 200 mg/day; start 1 week before travel, stop 4 weeks after travel	3 mg/kg, once daily; start 1 week before travel, stop 4 weeks after travel
Mefloquine	1 tab. = 250 mg base (~274 mg salt); initially 3 tab., 6–8 h later 2 tab., if >60 kg 6–8 h later 1 tab.	From 3 months and 5 kg: 15 mg/kg; 6–24 h later 10 mg/kg (or 25 mg/kg as single dose); >45 kg as adult	1 tab. = 250 mg base (~274 mg salt); 1 × 1 tab./week.; start 1 week before travel, stop 4 weeks after travel	From 3 months and 5 kg: 5 mg/kg; once per week; start 1 week before travel, stop 4 weeks after travel
Atovaquone–proguanil	1 tab. = 250 mg/100 mg; >40 kg: 1 × 4 tab./day for 3 days	250 mg/100 mg (=1 tab): 11–20 kg: 1 tab; 21–30 kg: 2 tab.; 31–40 kg: 3 tab.; >40 kg: 4 tab.; for 3 days	1 tab. = 250 mg/100 mg: 1 tab./day; start 1 day before travel, stop 1 week after travel	1 tab. Junior = 62,5 mg/25 mg; 11–20 kg: 1 tab.; 21–30 kg: 2 tab.; 31–40 kg: 3 tab.; >40 kg: 1 tab in adult dosing; start 1 day before travel, stop 1 week after travel

Dihydroartemisinine –piperaquine	1 tab = 40 mg/320 mg; 4 mg/kg/day dihydroartemisinin and 18 mg/kg/day piperaquine once per day for 3 days, with a therapeutic dose range of 2–10 mg/kg/day dihydroartemisinin and 16–26 mg/kg/dose piperaquine	1 tab = 40 mg/ 320 mg; 4 mg/kg/day dihydroartemisinin and 18 mg/kg/day piperaquine once per day for 3 days, with a therapeutic dose range of 2–10 mg/kg/day dihydroartemisinin and 16–26 mg/kg/dose piperaquine	Not effective	Not effective
Artemether –lumefantrine	1 tab. = 20 mg/120 mg; 4 tab. initially, 8 h later 4 tab., then 2 × 4 tab./day at day 2 and 3 (total dose 24 tab.)	1 tab. = 20 mg/240 mg; from 12 years and 35 kg dosing as adult	Not effective	Not effective
Doxycycline (monohydrate)	Only in combination with quinine: 3 mg/kg for 7–10 days; not for SBET	Contraindicated	1 × 100 mg/day; start 1 day before travel, stop 4 weeks after travel	From 8 years: 1.5 mg salt/kg/day; start 1 day before travel, stop 4 weeks after travel
Quinine	Only in complicated falciparum malaria: 3 × 10 mg quinine-hydrochloride/kg IV for 7–10 days; loading dose 7 mg quinine/kg for 30 min (not after mefloquine or quinine during the last 24 h), then 10 mg kg IV for 4 h; then 10 mg kg IV every 8 h; not for SBET	Only in complicated falciparum malaria: <2 years: initially 20 mg/kg for 4 h, then 10 mg/kg every 8 h in 5–10 mL 5% glucose/kg; >2 years: initially 20 mg/kg for 4 h, then 10 mg/kg every 12 h in 5–10 mL 5% glucose/kg; not for SBET	Not effective	Not effective
Primaquine	30 mg/day (0.5 mg base/kg) for 14 days	<1 year: 1–2 mg/day for 14 days; 1–3 years: 3–4 mg daily for 14 days; 4–12 years: 7.5 mg daily for 14 days; >12 years: as adult	Not effective	Not effective

prophylactic antimalarial that can be used during pregnancy. However, the drug has a significant potential for causing neuro-psychiatric side-effects, including severe psychosis and depression. The occurrence of these events is highly individual and very difficult to predict. Before long-term use, mefloquine should be tested for 3 weeks prior to travel in order to establish tolerance.

Atovaquone–proguanil is a comparatively new combination that has become established very rapidly as the chemoprophylaxis of choice for most travelers. Since it is already effective during the hepatic stage of falciparum malaria, it can be stopped comparably shortly after travel. Side-effects include nausea and vomiting.

Although not effective for the treatment of malaria, doxycycline can be used for chemoprophylaxis at an adult dose of 100 mg/day. Side-effects include phototoxicity, which occasionally poses a problem for travel to tropical countries. The use of primaquine for prophylaxis can be recommended for destinations with an overwhelming occurrence of vivax malaria.

A Cochrane analysis of eight clinical studies with a total of 4240 subjects confirmed that atovaquone–proguanil and doxycycline are tolerated best and that mefloquine is associated with neuro-psychiatric side-effects [43]. Chloroquine–proguanil showed significantly more side-effects, in particular gastrointestinal. Case reports about deaths in association with malaria chemoprophylaxis have only been involved mefloquine: in total, mefloquine accounted for 22 cases, including five suicides [43].

Stand-by emergency treatment (SBET)

Drug details can be found in Table 9.2. Stand-by emergency treatment (SBET) is described as the self-administration of antimalarial drugs by travelers. With this strategy, travelers are prescribed antimalarial medication which they carry during their journey. They are advised to use the medication when malaria is suspected and prompt medical attention is unavailable within 24 hours of onset of symptoms. This strategy is indicated as a potentially life-saving measure since malaria poses an emergency situation [40]. SBET is not intended to replace chemoprophylaxis in high-risk destinations such as sub-Saharan Africa or to detract from the importance of seeking a medical consultation when suspected malaria occurs. However, the world-wide increasing issue of counterfeit medication is of great concern for travelers. The concept of SBET ensures the availability of safe and effective medication when it is needed, since carriage of an antimalarial bought prior to travel from a safe source ensures reliable quality of the medication, in contrast to locally bought medication that could be counterfeit [41].

SBET can be recommended for travelers [4,42,44] who are:
- visiting an area with a minimal malaria risk and/or a remote area far from medical attention;
- expatriates or long-term travelers likely to have gaps in adherence to chemoprophylaxis;
- likely to have a changing itinerary with different malaria risks (e.g., backpackers);
- short-stay, frequent travelers (e.g., aircrews and business travelers);
- visiting destinations without qualified medical services and/or with the high likelihood of encountering counterfeit antimalarials.

According to WHO guidelines [40], drug options indicated for SBET are the same as the treatment options for uncomplicated malaria (Table 9.2): artemether–lumefantrine, dihydroartemisinin–piperaquine, mefloquine, atovaquone–proguanil, quinine with doxycycline or clindamycin or chloroquine (in areas without chloroquine resistance). Owing to their fast-acting mechanism with resulting rapid parasite clearance and disappearance of symptoms, artemisinin-based combinations are highly preferable in this setting. The WHO recommends oral artemisinin-based combination therapy (ACT) as standard treatment of uncomplicated malaria [45]. Artemisinin is an extract of the medical plant *Artemisia annua*, which together with its derivatives, artesunate and artemether, are the most effective antimalarial compounds to date [46–48]. Artemisinin derivatives are highly potent and capable of reducing the parasite biomass very fast. Another advantage of artemisinin derivatives is their ability to kill gametocytes, thus interrupting malaria transmission and making them the drugs of choice in epidemics. The artemisinin derivatives have a rapid onset of therapeutic effect, which makes their use particularly desirable in non-immune patients who may develop complicated malaria within very short time. However, they have a very short terminal elimination half-life of less than 2 hours [47,48]. Therefore, monotherapy should be avoided [45].

Artemether–lumefantrine (Riamet, Coartem) and dihydroartemisinin–piperaquine (Eurartesim) are the only artemisinin derivatives licensed for use in Europe. Artemether–lumefantrine is the most widely used ACT globally. It is well tolerated and highly efficacious in all endemic regions except for *P. falciparum* infections acquired in Cambodia and the border regions of Thailand with Myanmar, where multi-drug-resistant *P. falciparum* strains are prevalent [1,3]. The recommended treatment is a six-dose regimen over a 3-day period (Table 9.2). Artemether–lumefantrine has to be administered with fatty food in order to obtain optimal plasma drug concentrations [46]. This might be a disadvantage in a clinical setting, and in particular when the combination is used as SBET, since patients with malaria tend to suffer from nausea and will frequently decline food.

Dihydroartemisinin–piperaquine was approved by the European Medicines Agency in 2011 for the treatment of symptomatic, uncomplicated malaria in adults, children, and infants older than 6 months and/or above 5 kg. This combination is currently available as a fixed-dose combination with tablets containing 40 mg of dihydroartemisinin and 320 mg of piperaquine. Dihydroartemisinin–piperaquine should be taken fasting, a clear advantage since malaria patients are frequently nauseated and anorectic.

If the strategy of SBET is employed when counseling travelers visiting malarious areas, an antimalarial with high antiparasitic capacity should be prescribed as carry-on medication. A strong point in support of equipping travelers with a highly effective antimalarial treatment as part of their travel medical kit is the global proliferation of counterfeit antimalarials. ACTs are clearly superior to any other oral antimalarial in their fast reduction of parasite biomass and in decreasing clinical symptoms. Numerous trials and clinical experience have shown that ACTs are safe to use and that relevant side-effects are exceedingly rare. Although resistance against artemisinins in South-East Asia has been described, it has no impact on the clinical efficacy of ACTs. Hence they are the drugs of choice for travelers who need to decide upon their symptoms or by self-diagnosis via RDT whether they have to treat themselves against malaria.

References

1 Cibulskis RE, Aregawi M, Williams R, et al. Worldwide incidence of malaria in 2009: estimates, time trends, and a critique of methods. *PLoS Med* 2011; **8**(12): e1001142.

2 Murray CJ, Rosenfeld LC, Lim SS, et al. Global malaria mortality between 1980 and 2010: a systematic analysis. *Lancet* 2012; **379**: 413–431.

3 WHO. *World Malaria Report 2011*. Geneva: World Health Organization, 2011. http://www.who.int/malaria/world_malaria_report_2011/en/ (accessed 13 December 2012).

4 Schlagenhauf P, Petersen E. Standby emergency treatment of malaria in travelers. *Expert Rev Anti Infect Ther* 2012; **10**: 537–546.

5 Leder K, Tong S, Weld L, et al. GeoSentinel Surveillance Network. Illness in travelers visiting friends and relatives: a review of the GeoSentinel Surveillance Network. *Clin Infect Dis* 2006; **43**: 1185–1193.

6 Jelinek T, Schulte C, Behrens R, et al. for TropNetEurop. Clinical and epidemiological characteristics of falciparum malaria among travellers and immigrants with imported falciparum malaria in Europe: sentinel surveillance data from TropNetEurop. *Clin Infect Dis* 2002; **34**: 572–576.

7 Phillips-Howard PA, Bradley DJ, Blaze M, Hurn M. Malaria in Britain: 1977–86. *BMJ* 1988; **296**: 245–248.

8 Christen D, Steffen R, Schlagenhauf P. Deaths caused by malaria in Switzerland 1988–2002. *Am. J. Trop. Med. Hyg* 2006; **75**: 1188–1194.

9 Jelinek T, Behrens R, Bisoffi Z, et al. Recent cases of falciparum malaria imported to Europe from Goa, India, December 2006–January 2007. *Euro Surveill* 2007; **12**(1): E070111.1.

10 Checkley AM, Smith A, Smith V, et al. Risk factors for mortality from imported falciparum malaria in the United Kingdom over 20 years: an observational study. *BMJ* 2012; **344**: e2116.

11 Cullen KA, Arguin PM. Malaria surveillance – United States, 2011. *MMWR Surveill Summ* 2013; **62**(5): 1–17.

12 Askling HH, Nilsson J, Tegnell A, et al. Malaria risk in travelers. *Emerg Infect Dis* 2005; **11**: 436–441.

13 Seringe E, Thellier M, Fontanet A, et al.; French National Reference Center for Imported Malaria Study Group. Severe imported *Plasmodium falciparum* malaria, France, 1996–2003. *Emerg Infect Dis* 2011, **17**: 807–813.

14 Jelinek T, Larsen CS, Siikamäki H, et al. European cluster of imported falciparum malaria from Gambia. *Euro Surveill* 2008, **13**(51): pii: 19077.

15 Grobusch MP, Kremsner PG. Uncomplicated malaria. *Curr Top Microbiol Immunol* 2005, **295**: 83-104.

16 Mascarello M, Allegranzi B, Angheben A, et al. Imported malaria in adults and children: epidemiological and clinical characteristics of 380 consecutive cases observed in Verona, Italy. *J Travel Med* 2008, **15**: 229–236.

17 Legros F, Bouchaud O, Ancelle T, et al., for the French National Reference Centers for Imported and Autochthonous Malaria Epidemiology and Chemosensitivity Network. Risk factors for imported fatal *Plasmodium falciparum* malaria, France, 1996–2003. *Emerg Infect Dis* 2007; **13**: 883–888.

18 Muentener P, Schlagenhauf P, Steffen R. Imported malaria (1985–95): trends and perspectives. *Bull World Health Organ* 1999; **77**: 560–566.

19 D'Ortenzio E, Godineau N, Fontanet A, et al. Prolonged *Plasmodium falciparum* infection in immigrants, Paris. *Emerg Infect Dis* 2008; **14**: 323–326.

20 Bouchaud O, Cot M, Kony S, et al. Do African immigrants living in France have long-term malarial immunity? *Am J Trop Med Hyg* 2005; **72**: 21–25.

21 Krajden S, Panisko DM, Tobe B, et al. Prolonged infection with *Plasmodium falciparum* in a semi-immune patient. *Trans R Soc Trop Med Hyg* 1991; **85**: 731–732.

22 Greenwood T, Vikerfors T, Sjoberg M, et al. Febrile *Plasmodium falciparum* malaria 4 years after exposure in a man with sickle cell disease. *Clin Infect Dis* 2008; **47**: e39–e41.

23 Szmitko PE, Kohn ML, Simor AE. *Plasmodium falciparum* malaria occurring 8 years after leaving an endemic area. *Diagn Microbiol Infect Dis* 2009; **63**: 105–107.

24 Monge-Maillo B, Jiménez BC, Pérez-Molina JA, et al. Imported infectious diseases in mobile populations, Spain. *Emerg Infect Dis* 2009; **15**: 1745–1752.

25 Marangi M, Di Tullio R, Mens PF, et al. Prevalence of Plasmodium spp. in malaria asymptomatic African migrants assessed by nucleic acid sequence based amplification. *Malar J* 2009; **8**: 12.

26 Bowers KM, Bell D, Chiodini PL, et al. Inter-rater reliability of malaria parasite counts and comparison of methods. *Malar J* 2009; **8**: 267.

27 Petersen E, Marbiah NT, New L, Gottschau A. Comparison of two methods for enumerating malaria parasites in thick blood films. *Am J Trop Med Hyg* 1996; **55**: 485–489.

28 Flegg JA, Guerin PJ, White NJ, Stepniewska K. Standardizing the measurement of parasite clearance in falciparum malaria: the parasite clearance estimator. *Malar J* 2011; **10**: 339.

29 Chiodini PL, Bowers K, Jorgensen P, et al. The heat stability of *Plasmodium* lactate dehydrogenase-based and histidine-rich protein 2-based malaria rapid diagnostic tests. *Trans R Soc Trop Med Hyg* 2007; **101**: 331–337.

30 van Hellemond JJ, Rutten M, Koelewijn R, et al. Human *Plasmodium knowlesi* infection detected by rapid diagnostic tests for malaria. *Emerg Infect Dis* 2009; **15**: 1478–1480.

31 WHO. *Malaria Rapid Diagnostic Test Performance – Results of WHO Product Testing of Malaria RDTs: Round 3 (2010–2011)*. Geneva: World Health Organization, 2011. http://www.who.int/tdr/publications/tdr-research-publications/rdt_round3/en/index.html (accessed 13 December 2012).

32 Luchavez J, Baker J, Alcantara S, et al. Laboratory demonstration of a prozone-like effect in HRP2-detecting malaria rapid diagnostic tests: implications for clinical management. *Malar J* 2011; **10**: 286.

33 Gillet P, Scheirlinck A, Stokx J, et al. Prozone in malaria rapid diagnostics tests: how many cases are missed? *Malar J* 2011; **10**: 166.

34 Koita OA, Doumbo OK, Ouattara A, et al. False-negative rapid diagnostic tests for malaria and deletion of the histidine-rich repeat region of the hrp2 gene. *Am J Trop Med Hyg* 2012; **86**: 194–198.

35 Baker J, Gatton ML, Peters J, et al. Transcription and expression of *Plasmodium falciparum* histidine-rich proteins in different stages and strains: implications for rapid diagnostic tests. *PLoS One* 2011; **6**(7): e22593.

36 Grobusch MP, Alpermann U, Schwenke S, et al. False-positive rapid tests for malaria in patients with rheumatoid factor. *Lancet* 1999; **353**: 297.

37 Grobusch MP, Hänscheid T, Göbels K et al. Sensitivity of *P. vivax* rapid antigen detection tests and possible implications for self-diagnostic use. *Travel Med Infect Dis* 2003; **1**; 119–122.

38 Jelinek T. Malaria self-testing by travellers: opportunities and limitations. *Travel Med Infect Dis* 2004; **2**; 143–148.

39 Berg J, Breederveld D, Roukens AH, et al. Knowledge, attitudes, and practices toward malaria risk and prevention among frequent business travelers of a major oil and gas company. *J Travel Med* 2011;**18**; 395–401.

40 WHO. Malaria. In: *International Travel and Health*. Geneva: World Health Organization, 2012, Chapter 7.

41 Newton PN, Green MD, Fernández FM, et al. Counterfeit anti-infective drugs. *Lancet Infect Dis* 2006: **6**; 602–613.

42 Nothdurft HD, Jelinek T, Pechel SM, et al. Stand-by treatment of suspected malaria in travellers. *Trop Med Parasitol* 1995: **46**; 161–163.

43 Jacquerioz FA, Croft AM. Drugs for preventing malaria in travellers. *Cochrane Database Syst Rev* 2009; (**4**): CD006491.

44 Chen LH, Wilson ME, Schlagenhauf P. Controversies and misconceptions in malaria chemoprophylaxis for travelers. *JAMA* 2007: **297**; 2251–2263.

45 WHO. *Guidelines for the Treatment of Malaria*. Geneva: World Health Organization, 2011c. http://www.who.int/malaria/world_malaria_report_2010/en/index.html (accessed 28 January 2015).

46 Haynes RK. Artemisinin and derivatives: the future for malaria treatment? *Curr Opin Infect Dis* 2001; **14**: 719–726.

47 Woodrow CJ, Haynes RK, Krishna S. Artemisinins. *Postgrad Med J* 2005; **81**: 71–78.

48 Keating GM. Dihydroartemisinin/piperaquine. Review of its use in the treatment of uncomplicated *Plasmodium falciparum* malaria. *Drugs* 2012: **72**; 937–961.

CHAPTER 10

Respiratory disease

Regina LaRocque & Edward T. Ryan
Massachusetts General Hospital, Boston, MA, USA

Causative agents

In general, the etiologic agents of respiratory infections in travelers are similar to those in non-travelers (Table 10.1). Viral pathogens are the most common causative agents of respiratory infections, particularly upper respiratory tract infection. Coronavirus, adenovirus, rhinovirus, influenza virus, parainfluenza virus, human metapneumovirus, and respiratory syncytial virus are common viral causes of respiratory infection. Bacterial causes of respiratory infection include *Streptococcus pneumoniae*, *Mycoplasma pneumoniae*, *Haemophilus influenzae*, and *Chlamydophila pneumoniae*. Endemic mycoses, such as *Histoplasma capsulatum*, *Coccidioides immitis*, and *Paracoccidioides brasiliensis*, are rare but geographically restricted causes of lower respiratory infection. Tissue-migrating parasites, such as *Strongyloides stercoralis*, hookworm, and *Ascaris lumbricoides*, can cause pulmonary symptoms (Loeffler syndrome) and may be acquired during travel to the developing world. *Paragonimus westermani* is a lung fluke that occurs in the Far East, the Americas and West Africa.

Respiratory pathogens associated with outbreaks

Influenza

Influenza is the most important viral respiratory infection of travelers, and is also among the most common vaccine-preventable illnesses among travelers [1,2]. Travelers acquire influenza sporadically, but also from outbreaks on-board ships and airplanes and in tour groups. Influenza is a particular concern among pilgrims to the Hajj [3,4]. International travelers play a key role in the global spread of influenza, as exemplified by the rapid worldwide dissemination of influenza A/H1N1 in 2009, in which all cases in countries other than Mexico were imported. Of note, influenza peaks in different months in the northern and southern hemispheres; February (winter in the northern hemisphere) is usually the peak month in the United States, and August (winter in the southern hemisphere) in Australia. Influenza transmission can occur year round in tropical climates.

Essential Travel Medicine, First Edition.
Edited by Jane N. Zuckerman, Gary W. Brunette and Peter A. Leggat.
© 2015 John Wiley & Sons, Ltd. Published 2015 by John Wiley & Sons, Ltd.

Table 10.1 Etiologic agents of upper and lower respiratory infections in travelers.

	Viruses	Bacteria	Fungi	Parasites
Upper respiratory tract infection	Coronavirus Adenovirus Rhinovirus Influenza A and B viruses Parainfluenza virus Human metapneumovirus Respiratory syncytial virus Human immunodeficiency virus (pharyngitis)	Group A Streptococcus (pharyngitis) Corynebacterium diphtheriae (pharyngitis) Streptococcus pneumoniae Mycoplasma pneumoniae Haemophilus influenzae Moraxella catarrhalis		
Lower respiratory tract infection	Influenza A and B viruses Measles Hantavirus SARS-coronavirus MERS-coronavirus Respiratory syncytial virus Varicella	Streptococcus pneumoniae Mycoplasma pneumoniae Staphylococcus aureus Haemophilus influenzae Chlamydophila pneumoniae Mycobacterium tuberculosis Chlamydophila psittaci Coxiella burnetii Burkholderia pseudomallei Yersinia pestis Bacillus anthracis (mediastinitis)	Histoplasma capsulatum Coccioides immitis Cryptococcus neoformans Paracoccidioides brasiliensis	Strongyloides stercoralis Hookworm Ascaris lumbricoides (Loeffler syndrome) Paragonimus westermani (lung fluke) Dirofilariasis (lung nodule) Schistosoma spp. [Katayama fever (acute) and pulmonary fibrosis (late)] Tropical pulmonary eosinophilia (lymphatic filariasis)

SARS

Severe acute respiratory syndrome (SARS) is a novel respiratory infection that first appeared in China in 2002. Subsequent studies demonstrated SARS to be a zoonosis, and the causative agent, SARS coronavirus (SARS-CoV), was associated with civets and bats. The disease spread within the course of weeks in early 2003 in travelers from China to Hong Kong, Vietnam, Singapore, and Canada [5]. In-flight transmission of SARS was specifically documented [6]. By the end of the epidemic, SARS caused 8273 cases and 775 deaths in multiple countries, with a case fatality rate of 9.6% [7].

MERS

In September 2012, another novel coronavirus infection, Middle East respiratory syndrome (MERS), was reported in a man in Saudi Arabia with pneumonia and acute kidney injury [8]. More than 100 laboratory-confirmed cases of Middle East respiratory syndrome coronavirus (MERS-CoV) have subsequently occurred. To date, the majority of cases have been in Saudi Arabia, but cases have occurred in several other countries in the Middle East. Travelers returning to Tunisia, Germany, Italy, the United Kingdom, and France from the Middle East have also become ill with the disease. MERS-CoV appears to be related to several bat coronaviruses, with bridge transmission possibly involving camels [9]. Human-to-human transmission occurs [10]. In 2013, the Ministry of Health of Saudi Arabia recommended that individuals with higher risk of complications from MERS (e.g., extremes of age, chronic medical conditions, immunosuppression, pregnancy) postpone their plans to travel to Saudi Arabia for Hajj or Umrah due to the outbreak of MERS-CoV.

Legionella species

Legionella pneumophila is the most common infecting species in the Legionellaciae family and can cause community-acquired pneumonia (Legionnaires' disease) or an acute, self-limited febrile syndrome (Pontiac fever). Approximately 20% of reported cases of Legionnaires' disease in the United States are associated with travel [11]. *Legionella* multiplies within water systems, often within free-living amoebae, and can form biofilms in cooling towers, water pipe fittings, and shower heads. Aerosolized bacteria from contaminated hotel water and air conditioning or ventilatory systems are common sources of infection among travelers [12]. Outbreaks on cruise ships have also been described [13].

Others

Other respiratory diseases that have caused outbreaks of infection among travelers include *Coxiella burnettii* (Q fever) [14], *Histoplasma capsulatum* [15–17], measles [18], varicella [19], and diphtheria [20]. Exposure to *Mycobacterium tuberculosis* can also occur during travel, particularly long-term travel [21–23].

Risk in travelers

Respiratory infections are a leading cause of illness in travelers [24]. Among ill travelers seeking care at clinical sites in the GeoSentinel Surveillance Network from June 1996 to August 2004, the overall rate of respiratory disorders was 77/1000, with a range from 45/1000 among travelers to the Caribbean to 97/1000 among travelers to South-East Asia [25]. These rates are likely to be underestimates, since travelers with mild or moderate respiratory symptoms may not seek medical care. Overall, respiratory infections were diagnosed in 7.8% of ill returned travelers in GeoSentinel, and upper respiratory infection comprised the majority of these cases [26]. Prolonged travel, travel to visit friends and relatives, and travel during the northern hemisphere winter were associated with an increased likelihood of influenza, and male gender and increasing age were associated with lower respiratory tract infection in this cohort.

Travelers may also play an important role in the global transmission of respiratory infections. In recent years, transmission of SARS and influenza A/H1N1 has been closely linked with international air travel.

Clinical manifestations

Respiratory infection may involve the upper respiratory tract (rhinitis, sinusitis, otitis, pharyngitis, tracheitis), the lower respiratory tract (bronchitis, pneumonia), or both. Most viral upper respiratory illnesses involve sneezing, rhinorrhea, sore throat, cough, low-grade fever, headache, and malaise. Acute bacterial rhinosinusitis is a rare complication in adults with upper respiratory infection. Symptoms suggestive of pneumonia include productive cough, chest pain, and shortness of breath. Chest examination may identify crepitation or rhonchi, and chest imaging can be useful to confirm the presence of lobar consolidation and evaluate for associated complications such as empyema, pneumothorax, or cavitation.

Diagnosis

Most upper respiratory tract infections are caused by viruses. Identifying a specific etiologic agent may be difficult and is often not clinically necessary. Molecular methods are available to identify a number of respiratory viruses, including influenza, parainfluenza, adenovirus, human metapneumovirus, and respiratory syncytial virus. Rapid tests are available to identify pharyngitis due to Group A streptococcus.

Identifying a causative pathogen is more desirable in individuals with lower respiratory tract infections, such as pneumonia. Microbiologic culturing of sputum and blood is commonly performed, but may lack sensitivity. Urine antigen tests are available for the diagnosis of *L. pneumophila* and *S. pneumoniae*. Pulmonary embolism should also be considered in travelers who present with dyspnea, cough and/or pleurisy and fever. Pulmonary findings and eosinophilia in a traveler should raise the diagnostic suspicion of Loeffler syndrome or other geographically restricted causes of pulmonary infection (Table 10.2).

Table 10.2 Causes of pulmonary findings with peripheral blood eosinophilia.

Loeffler syndrome (acute *Ascaris lumbricoides*, *Strongyloides stercoralis*, hookworm infection)
Mycobacterium tuberculosis
Coccidioides immitis
Paragonimus spp.
Visceral larva migrans
Katayama fever (acute *Schistosoma* spp. infection)
Dirofilaria immitis
Tropical pulmonary eosinophilia (lymphatic filariasis)

Treatment

Most viral upper respiratory tract infections are uncomplicated and resolve with supportive treatment. A number of over-the-counter medications are also available to treat common symptoms of viral upper respiratory tract infection. Individuals with pharyngitis due to Group A streptococcus should be treated with penicillin or amoxicillin to decrease the likelihood of sequelae such as glomerulonephritis and rheumatic fever. Otitis media and sinusitis complicating air travel are most commonly of viral origin, but antibiotics may be prescribed if bacterial infection is suspected. Active initiatives to limit the use of antibiotics for upper respiratory infections are ongoing in Europe and the United States (CDC Get Smart: http://www.cdc.gov/getsmart/).

For travelers with signs or symptoms of pneumonia, antibiotics should be targeted at the common community-acquired pathogens, including *S. pneumoniae, M. pneumoniae, C. pneumoniae,* and *Legionella.* Guidelines are available to assist with the selection of antibiotics for the treatment of pneumonia [27]. A thorough travel and exposure history, and also knowledge of the traveler's underlying medical conditions, is useful for targeting therapy, as a specific etiologic agent is not always identified.

Prevention

Direct airborne transmission of pathogens on aircraft is unusual because of frequent air recirculation and filtration, although sporadic cases have occurred, particularly when there is a prolonged ground delay with closed doors [28,29]. Partly as a result of such outbreaks, it is now recommended that aircraft ventilation be supplied when a delay is longer than 30 minutes. Transmission by direct contact or droplets can occur between passengers who are seated adjacent to each other. Fomites, such as seat belts on planes and handrails on cruise ships, may also play a role in the spread of respiratory infections in travelers.

Hand hygiene, which includes frequent handwashing and avoiding touching one's mouth, nose, and eyes, is essential to preventing the transmission of agents associated with respiratory infection during travel. The use of alcohol-based hand sanitizers has also been associated with decreased transmission of respiratory viruses [30,31], and travelers should be instructed to sneeze or cough into disposable tissues or their flexed elbow. Travelers should postpone travel if they are coughing or are acutely ill and febrile.

Yearly influenza immunization is recommended for all individuals older than 6 months [32]. Travelers in particular should be vaccinated against influenza before departure if they have not previously received the seasonal vaccine. Travelers should also be appropriately immunized for measles and *Neisseria meningitidis,* which are also spread via the respiratory route. Some providers supply a prescription for neuraminidase inhibitors for empiric self-treatment of influenza by travelers during outbreaks, if influenza vaccine is unavailable or contraindicated or for patients with severe comorbid conditions. The use of masks to prevent respiratory infection during travel is not clearly supported by data, although anecdotal evidence suggests they may be protective [33].

References

1 Boggild AK, Castelli F, Gautret P, et al. Vaccine preventable diseases in returned international travelers: results from the GeoSentinel Surveillance Network. *Vaccine* 2010; **28**: 7389–7395.

2 Luna LK, Panning M, Grywna K, et al. Spectrum of viruses and atypical bacteria in intercontinental air travelers with symptoms of acute respiratory infection. *J Infect Dis* 2007; **195**: 675–679.

3 Benkouiten S, Charrel R, Belhouchat K, et al.. Circulation of respiratory viruses among pilgrims during the 2012 Hajj pilgrimage. *Clin Infect Dis* 2013; **57**: 992–1000.

4 Gautret P, Parola P, Brouqui P. Relative risk for influenza like illness in French Hajj pilgrims compared to non-Hajj attending controls during the 2009 influenza pandemic. *Travel Med Infect Dis* 2013; **11**: 95–97.

5 Peiris JS, Yuen KY, Osterhaus AD, Stohr K. The severe acute respiratory syndrome. *N Engl J Med* 2003; **349**: 2431–2441.

6 Olsen SJ, Chang HL, Cheung TY, et al. Transmission of the severe acute respiratory syndrome on aircraft. *N Engl J Med* 2003; **349**: 2416–2422.

7 WHO. *Summary of Probable SARS Cases with Onset of Illness from 1 November 2002 to 31 July 2003.* Geneva: World Health Organization, 2004.

8 Zaki AM, van Boheemen S, Bestebroer TM, et al. Isolation of a novel coronavirus from a man with pneumonia in Saudi Arabia. *N Engl J Med* 2012; **367**: 1814–1820.

9 Reusken CB, Haagmans BL, Muller MA, et al. Middle East respiratory syndrome coronavirus neutralising serum antibodies in dromedary camels: a comparative serological study. *Lancet Infect Dis* 2013; **13**: 859–866.

10 Assiri A, McGeer A, Perl TM, et al.Hospital outbreak of Middle East respiratory syndrome coronavirus. *N Engl J Med* 2013; **369**: 407–416.

11 Centers for Disease Control and Prevention (CDC). Surveillance for travel-associated legionnaires disease – United States, 2005–2006. *MMWR Morb Mortal Wkly Rep* 2007; **56**: 1261–1263.

12 Centers for Disease Control and Prevention (CDC). Legionnaires disease associated with potable water in a hotel – Ocean City, Maryland, October 2003–February 2004. *MMWR Morb Mortal Wkly Rep* 2005; **54**: 165–168.

13 Centers for Disease Control and Prevention (CDC). Cruise-ship-associated Legionnaires disease, November 2003–May 2004. *MMWR Morb Mortal Wkly Rep* 2005; **54**: 1153–1155.

14 Ta TH, Jimenez B, Navarro M, et al. Q Fever in returned febrile travelers. *J Travel Med* 2008; **15**: 126–129.

15 Cottle LE, Gkrania-Klotsas E, Williams HJ, et al. A multinational outbreak of histoplasmosis following a biology field trip in the Ugandan rainforest. *J Travel Med* 2013; **20**: 83–87.

16 Morgan J, Cano MV, Feikin DR, et al. A large outbreak of histoplasmosis among American travelers associated with a hotel in Acapulco, Mexico, spring 2001. *Am J Trop Med Hyg* 2003; **69**: 663–669.

17 Centers for Disease Control and Prevention (CDC). Outbreak of histoplasmosis among travelers returning from El Salvador – Pennsylvania and Virginia, 2008. *MMWR Morb Mortal Wkly Rep* 2008; **57**: 1349–1353.

18 Centers for Disease Control and Prevention (CDC). Measles – United States, 2011. *MMWR Morb Mortal Wkly Rep* 2012; **61**: 253–257.

19 Mitruka K, Felsen CB, Tomianovic D, et al. Measles, rubella, and varicella among the crew of a cruise ship sailing from Florida, United States, 2006. *J Travel Med* 2012; **19**: 233–237.

20 Centers for Disease Control and Prevention (CDC). Fatal respiratory diphtheria in a U.S. traveler to Haiti – Pennsylvania, 2003. *MMWR Morb Mortal Wkly Rep* 2004; **52**: 1285–1286.

21 Visser JT, Narayanan A, Campbell B. Strongyloides, dengue fever, and tuberculosis conversions in New Zealand police deploying overseas. *J Travel Med* 2012; **19**: 178–182.

22 Hunziker T, Berger C, Staubli G, et al. Profile of travel-associated illness in children, Zurich, Switzerland. *J Travel Med* 2012; **19**: 158–162.

23 Cobelens FG, van Deutekom H, Draayer-Jansen IW, et al. Risk of infection with *Mycobacterium tuberculosis* in travellers to areas of high tuberculosis endemicity. *Lancet* 2000; **356**: 461–465.

24 O'Brien D, Tobin S, Brown GV, Torresi J. Fever in returned travelers: review of hospital admissions for a 3-year period. *Clin Infect Dis* 2001; **33**: 603–609.

25 Freedman DO, Weld LH, Kozarsky PE, et al. Spectrum of disease and relation to place of exposure among ill returned travelers. *N Engl J Med* 2006; **354**: 119–130.

26 Leder K, Sundararajan V, Weld L, et al. Respiratory tract infections in travelers: a review of the GeoSentinel surveillance network. *Clin Infect Dis* 2003; **36**: 399–406.

27 Mandell LA, Wunderink RG, Anzueto A, et al. Infectious Diseases Society of America/ American Thoracic Society consensus guidelines on the management of community-acquired pneumonia in adults. *Clin Infect Dis* 2007; **44**(Suppl 2): S27–S72.

28 Moser MR, Bender TR, Margolis HS, et al. An outbreak of influenza aboard a commercial airliner. *Am J Epidemiol* 1979; **110**: 1–6.

29 Zitter JN, Mazonson PD, Miller DP, et al. Aircraft cabin air recirculation and symptoms of the common cold. *JAMA* 2002; **288**: 483–486.

30 Lee GM, Salomon JA, Friedman JF, et al. Illness transmission in the home: a possible role for alcohol-based hand gels. *Pediatrics* 2005; **115**: 852–860.

31 Sandora TJ, Taveras EM, Shih MC, et al. A randomized, controlled trial of a multifaceted intervention including alcohol-based hand sanitizer and hand-hygiene education to reduce illness transmission in the home. *Pediatrics* 2005; **116**: 587–594.

32 Influenza Division, National Center for Immunization and Respiratory Diseases, CDC. Prevention and control of seasonal influenza with vaccines. *MMWR Recomm Rep* 2013; **62**(RR-07): 1–43.

33 Zhang L, Peng Z, Ou J, et al. Protection by face masks against influenza A(H1N1)pdm09 virus on trans-Pacific passenger aircraft, 2009. *Emerg Infect Dis* 2013; **19**: 1403–1410.

CHAPTER 11

Sexually transmitted infections

Alberto Matteelli[1], Anna Cristina C. Carvalho[2], & Patricia Schlagenhauf[3]

[1] Spedali Civili Hospital, University of Brescia, Brescia, Italy
[2] Oswaldo Cruz Institute (IOC), Rio de Janeiro, Brazil
[3] University of Zürich Centre for Travel Medicine, Zürich, Switzerland

Introduction

Historically, travel and the spread of sexually transmitted infections (STIs) are closely linked. Syphilis is thought to have been introduced into Europe from the Americas by Columbus and the conquistadors [1]. The international spread of HIV was and is facilitated by travel and human mobility. Travelers are likely to have casual travel sex. Travel is considered to be a risk factor for the acquisition of a broad range of STIs because it interferes with sexual practices by physical separation of partners and by removing social taboos that inhibit sexual freedom [2–4]. Increased sexual promiscuity and casual sexual relationships are likely to occur during travel because people have the opportunity to escape the confines of standardized behaviors commonly regarded as acceptable by their society. A systematic review showed a high-pooled prevalence of travel-related casual sex of over 20% [5] and over 49% of these encounters were unprotected sexual intercourse. Travelers may be active as "sex tourists" and impact destination populations and partners in the countries of origin. Risky behavior of HIV-positive persons during travel has been described [6] and includes discontinuation of antiretroviral therapy (ART) and inconsistent use of condoms with new partners. The phenomenon of "epidemiological synergy" suggests that having an STI increases the probability of acquiring or transmitting a concomitant HIV infection [7]. Travel-associated infections allow for the ease of movement of resistant strains, as exemplified by the spread of quinolone-resistant *Neisseria gonorrhoeae* from South-East Asia into the United States and Europe.

STIs encompass a wide range of conditions and are responsible for several acute and chronic medical problems. These include lower and upper genital tract infections, their complications in women (pelvic inflammatory disease, infertility, ectopic pregnancy, and chronic pelvic pain), chronic liver diseases and cancer caused by hepatitis B (HBV) and C (HCV) infection, genital cancer due to several types of human papillomavirus (HPV), and AIDS, caused by the human immunodeficiency virus (HIV). In addition, the role of several STIs in amplifying the risk of acquisition or transmission of HIV itself is fully recognized [8], making prevention of infection with STIs a mainstay of HIV–AIDS prevention.

Essential Travel Medicine, First Edition.
Edited by Jane N. Zuckerman, Gary W. Brunette and Peter A. Leggat.
© 2015 John Wiley & Sons, Ltd. Published 2015 by John Wiley & Sons, Ltd.

STI exposure associated with travel and migration

Published reports on travel-associated STIs focus on risk behaviors and demonstrate increased exposure to STIs, which can be attributed to a combination of the high rate of casual sex and low rate of condom use [2]. A recent systematic review reported a pooled prevalence of travel-associated casual sex to be 20.4% [95% confidence interval (CI) 14.8–26.7%], with almost 50% of these encounters being unprotected intercourse [5].

Casual sex occurs even more frequently among long-term overseas travelers [9–11]. This subgroup of travelers typically includes European expatriates in Africa [12,13] and American Peace Corp Volunteers [14]. One case–control study reported that British workers at an international holiday destination were five times more likely to have casual sex and three times more likely to have unprotected intercourse compared with British visitors to the resort [15]. Military personnel stationed abroad represent an additional population with documented high rates of STI exposure [16,17].

The term "sex tourist" is used to identify travelers whose reason for travel is to reach destinations where sex is for sale. An increased demand for sex by tourists often matches an increased offer of sexual services at destination sites, and commercial sex with foreigners represents, in many low-income countries, a way to increase national revenues and to allow individuals to contribute significantly to their family's survival. These networks bridge high-risk groups, the general population, and travelers with the potential to amplify the spread of STIs and HIV [18]. Sex tourism has traditionally been concentrated in relatively few places. Thailand has been a sex tourism destination for Japanese, European, American, and Australian travelers [19] because of its large number of sex workers. However, formal and informal prostitution is likely to be present in most tourist destinations, acting as a driving force for the constitution of a local core population with high prevalence of STIs [20].

Finally, it is important to mention the recent phenomenon of migrant sexual workers as a population group that is highly vulnerable to STIs in Western Europe. Women from poor countries are trafficked and illegally introduced in Europe, are forced to work as prostitutes, and almost invariably suffer sexual violence. A high prevalence of syphilis, gonorrhoea, and *Chlamydia tracomatis* in female sex workers from Eastern Europe [21–23] and of HIV among those from Sub-Saharan Africa have been described [24]. Male sex workers from Latin America, including transvestites and transsexuals, represent another category of sexual worker with particularly high prevalences of STIs and HIV infection [24,25]. Political and social interventions to fight the racket of illegal migration and campaigns to promote condom use and screening of STIs have been advocated to reduce the burden and the spread of STIs associated with migrant sexual workers.

Factors associated with increased exposure

Because new and casual sexual partnership are common during foreign travel, it is important to understand if sexual behavior changes during travel and to

Table 11.1 Demographic and behavioral characteristics associated with higher frequency of casual sex during travel.

Characteristic	Ref.
Male gender	[10, 11, 2–32]
Younger age	[11, 16, 27, 29, 30, 33–35]
Single status	[10, 11, 16, 29, 30, 33]
Traveling without a partner	[11, 26, 29–31]
Business travelers	[11]
Being a man who has sex with men (MSM)	[29, 30, 36]
History of practicing casual sex in the home country	[11, 12, 27, 31, 34–38]
History of previous STI diagnosis	[9, 35]
History of visiting an STI clinic	[39]
Being a casual user of illicit drugs	[34, 37]
Being an abuser of alcohol	[5, 13, 14, 20]
The destination area	[30, 33, 34]
Visited the same destination more than twice	[26]
Earlier coitarche in women	[38]

identify objective criteria that can identify high-risk travelers for targeted preventive interventions.

A number of studies have identified demographic and behavioral characteristics associated with casual sex during travel (Table 11.1). Richens reviewed and listed the main predictors of sexual intercourse while traveling: being a male and a young traveler, traveling alone or with a peer but without a regular partner, high alcohol consumption and recreational drug use, long-duration travel, repeated visits to the same location, early coitarche, frequent casual sex at home, high number of lifetime sexual partner, and frequent extramarital sex relations were all included [40].

Travel-associated STIs

Theoretically, STI risk in travelers is a product of the number of sexual partners, the use (or lack of use) of protective measures, and the prevalence of STIs in the contact population of the destination country. The last factor is influenced by the uneven global distribution of STIs, with a marked concentration of the disease burden in resource-limited settings [41]. Considering the dynamic interplay among pathogens, human behaviors, and control efforts, resource-poor countries almost invariably fall in the hyperendemic phase for STIs, implying that these diseases have high incidence in the general population [42].

Remarkably, prospective data on the incidence of STIs among travelers are unavailable, and there is sparse information on the extent of travel-related STI morbidity. The rate of STIs in UK people who had new sexual partners abroad has been estimated at 18.2% for women and 35.2% for men over a 5-year period [35]. In Sweden, a significant increase in the prevalence of *Chlamydia trachomatis, Neisseria gonorrhoeae*, and genital warts has been associated with women who have casual travel sex abroad [43]. In the meta-analysis by Vivancos et al. [5], the estimated pooled unadjusted odds ratio (OR) for acquiring an STI associated with casual travel sex was 3.09 (95% CI 2.44–3.92). The risk was higher in men than in women.

Information on the range of STIs in travelers is usually limited to small case series from individual centers [44]. Recently, data on ill travelers visiting GeoSentinel clinics worldwide from June 1996 through November 2010 were analyzed to describe the disease range and demographic and geographic factors associated with the acquisition of travel-related STIs [32]. The final analysis included 112,180 ill travelers: patients seen after travel ($n = 64,335$), patients seen during travel ($n = 38,287$), and immigrant patients ($n = 9558$). A total of 974 patients had an STI diagnosis (with a total of 1001 STI diagnoses), giving a STI proportion of 0.9%. Demographic and trip characteristics of travelers with an STI, by traveler category, are summarized in Table 11.2.

Figure 11.1 presents the specific STI diagnoses among ill travelers, according to clinical setting in the GeoSentinel cohort. Non-gonococcal/unspecific urethritis was the most frequent diagnosis overall. Syphilis was also a frequent diagnosis among travelers and immigrants: this observation is in line with the evidence of a global re-emergence of the disease [45]. Exotic STIs (lymphogranuloma venereum, chancroid, and donovanosis) were infrequent or not represented at all. The type of STIs differed according to traveler group: the most frequent STI diagnoses in patients seen after travel were non-gonococcal/unspecified urethritis (30%) and acute HIV infection (27%). Non-gonococcal/unspecified urethritis (21%), epididymitis (15%), and cervicitis (12%) were the predominant STIs in patients seen during travel, and syphilis among immigrant travelers (68%). The most frequent (top five) STIs diagnosed in the GeoSentinel cohort according to clinical setting and sex are presented in Table 11.3. Among ill travelers seen after travel, logistic regression analyses showed a significant association between STI diagnosis and male gender, traveling to visit friends and relatives, travel duration of less than 1 month, and having no pretravel health consultation. In the GeoSentinel analysis, the proportionate morbidity ratio ranged from 6.6 per 1000 in returning ill travelers to 16.8 per 1000 in immigrants seen in GeoSentinel clinics. Whenever comparative analyses were carried out, the highest STI proportionate morbidity was reported in those born in low-income countries and living in high-income countries who traveled to their region of birth to visit friends and relatives (immigrant VFR) [46,47].

Travelers with genital symptoms are likely to seek care at other venues (STI clinics, primary care providers) rather than at travel medicine clinics; investigations conducted at the latter sites likely underestimate the true burden of STIs among international travelers. In small prospective studies on health problems of ill travelers, no STI cases were reported [48–50]. In one study in the UK, the incidence of STIs among people with a recent history of travel at a genitourinary medicine clinic in London was similar to that in people who did not travel at all (19% vs. 23%), and the maximum attributable fraction of new STIs that could have resulted from a new partnership abroad was 12% [39].

Still, there are several examples of the public health impact of travel-related STIs: prognosis, diagnosis, and treatment of HIV infection in Western countries are affected by the importation of non-B clades [51], syphilis outbreaks in northern Europe are often introduced from Russia [52], and quinolone-resistant *N. gonorrhoeae* strains

Table 11.2 Demographic and trip characteristics of ill travelers with an STI, by traveler category in GeoSentinel (*N* = 974 travelers).

Characteristic	Seen after travel (*n* = 424)	Seen during travel (*n* = 389)	Immigration travel (*n* = 161)
Age (years) (mean ± SD)	40.2 (12.9)	34.7 (11.3)	37.7 (14.1)
Gender ratio (M:F)	2.45	1.92	1.39
Exposure region Top 5 (%)	South-East Asia: 106 (22%)	South Central Asia: 130 (33%)	Sub-Saharan Africa: 79 (49%)
	Sub-Saharan Africa: 103 (22%)	Unknown region[a]: 125 (32%)	North Africa: 18 (11%)
	Unknown regions[a]: 53 (11%)	North-East Asia: 72 (19%)	South America: 16 (10%)
	South America: 39 (8%)	South-East Asia: 30 (8%)	South-East Asia: 14 (9%)
	Western Europe: 30 (6%)	South America: 8 (2%)	Eastern Europe: 10 (6%)
Duration of trip	<1 month: 290 (70%)	<1 month: 91 (44%)	NA
Patient setting	Inpatient: 80 (19%)	Inpatient: 17 (4%)	Inpatient: 37 (23%)
	Outpatient: 337 (79%)	Outpatient: 372 (96%)	Outpatient: 123 (76%)
	Missing: 7 (2%)		Missing: 1 (1%)
Reason for travel	Tourism: 213 (50%)	Business: 243 (63%)	NA
	VFR: 93 (22%)	Tourism: 107 (28%)	
	Business: 74 (17%)	Missionary/volunteer: 25 (6%)	
	Missionary/volunteer: 38 (9%)	Student: 10 (3%)	
	Others: 5 (1%)	Others: 4 (1%)	

[a]Unknown includes travelers whose itinerary was too complex to assign a region of likely exposure.

NA, not applicable; SD, standard deviation; VFR, visiting friends and relatives.

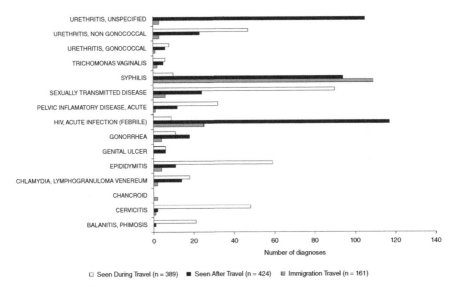

Figure 11.1 Distribution of specific STI diagnoses among ill travelers, according to clinical setting in GeoSentinel (*N* = 1001 diagnoses, travelers can have more than one STI diagnosis).

spread into the United States and Europe from South-East Asia, prompting changes in therapeutic recommendations for gonorrhoea [53].

Pre-travel interventions

Despite increasing evidence of significant exposure among travelers, STI prevention has a low profile among travel clinic practices. This is possibly due to the synergism between low perception of the consequences, and the difficulties of prevention and care of travel-associated STIs. The prevention of STI morbidity and the reduction of transmission of agents unfortunately do not rely on delivering a vaccine shot or prescribing preventive pills. It is based on primary prevention interventions (education, condom promotion, and counseling for promotion of safe behaviors) and on early recognition of the infection and its effective treatment to prevent complications. Primary prevention represents the only effective option for many viral STIs that are currently incurable (including HIV, HBV, herpes simplex virus, and human papillomavirus infections).

When celibacy and sexual monogamy are not acceptable options for the traveler, safe-sex practices must be recommended, including a limitation of the number of new sexual partners and the consistent and proper use of latex condoms during sexual activity. Correct condom use should be explained and, if possible, demonstrated. Counseling, aiming at facilitating modifications of behaviors, should focus on the nature and consequences of STIs, the ways to prevent them, and factors that may prevent the adoption of safe behaviors (including alcohol and drug use).

Counseling and education for the prevention of travel-related diseases are not unique to STIs (others include swimming in rivers and schistosomiasis, insect bites

Table 11.3 Top five STIs diagnosed among ill travelers, according to clinical setting and gender, in GeoSentinel (N = 1001 diagnoses, 974 travelers; travelers can have more than one STI diagnosis).

Gender	Seen after travel (n = 424)		Seen during travel (n = 389)		Immigration travel (n = 161)	
	Diagnosis	n (%)	Diagnosis	n (%)	Diagnosis	n (%)
Female	Urethritis	48 (38)	Cervicitis	48 (36)	Syphilis	49 (72)
	HIV	27 (21)	PID, acute	31 (23)	HIV	11 (16)
	Syphilis	18 (14)	STD	25 (19)	Gonorrhea	2 (3)
	PID, acute	12 (9)	Urethritis	9 (7)	Cervicitis	1 (1)
	Trichomonas vaginalis	5 (4)	*Trichomonas vaginalis*	6 (4)	PID, acute	1 (1)
Male	HIV	89 (29)	Urethritis	73 (27)	Syphilis	60 (64)
	Urethritis	79 (26)	STD	65 (24)	HIV	14 (15)
	Syphilis	76 (25)	Epididymitis	59 (22)	STD	5 (5)
	Gonorrhea	20 (6)	Balanitis, phimosis	21 (8)	Epididymitis	4 (4)
	STD	20 (6)	Gonorrhea	18 (7)	Urethritis	4 (4)

HIV, acute infection (febrile); PID, pelvic inflammatory disease; STD, sexually transmitted disease; Urethritis, non-gonococcal and unspecified urethritis; Gonorrhoea, gonococcal urethritis and other forms of gonorrhea.

and dengue, and prevention of road accidents), but they are specifically challenging because they touch the intimate sphere of sexual life.

STI preventive interventions need to be delivered at appropriate sites. Informative leaflets can be distributed to travelers at the airport: the results from one study, however, show that promotional information displayed in the departure lounge of an international airport is unable to modify the sexual behavior of travelers [10]. Another study showed that such leaflets are consulted significantly more frequently by subjects who will thereafter practice casual sex during travel compared with those who will not [26].

Counseling and education can also be carried out by direct contact during pre-travel consultations. Because pre-travel face-to-face education of all travelers is not feasible and, in many instances, is not necessary, education and counseling to prevent STI acquisition should target the subgroup of travelers who are actually likely to engage in risky behaviors. Unfortunately, effective algorithms for the identification of target travelers have not been documented.

Overall, there is no evidence that pre-travel educational interventions can reduce sexual exposure and the risk of STIs during travel. A systematic review and meta-analysis of the relation between pre-travel STI advice for travelers and sexual risk behavior abroad could not find evidence of any intervention with demonstrated efficacy [54]. In particular, the only randomized controlled trial showed that a motivational intervention was not superior to standard STI advice in reducing casual sex or promoting condom use [55]. Results from observational studies are similarly disappointing: among people who attended a travel clinic before departure, recall of reading a leaflet on STIs given at the clinic was independently associated with having casual travel sex; however, those who read the leaflet were also more likely to consistently use condoms [31]. Moreover, in a questionnaire survey reported by Gillies et al. [56], most people who had sexual intercourse abroad with a new partner were carrying condoms, but more than half "forgot" to use them at least once. In the study reported by Gagneux et al. [26], the majority of Swiss travelers stated at the time of departure that they would use condoms during casual sex, but the proportion of subjects who later reported condom use was significantly lower. Long-term travelers may be easier to target. After being exposed to intensive education and counseling on HIV, the Peace Corps volunteers who served in Africa in the second half of the 1980s showed a reduction in the rate of all reported STI infections from 131 to 68 per 1000 population per year. Of 282 volunteers deployed in Zaire during 1985–1988, none displayed seroconversion for HIV, and the seroprevalence of any markers for HBV was similar to that of healthy Americans who were matched for age [57].

STIs are diagnosed in travelers seen during travel at least as frequently as in those who have returned home [32]. Diseases such as gonorrhoea, which have a very short incubation period, are likely to appear before the end of the travel: the "information" package to be given to departing travelers at risk for STIs should include tools to recognize signs and symptoms of infection, the recommendation to seek healthcare early during travel, and to repeat a thorough screening after returning home.

Vaccines and chemoprophylaxis for STI agents

The only available vaccines for STIs are those against HBV and HPV. Travelers who are good candidates for HBV vaccination among attendees of travel clinics are frequent travelers, sex tourists, and military and non-government organization employees. The combined hepatitis A and B vaccine may be particularly suitable for travelers who need both vaccines. HBV vaccination should always be coupled with education to strengthen the concept that other STIs, like HIV, are not preventable in the same way.

Travelers do not appear to be an appropriate target for the newly marketed HPV vaccine, which is mostly effective when individuals have not yet started their sexually active life.

Chemoprophylactic use of antibiotics, before or immediately after sexual intercourse, is not recommended and should be discouraged. The use of chemoprophylaxis would confer a false and dangerous sense of protection, especially because such chemoprophylaxis provides no protection against viral agents.

Candidal vaginitis is not usually considered a true STI. However, recurrent candidal vulvovaginitis is a medical problem for some women. It has been reported that travel may trigger candida recurrences [58]. Women with known problems of recurrent candidal vulvovaginitis may have increased problems in warm and humid tropical environments and should carry therapeutic drugs that may be used in case infection develops. In this setting, oral regimens are preferable, for cosmetic reasons, to vaginal creams. Male partners of women with recurrent vulvovaginal candidiasis may experience increased frequency of sexually transmitted episodes of candidal balanitis.

Post-travel interventions

The incubation period of STIs may vary considerably, hence clinical signs may arise during or after travel. Some infections, such as gonorrhoea, are more likely to present warning symptoms (at least in males, presenting as urethritis), but others, such as *C. trachomatis* infection, usually remain asymptomatic. Viral infections such as HIV, herpes simplex virus, HBV, or HPV may only be recognized at the time they cause AIDS, or cervical or hepatic cancer.

Screening of asymptomatic travelers who had casual sex abroad could be encouraged, but the feasibility and cost-effectiveness of these interventions are virtually unexplored research fields. Subjects who report consistent condom use should still be offered screening because the capacity of individual travelers to judge the appropriateness of condom use has never been investigated. The appropriate timing of screening is unknown. For *C. trachomatis* and gonococcal infections, early diagnostic tests would be desirable, whereas for viral infections, screening should be conducted a few months after travel. Although there is no evidence base to guide STI screening, it seems reasonable to search for antibodies to HIV, HBV, and syphilis on serum samples and to detect *C. trachomatis* and *N. gonorrhoeae* nucleic acids by polymerase chain reaction (PCR) techniques on urine samples.

Treatment of STIs should be of high quality and carefully standardized on the basis of available guidelines [59]. Travelers who have developed genital symptoms and obtained care during travel should be encouraged to seek medical attention in their home country to define whether optimal care practices were followed and to provide screening for possible concomitant asymptomatic infections.

References

1 Desowitz RS. *Who Gave Pinta to the Santa Maria? Torrid Diseases in a Temperate World*. New York: W.W. Norton, 1997.

2 Matteelli A, Carosi G. Sexually transmitted diseases in travellers. *Clin Infect Dis* 2001; **32**: 1063–7.

3 Hynes NA. Sexually transmitted diseases in travellers. *Curr Infect Dis Rep* 2005; **7**: 132–137.

4 Memish ZA, Osoba AO. International travel and sexually transmitted diseases. *Trav Med Infect Dis* 2006; **4**: 86–93.

5 Vivancos R, Abubakar I, Hunter PR. Foreign travel, casual sex, and sexually transmitted infections: systematic review and metanalysis. *Int J Infect Dis* 2010; **14**: e842–e851.

6 Salit IE, Sano M, Boggild AK, Kain KC. Travel patterns and risk behaviour of HIV-positive people travelling internationally.*CMAJ* 2005; **172**: 884–888.

7 Adolf R, Bercht F, Aronis ML, et al. Prevalence and risk factors associated with syphilis in a cohort of HIV positive individuals in Brazil. *AIDS Care* 2012; **24**: 252–228.

8 Cohen MS. Sexually transmitted diseases enhance HIV transmission: no longer a hypothesis. *Lancet* 1998; **351**(Suppl 3): S5–S7.

9 Hawkes S, Hart GJ, Johnson AM, et al. Risk behavior and HIV prevalence in interregional travelers. *AIDS* 1994; **8**: 247–252.

10 Gehring TM, Widmer J, Kleiber D, Steffen R. Are preventive HIV interventions at airports effective? *J Travel Med* 1998; **5**: 205–209.

11 Bloor M, Thomas M, Hood K, et al. Differences in sexual risk behaviour between young men and women travelling abroad from the UK. *Lancet* 1998; **352**: 1664–1668.

12 Bonneaux L, van der Suyft P, Tallman H, et al. Risk factors for HIV infections among Europeans expatriates in Africa. *BMJ* 1988; **297**: 581–584.

13 Houweling H, Coutinho RA. Risk of HIV infection among Dutch expatriates in Africa in sub-Saharan Africa. *Int J STD AIDS* 1991; **2**: 252–257.

14 Moore J, Beeker C, Harrison JS, et al. HIV risk behaviour among Peace Corps Volunteers. *AIDS* 1995; **9**: 795–799.

15 Hughes K, Bellis MA. Sexual behaviour among casual workers in an international nightlife resort: a case control study. *BMC Public Health* 2006; **6**: 39.

16 Hopperus-Buma APCC, Veltink RL, Van Ameijden EJC, et al. Sexual behavior and sexually transmitted diseases in Dutch marines and naval personnel on a United Nations mission in Cambodia. *Genitourin Med* 1995; **71**: 172–175.

17 Malone JD, Hyams KC, Hawkins RE, et al. Risk factors for sexually-transmitted diseases among deployed U.S. military personnel. *Sex Transm Dis* 1993; **20**: 294–298.

18 Bauer IL.Romance tourism or female sex tourism? *Travel Med Infect Dis* 2014; **12**(1): 20–29.

19 Mulhall BP. Sex and travel: studies of sexual behaviours, disease and health promotion in international travelers: a global review. *Int J STD AIDS* 1996; **7**: 455–465.

20 Cabada MM, Echevarria JI, Seas C, Gotuzzo E. High prevalence of sexually transmitted infections among young Peruvians who have sexual intercourse with foreign travelers in Cuzco. *J Travel Med* 2009; **16**: 299–303.

21 Matteelli A, Beltrame A, Carvalho AC, et al. *Chlamydia trachomatis* genital infection in migrant female sex workers in Italy. *Int J STD AIDS* 2003; **14**: 591–595.

22 Platt L, Grenfell P, Bonell C, et al. Risk of sexually transmitted infections and violence among indoor-working female sex workers in London: the effect of migration from Eastern Europe. *Sex Transm Infect* 2011; **87**: 377–384.

23 Zermiani M, Mengoli C, Rimondo C, et al. Prevalence of sexually transmitted diseases and hepatitis C in a survey of female sex workers in the north-east of Italy. *Open AIDS J* 2012; **6**: 60–64.

24 Gutiérrez M, Tajada P, Alvarez A, et al. Prevalence of HIV-1 non-B subtypes, syphilis, HTLV, and hepatitis B and C viruses among immigrant sex workers in Madrid, Spain. *J Med Virol* 2004;**74**: 521–527.

25 Spizzichino L, Zaccarelli M, Rezza G, et al. HIV infection among foreign transsexual sex workers in Rome: prevalence, behavior patterns, and seroconversion rates. *Sex Transm Dis* 2001; **28**: 405–411.

26 Gagneux OP, Blochliger CU, Tanner M, Hatz C. Malaria and casual sex: what travelers know. *J Travel Med* 1996; **3**: 14–21.

27 Abdullah AS, Fielding R, Hedley AJ. Travel, sexual behaviour, and the risk of contracting sexually transmitted diseases. *Hong Kong Med J* 1998; **4**: 137–144.

28 Daniels DG, Kell P, Nelson MR, et al. Sexual behaviour amongst travellers: a study of genitourinary medicine clinic attenders. *Int J STD AIDS* 1992; **3**: 437–438.

29 Cabada MM, Echevarria JI, Seas CR, et al. Sexual behavior of international travelers visiting Peru. *Sex Transm Dis* 2002; **29**: 510–513.

30 Cabada MM, Montoya M, Echevarria JI, et al. Sexual behavior in travelers visiting Cuzco. *J Travel Med* 2003; **10**: 214–218.

31 Croughs M, Van Gompel A, de Boer E, Van Den Ende J. Sexual risk behavior of travelers who consulted a pretravel clinic. *J Travel Med* 2008; **15**: 6–12.

32 Matteelli A, Schlagenhauf P, Carvalho AC, et al.; GeoSentinel Surveillance Network. Travel-associated sexually transmitted infections: an observational cross-sectional study of the GeoSentinel surveillance database. *Lancet Infect Dis* 2013; **13**: 205–213.

33 Batalla-Duran E, Oakeshott P, Hay P. Sun, sea and sex? Sexual behaviour of people on holiday in Tenerife. *Fam Pract* 2003; **20**: 493–494.

34 Bellis MA, Hughes K, Thomson R, Bennett A. Sexual behaviour of young people in international tourist resorts. *Sex Transm Infect* 2004; **80**: 43–47.

35 Mercer CH, Fenton KA, Wellings K, et al. Sex partner acquisition while overseas: results from a British national probability survey. *Sex Transm Infect* 2007; **83**: 517–522.

36 Bellis MA. Ibiza uncovered: changes in substance use and sexual behaviour amongst young people visiting an international night-life resort. *Int J Drug Policy* 2000; **11**: 235–244.

37 Egan CE. Sexual behaviours, condom use and factors influencing casual sex among backpackers and other young international travellers. *Can J Hum Sex* 2001; **10**: 41–58.

38 Arvidson M, Hellberg D, Nilsson S, Mardh PA. Sexual risk behaviour in Swedish women with experience of casual travel sex abroad. *Ital J Gynecol Obstet* 1996; **2**: 73–76.

39 Hawkes S, Hart GJ, Bletsoe E, et al. Risk behaviour and STD acquisition in genitourinary clinic attendees who have traveled. *Genitourin Med* 1995; **71**: 351–354.

40 Richens J. Sexually transmitted infections and HIV among travellers: a review. *Travel Med Infect Dis* 2006; **4**: 184–195.

41 Gerbase AC, Rowley JT, Mertens TE. Global epidemiology of sexually transmitted diseases. *Lancet* 1998; **351**(Suppl 3): 2–4.

42 Wasserheit JN, Aral SO. The dynamic topology of sexually transmitted disease epidemics: implications for prevention strategies. *J Infect Dis* 1996; **174**(Suppl 2): S201–S213.

43 Mardh PA, Arvidson M, Hellberg D. Sexually transmitted diseases and reproductive history in women with experience of casual travel sex abroad. *J Travel Med* 1996; **3**: 138–142.

44 Ansart S, Hochedez P, Perez L, et al. Sexually transmitted diseases diagnosed among travellers returning from the tropics. *J Travel Med* 2009; **16**: 79–83.

45 Hook EW, Peeling J, Dolin R. Syphilis control – a continuing challenge. *N Engl J Med* 2004; **351**: 122–124.

46 Leder K, Tong S, Weld L, et al., for the GeoSentinel Surveillance Network. Illness in travellers visiting friends and relatives: a review of the GeoSentinel surveillance network. *Clin Infect Dis* 2006; **43**: 1185–1193.

47 Fenner L, Weber R, Steffen R, Schlagenhauf P. Imported infectious diseases and purpose of travel, Switzerland. *Emerg Infect Dis* 2007; **13**: 217–221.

48 Hochedez P, Visentini P, Ansart S, Caumes E. Changes in the pattern of health disorders diagnosed among two cohorts of French travellers to Nepal, 17 years apart. *J Travel Med* 2004; **11**: 341–346.

49 Hill DR. Health problems in a large cohort of Americans traveling to developing countries. *J Travel Med* 2000; **7**: 259–266.

50 Winer L, Alkan M. Incidence and precipitating factors of morbidity among Israeli travellers abroad. *J Travel Med* 2002; **9**: 227–232.

51 Perrin L, Kaiser L, Yerly S. Travel and spread of HIV-1 genetic variants. *Lancet Infect Dis* 2003; **3**: 22–27.

52 Hiltunen-Back E, Haikala O, Koskela P, et al. Epidemics due to imported syphilis in Finland. *Sex Transm Dis* 2002; **12**: 746–751.

53 Centers for Diseases Control and Prevention. Increases in fluorquinolone-resistant *Neisseria gonorrhoeae* among men who have sex with men – United States 2003, and revised recommendations for gonorrhea treatment, 2004. *MMWR Morbid Mortal Wkly Rep* 2004; **53**: 335–338.

54 Croughs M, Remmen R, Van den Ende J. The effect of pre-travel advice on sexual risk behavior abroad; a systematic review. *J Travel Med* 2014; **21**: 45–51.

55 Senn N, de Vallière S, Berdoz D, Genton B. Motivational brief intervention for the prevention of sexually transmitted infections in travelers: a randomized controlled trial. *BMC Infect Dis* 2011; **11**: 300.

56 Gillies P, Slack R, Stoddart N, Conway S. HIV-related risk behavior in UK holiday-makers. *AIDS* 1992; **5**: 339–341.

57 Cappello M, Bernard KW, Jones B, et al. Human immunodeficiency virus infection among Peace Corps volunteers in Zaire. *Arch Intern Med* 1991; **151**: 1328–1330.

58 Mardh PA, Hira S. Sexually transmitted diseases. In: Du Pont HL, Steffen R (eds.) *Textbook of Travel Medicine*. Hamilton, ON: BC Decker, 1997, pp. 193–199.

59 Centers for Disease Control and Prevention. Sexually transmitted diseases treatment guidelines, 2010. *MMWR Morb Mortal Wkly Rep* 2010; **59**(RR-12): 1–110.

CHAPTER 12

Tropical skin infections

Francisco Vega-López & Sara Ritchie
University College London Hospitals – NHS Trust, London, UK

Bacterial infections

Pyogenic infections

Pyogenic infections range through impetigo, folliculitis, furunculosis, or cellulitis, and the diagnosis is usually clinical. Bacteriological swabs with antibiotic sensitivity profile should be requested if available. Mild infections are successfully treated with bathing or soaking the affected skin in potassium permanganate solution (1:10,000 dilution in water). Mild superficial infections respond well to antiseptic creams and ointments containing cetrimide, chlorhexidine, fucidic acid, or mupirocin. More severe infections require systemic β-lactam or macrolide antibiotics. Recurrent infections may require an antimicrobial soap substitute and screening and eradication of MRSA (methicillin-resistant *Staphylococcus aureus*). PVL (Panton–Valentine leukocidin) is a particularly virulent toxin produced by some species of *S. aureus*. Testing for this should be requested in severe, poorly responsive, or recurrent skin infections. Necrotizing soft tissue infections can have a high mortality and pose one of the few dermatologic emergencies.

Treponemal infections

Spirochete infections include venereal syphilis, non-venereal endemic syphilis, yaws, and pinta. Primary syphilis presents up to 3 months after infection, typically with a single, painless chancre. Secondary syphilis can present up to 6 months after infection with a generalized erythematous maculopapular rash. These lesions may evolve into nodules or plaques. Annular or circinate lesions may be seen. The mucous membranes are often involved, and there is frequently palmoplantar involvement. Late syphilis can produce noduloulcerative lesions and gummas. Primary syphilis can be diagnosed by dark-ground microscopy from a chancre. Secondary or late syphilis is confirmed by serology. All of the treponemal infections cause positive serology which may be indistinguishable from syphilis. The treatment of choice is penicillin, and allergic individuals respond to tetracyclines or erythromycin.

Essential Travel Medicine, First Edition.
Edited by Jane N. Zuckerman, Gary W. Brunette and Peter A. Leggat.
© 2015 John Wiley & Sons, Ltd. Published 2015 by John Wiley & Sons, Ltd.

Mycobacterial infections

The clinical appearance of skin lesions in cutaneous tuberculosis depends on the route of entry of the organism and the immune status of the patient. In lupus vulgaris, there is direct extension of underlying tuberculous foci causing crusted or scaly plaques or ulcers, often on the face, nose, or ears. Scrofuloderma is breakdown of the skin directly overlying tuberculosis-infected lymph nodes. Atypical mycobacterial skin infection should be considered in travel-related ecthyma which is suppurating or ulcerative, and is unresponsive to penicillins or second-generation macrolides. Mycobacterial infection should also be considered with a history of keeping tropical fish, or after injury or abrasion of the skin from coral.

If mycobacterial infection is suspected, skin biopsies should be taken for histology and microbiology. Histology may show caseating granulomata. Culture is the gold standard investigation, but can take a number of weeks to become positive, and has low sensitivity in paucibacillary cases. Polymerase chain reaction (PCR) may be more sensitive; however ,PCR, microscopy, and culture can each be negative. In the context of strong clinical suspicion, a trial of antituberculous therapy may be considered. All forms of skin tuberculosis respond to standard WHO antituberculosis regimens with four drugs for 2 months, followed by dual therapy for 4 months. Atypical mycobacteria should be treated with at least two antituberculous drugs.

Leprosy should be considered in individuals with a history of living for several years in endemic areas. Leprosy can affect the skin and peripheral nerves. Clinical features on the skin are determined by the host immune response. In paucibacillary leprosy, up to four skin lesions may be apparent clinically, which are usually anesthetic, and bacilli may not be seen on slit skin smear. In multibacillary leprosy, skin lesions may be diffuse, and nerve damage occurs late, giving lesions that may be only slightly anesthetic, but may eventually cause a glove-and-stocking anesthesia. In these cases, bacilli are usually seen on microscopy. The patient should also be examined for signs of nerve damage and for signs of reversal reactions. The patient may be in reversal at diagnosis, which would be suggested by erythema or edema in the skin lesions, or by nerve tenderness. The investigation of choice is slit skin smear to look for acid-fast bacilli. Biopsy may show granulomata. PCR is very sensitive. The WHO recommends a two-drug regimen for paucibacillary leprosy and a three-drug regimen for multibacillary leprosy.

Fungal infections

Superficial fungal infection

Superficial fungal infection can be caused by dermatophytes or malassezia. Dermatophyte infections may manifest as single or multiple coalescing circinate or annular plaques with erythema and variable degrees of scaling. Scalp infections in children can manifest with the kerion clinical form with patches of non-scarring alopecia and boggy inflammation of the skin. The commensal yeast *Malassezia* can cause a superficial infection called pityriasis versicolor, which is characterized by small coalescing patches or plaques showing hyper- or hypopigmentation. Dermatophytes respond to triazole compounds, terbinafine, or griseofulvin. Localized infections require topical therapy for 3–8 weeks. Oral antifungals are indicated in severe or disseminated skin infections, tinea capitis, and onychomycosis. Tinea capitis in children requires oral terbinafine (or griseofulvin) 15–20 mg/kg for 6–8 weeks. Malasseziosis responds to topical selenium–sulfur shampoo or azole antifungals.

Subcutaneous fungal infection

Sporotrichosis is a worldwide fungal infection that can occur after exposure to abrasions from thorns or splinters. It classically disseminates into proximal satellite lesions via the lymphatic system, called sporotrichoid spread. Definitive diagnosis of sporotrichosis is based on identification in culture. Microscopy, histopathology, or serology may allow an earlier presumptive diagnosis.

Mycetoma, or madura foot, comprises a clinical triad of a subcutaneous mass, sinus tract formation, and granular discharge affecting particularly one foot. It includes both fungal eumycetoma and bacterial actinomycetoma, and can occur within the "mycetoma belt" from 15°S to 30°N of the equator. The infection is acquired by direct inoculation, and local agricultural workers at highest risk. Correct species identification is important for management, from deep-tissue biopsy, cultures, serology, or PCR. X-ray, ultrasound scan (USS), computed tomography (CT), or magnetic resonance imaging (MRI) may detect underlying bone involvement. Antimicrobial or surgical therapy is usually protracted.

Deep fungal infection

A number of fungi can cause deep fungal infection of the skin, including coccidioidomycosis, paracoccidioidomycosis, and histoplasmosis. In travelers these pose a particular risk in the context of immunosuppression. Coccidioidomycosis is acquired through inhalation of infective spores in subtropical desert regions of the world, most commonly in urban areas in the Americas. The skin becomes involved in a small proportion of cases, and lesions manifest as erythematous, verrucous, scarring, or scaling nodules. Paracoccidioidomycosis occurs only in the American continent, particularly in Mexico and Central and South America. It predominantly affects male agricultural workers, in rural rainforest areas. Infection is via inhalation or direct inoculation into the skin. It may present years after an individual has left an endemic region, with painful nodular, hemorrhagic, ulcerated, or verrucous lesions. The skin in affected in most cases, but it is also a systemic disease, which can affect the pulmonary, endocrine, or neurologic system. In addition to skin biopsies, a chest radiograph and lumbar puncture are necessary in all cases. Treatment requires specialist doctors in dermatology or infectious diseases.

Parasitic and ectoparasitic infections

Cutaneous leishmaniasis

Cutaneous leishmaniasis should be considered in anyone who has been to a country of endemicity who presents with slowly progressive skin lesions unresponsive to antibiotics. The protozoa is transmitted by sandflies, and is endemic in 88 countries, including all countries bordering the Mediterranean. The incubation period can be as short as 15 days, but is commonly around 4–8 weeks. Clinical manifestations include nodules covered with crust, or ulceration with a raised border. The differential diagnosis of lymphangitic forms may include atypical mycobacterial infection, or subcutaneous fungal infection. Classification in geographic terms as Old World or New World is important to guide diagnosis and treatment. The infecting species must be determined in order to guide choice of treatment. Investigation includes skin biopsies for histology to look for granulomata, direct microscopy with Giemsa stain to reveal amastigotes, culture in NNN medium, and genetic analysis by PCR techniques. Antimonials are the first-line treatment, and can be injected intralesionally at weekly intervals for many Old World infections. Severe, mucosal, or New World infections may need parenteral treatment. In HIV coinfection, leishmaniasis can present atypically, be more severe, or may present as immune reconstitution.

Schistosomiasis
Cercarial dermatitis should be considered in a traveler who develops an itchy papular rash soon after swimming in a freshwater lake in endemic countries. Cercarial dermatitis is caused by penetration of the skin by the free-living larval stages of the helminth schistosomiasis, which lives part of its life cycle in freshwater snails. It occurs within hours of infection, resolves within 10 days, and is a clinical diagnosis. Schistosomiasis occurs in Sub-Saharan Africa, South-East Asia, and also parts of Brazil and Venezuela. Treatment with praziquantel should be offered. At this stage, serology may be negative, and in addition urine and stool may be also be negative in the first 8 weeks after infection. Screening should be delayed till 3 months after exposure.

Onchocerciasis
Onchocerciasis is a filarial helminth endemic across equatorial Africa that can have chronic dermatological manifestations. Following an incubation period of approximately 1 year, the adult worms live freely in the skin or within fibrotic nodules called onchocercomata. Skin lesions can also present with lichenification and dyschromia. Diagnosis is by microscopy for microfilariae from skin snips taken from the back, hips, and thighs, skin-snip PCR, serology, or antigen dipstick tests.

Strongyloidiasis
Strongyloidiasis is a common, worldwide helminth infection transmitted via skin contact with infected soil or sand. It can present with the typically fast-moving rash of larva currens, which travels at several centimeters per hour. It is diagnosed serologically, and can be treated with the anthelmintic ivermectin, as a single dose of 200 µg/kg according to body weight (or multiple doses in the context of immunosuppression). Ivermectin should be avoided in pregnancy.

Cutaneous larva migrans
Cutaneous larva migrans results from the accidental penetration of the human skin by hookworm larvae. It is a common worldwide infection that can occur after barefoot contact with infected sand or soil. It causes a creeping erythematous, serpiginous larval track which moves at the rate of 1–2 cm per day, and the diagnosis is

clinical. Treatment is with albendazole 400–800 mg (according to body weight) daily for 3 days, or ivermectin 200 µg/kg stat dose.

Tungiasis

Tungiasis, or the sandflea, commonly affects one foot and is caused by the burrowing flea *Tunga penetrans*. The fleas usually penetrate the soft skin on the toe-web spaces. A crateriform single nodule develops with a central hemorrhagic punctum. Cryotherapy, curettage, surgical excision, or application of Vaseline and then careful removal of the flea and eggs with a sterile needle are curative.

Myiasis

Several worldwide fly larvae are capable of colonizing the human skin, which can cause myiasis. These can manifest as boils. The treatment of choice for myiasis is the mechanical removal or surgical excision of the larvae. Lesions can be covered by Vaseline to suffocate the larvae, which can subsequently be extracted via a cruciform incision.

Ticks

Tropical infections transmitted by ticks include spotted fever, tick typhus, and relapsing fever, among others. The bite characteristically produces an eschar. It is important to consider rickettsial infection in any traveler returning from an African game park who has a febrile illness with a petechial rash. Empirical antibiotic therapy should be started early before awaiting confirmation of diagnosis. The drugs of choice for treatment of rickettsial infection are doxycycline (100 mg BID) or tetracycline (500 mg QDS). Antibiotics should be continued for at least 3 days after the patient becomes afebrile to prevent recrudescence.

Viral skin infections

Viral infections that are prevalent globally include molluscum contagiosum in children, the wart virus, and herpesviruses. In an infected individual, herpes simplex virus can cause grouped vesicles at any site of skin injury, which can subsequently intermittently recur at this same site. Varicella zoster virus should be considered with blisters in a dermatomal distribution. Patients with HIV infection commonly suffer from a variety of skin conditions. The frequency and number of infectious skin disorders increase with progressing AIDS-established illness, to include cytomegalovirus, severe dermatophyte infections, cutaneous cryptococcosis, and Kaposi sarcoma. For a fully extensive list, separate texts on HIV dermatology should be consulted.

Bibliography

1 Demos M, McLeod MP, Nouri K. Recurrent furunculosis: a review of the literature. *Br J Dermatol* 2012; **167**: 725–732.

2 Abdalla CMZ, Prado de Oliveira ZN, et al. Polymerase chain reaction compared to other laboratory findings and to clinical evaluation in the diagnosis of cutaneous tuberculosis and atypical mycobacteria skin infection. *Int J Dermatol* 2009; **48**: 27–35.

3 Ustianowski A, Lawn SD, Lockwood DN. Interactions between leprosy and HIV: a paradox. *Lancet Infect Dis* 2006; **6**: 350–360.

4 Bastos de Lima Barros M, de Almeida Paes R, Oliveira Schubach A. *Sporothrix schenckii* and sporotrichosis. *Clin Microbiol Rev* 2011; **24**: 633–654.

5 Ameen M, Arenas R. Emerging therapeutic regimes for the management of mycetomas. *Expert Opin Pharmacother* 2008; **9**: 2077–2085.

6 Parola P, Paddock CD, Raoult D. Tick-borne rickettsioses around the world: emerging diseases challenging old concepts. *Clin Microbiol Rev* 2005; **18**: 719–756.

7 Goto H, Lindoso JAL. Current diagnosis and treatment of cutaneous and mucocutaneous leishmaniasis. *Expert Rev Anti Infect Ther* 2010; **8**: 419–433.

8 Stingl P. Onchocerciasis: developments in diagnosis, treatment and control. *Int J Dermatol* 2009; **48**: 393–396.

9 Udall DN. Recent updates on onchocerciasis: diagnosis and treatment. *Clin Infect Dis* 2007; **44**: 53–60.

10 Hoerauf A, Specht S, Marfo-Debrekyei Y, et al. Efficacy of 5-week doxycycline treatment on adult *Onchocerca vulvulus. Parasitol Res* 2009; **104**: 437–447.

11 Boussinesq M. *Loiasis. Ann Trop Med Parasitol* 2006; **100**: 715–731.

12 Herman JS, Chiodini PL. Gnathostomiasis, another emerging imported disease. *Clin Microbiol Rev* 2009; **22**: 484–492.

CHAPTER 13

Rabies

Mary J. Warrell
Oxford Vaccine Group, Oxford, UK

Introduction

Human rabies encephalitis is caused by viruses of canine origin in over 99% of instances, and this has always been fatal. All rabies deaths are due to failure to give adequate prophylaxis.

For travelers, there are two possible strategies to prevent rabies: to wait until bitten by a suspect rabid animal and then start full post-exposure treatment, or alternatively to have vaccine before encountering a rabid mammal (pre-exposure), with a booster course after possible exposure. In previously unvaccinated people, immediate complete post-exposure vaccination with rabies immunoglobulin (RIG) is very successful, but delay or inadequate treatment can prove fatal. However, no rabies deaths have been reported in previously immunized patients if booster vaccination was given after exposure. Rabies is entirely preventable.

The inaccessibility and cost of rabies vaccines often discourage prophylaxis. There is now evidence to change practice to use less vaccine for all regimens, with fewer visits for post-exposure treatment. The expensive current intramuscular (IM) route of delivery could be changed to intradermal (ID) injection as the standard route not only for pre-exposure, but also for both primary and booster post-exposure regimens. A simple plan for economical ID vaccine prophylaxis has emerged.

Epidemiology

Globally, the domestic dog is the most important reservoir species and is the dominant vector in Asia, Africa, and some areas of Latin America. Wild mammals are the predominant reservoirs in North America, Europe, parts of southern Africa, and the Caribbean. Rabies infects mammals and can be transmitted to domestic animals, including cats, and to humans. Rabies (species 1) infects terrestrial mammalian reservoir species and bats in the Americas. Western Europe and Australia are free from rabies in terrestrial mammals, but harbor rabies-related lyssaviruses in bats. These viruses cause fatal rabies-like encephalitis in humans and also occur in Africa and Asia, but not in the Americas.

Essential Travel Medicine, First Edition.
Edited by Jane N. Zuckerman, Gary W. Brunette and Peter A. Leggat.
© 2015 John Wiley & Sons, Ltd. Published 2015 by John Wiley & Sons, Ltd.

Human rabies mortality has not been determined reliably in tropical areas where about 99% of the global deaths occur. The estimate of the World Health Organization (WHO) of 55,000 deaths annually was inferred from the incidence of human dog bites. The highest mortality is in South Asia.

In Europe, the annual mortality is fewer than 10, predominantly in Russia and Ukraine; 10% are imported. In the United States, where about three cases are diagnosed annually, 95% of indigenous infections derive from insectivorous bat rabies virus, but 43% of such victims denied contact with a bat.

Clinical manifestation, diagnosis, and treatment

The incubation period is highly variable but is usually 20–90 days. Travel in a rabies-endemic area and animal contact point to the diagnosis. Prodromal itching or parasthesiae at the site of the bite are followed by symptoms of furious rabies (hydrophobia, aerophobia, encephalitis) or paralytic rabies (ascending flaccid paralysis). Features suggest stimulation of the autonomic nervous system: salivation, lacrimation, fluctuating temperature and blood pressure. Without treatment, death usually ensues within a few days, but patients with paralytic rabies can survive for 1 month. If life is prolonged by intensive care, multisystem complications include cardiac and pulmonary disturbance, cerebral edema, and diabetes insipidus.

No unvaccinated patient is known to have survived rabies encephalitis resulting from infection by a terrestrial mammal. Of 10 survivors, only three recovered without major neurologic sequelae: two were vaccinated, after being bitten by a dog or bat, and a single unvaccinated patient recovered from an American bat infection.

Rapid diagnosis depends on identification of antigen by reverse transcriptase polymerase chain reaction (RT-PCR) in skin, saliva, or cerebrospinal fluid (CSF), or immunofluorescence (IF) staining of a skin biopsy or post-mortem brain. Viral isolation is ideal. In unvaccinated patients, detection of rabies-neutralizing antibody is diagnostic.

There is no proven effective specific treatment of rabies encephalitis. Rabies of canine origin remains 100% fatal in unvaccinated patients. Intensive care should be considered for previously vaccinated patients, or if infected by American bat rabies virus. In most cases, palliation is recommended. Close contacts should be vaccinated as reassurance.

Rabies vaccines

Three tissue culture rabies vaccines, accredited by the WHO, are widely exported, but availability is variable in developing countries:
- Human diploid cell vaccine (HDCV) (Imovax Rabies Vaccine, Sanofi Pasteur). IM dose is 1 mL.
- Purified chick embryo cell (PCEC) vaccine (Rabipur/RabAvert, Novartis). IM dose is 1 mL.
- Purified Vero cell vaccine (PVRV) (Verorab, Sanofi Pasteur). IM dose is 0.5 mL. This is not licensed in the United Kingdom or United States.

All these vaccines are interchangeable. Sanofi might soon introduce a new purified serum-free Vero rabies vaccine, which is now in phase 3 clinical trials.

Other vaccines include a purified duck embryo vaccine (PDEV) (Vaxirab, Zydus Cadila), approved by the WHO, manufactured originally in Switzerland and now in India. Tissue culture vaccines are also produced in India, China, Japan, and Russia but they have not been accredited by the WHO.

Nervous tissue rabies vaccines made from sheep, goat, or suckling mouse brains are being phased out but are still manufactured in a few countries.

The side-effects of rabies tissue culture vaccines [1,2] include mild inflammation and pain at injection sites. Local irritation is more common after ID injections. Generalized symptoms include headache, malaise, fever, and a rash distant from the injection site. Allergic reactions occur occasionally after the first or subsequent doses. Anaphylaxis has very rarely been reported. Cases of neurologic illness have occasionally followed injection of tissue culture vaccines but the incidence after rabies vaccines is no greater than after other commonly used vaccines. Many pregnant women have been vaccinated without problems. Post-exposure treatment should be given to pregnant women. As vaccines are not generally recommended in pregnancy, pre-exposure immunization should be delayed if possible.

The usual route of injection is IM into the deltoid or anterolateral thigh in children, but not into the gluteal region where it is less immunogenic. The ID injection delivers vaccine to the dermal antigen-presenting cells. It is immunogenic and more economical for both pre- and post- exposure regimens [3]. ID immunization usually involves sharing vials of vaccine between patients. ID regimens are recommended for use in some countries but, if not approved by national authorities, the physician bears the responsibility for giving the vaccine. Wastage can be avoided by planning pre-exposure immunization of groups on a single day. Strict aseptic procedure is essential. A new syringe and needle must be used for each patient. Lyophilized rabies vaccines do not contain preservatives, so once reconstituted, they must be refrigerated and used within 6–8 hours [4].

Pre-exposure prophylaxis

Who might benefit from pre-exposure vaccination?

Rabies immunization is recommended for anyone at risk of contact with a rabid mammal. Asia, Africa, and parts of Latin America are enzootic for dog rabies, the major cause of human deaths, and some wild mammal species are also rabies reservoirs both in these areas and in North America and Eastern Europe. Several bat species harbor rabies-related lyssaviruses, which are widespread and have caused fatal encephalitis in humans. Contact with a bat anywhere in the world should be assessed as a possible risk. Travelers should avoid dogs, cats, and wild mammals in enzootic areas. Pre-exposure vaccination is only required once in a lifetime. It should be strongly recommended for travelers to, and residents of, dog rabies-infected countries, and for those at risk though occupation or leisure activities [4].

- *Pre-exposure vaccine regimen* (three visits, one month) (Tables 13.1 and 13.2)
  Days 0, 7, and 28: one dose IM or 0.1 mL ID is given in the deltoid area.

Table 13.1 Intramuscular rabies vaccine regimens.

Vaccine IM regimen	Days of injection (No. of sites injected if >1)	Visits	Total vials
Pre-exposure			
IM	0, 7, 28	3	3
Post-exposure (+ RIG day 0)			
IM five-dose standard	0, 3, 7, 14, 28	5	5
IM "2-1-1" Zagreb	0 (x2), 7, 21	3	4
Post-exposure if previous immunization			
IM	0, 3	2	2

Table 13.2 Simplified robust scheme for economical intradermal rabies prophylaxis.

Vaccine ID regimen	Days of injection (No. of sites injected if >1)	Visits	Total vials
Pre-exposure			
ID[a]	0, 7, 28	3	0.3 mL
Post-exposure (+ RIG day 0)			
Four-site ID[b]	0 (x4)[c], 7 (x2), 28	3	<2 If no vial sharing. max. 3
Post-exposure if previous immunization			
ID	0 (x4)[c]	1	1

[a]ID doses are all 0.1 mL/site of injection.
[b]ID doses are 0.2 mL/site of injection for vaccine 1.0 mL/ampoule (PCECV), or 0.1 mL/site for vaccine 0.5 mL/ampoule (PVRV).
[c]Use whole ampoule.

The timing of the final dose can be delayed or advanced to day 21. To reduce the cost, this vaccine can be injected ID [4]. If chloroquine is being used (e.g., for malaria prophylaxis) the vaccine must be given IM. ID pre-exposure vaccination is also contraindicated with other immunosuppressive drugs or diseases.

The economical ID route can be used by any doctor willing to take responsibility for the treatment, and some government health agencies, including in Canada, Australia, and New Zealand, recommend the method with serologic testing 2–4 weeks later. The ID route is not recommended at present in the United States. The UK regulations permit ID injection by suitably qualified and experienced healthcare professionals with warnings about the prescriber's responsibility and the risk of contamination of vials, but without a requirement for serologic tests [5].

If there is insufficient time for a full vaccine course before travel, one or two doses can be give,. Having had any vaccine previously is better than none if one is exposed to rabies. The course can be completed later. In the event of exposure, unless three doses have been given, a full post-exposure course is required. There is no need to restart a course after partial vaccination. For emergency pre-exposure immunization, a first dose of four ID injections has been recommended previously in the United Kingdom [3,6]. This is followed with a second and third single-site 0.1 mL ID or IM dose.

Booster doses of pre-exposure vaccine

No boosters are normally needed for travelers. It is assumed that they will have access to vaccine for booster post-exposure treatment if needed. A booster dose IM or ID 1–2 years after the primary course prolongs the immune response [7], and so an optional single booster would be an appropriate precaution for those who foresee repeated journeys to dog rabies-enzootic areas. People going to remote places where post-exposure treatment might be delayed would be wise to have a booster dose before departure if their last dose was more than 5 years previously.

For those at occupational or other high risk of infection, booster doses are recommended at intervals from 6 months to 5 years depending on the likelihood of exposure [4,5,8].

Serology

Unnecessary booster vaccination can be avoided by measuring the level of rabies-neutralizing antibody. Many people will still have detectable immunity. About 3% of the population are relatively "low responders," with consistently low rabies antibody levels, but the clinical significance of this is unknown.

If antibody is present (>0.5 IU/mL), no booster is needed, and vaccine is not wasted. The cost and availability of serology vary in different countries.

Post-exposure prophylaxis

If a rabid mammal bite, scratch, or lick on a mucous membrane is suspected or proven, wound cleaning, rabies vaccination, and maybe RIG are urgent. However, it is never too late to start treatment. Rapid induction of immunity demands a larger antigenic stimulus, and hence more vaccine than for pre-exposure prophylaxis. For those who have not had a previous complete course of vaccine, the induction of antibody takes at least 1 week and so passive immunization with RIG is used to provide immediate neutralizing antibody at the site of inoculation.

In all cases, wash the wound thoroughly with soap or detergent and water and, ideally, apply povidone iodine [4]. Then decide which vaccine regimen is most suitable [3].

Booster post-exposure vaccination for previously vaccinated people

Provided that a complete pre- or post-exposure course of a tissue culture vaccine has been given previously, or if a serum rabies-neutralizing antibody level of >0.5 IU/mL has ever been recorded, RIG treatment is not necessary but a short booster vaccine course is essential. If there is any uncertainty about past vaccination, give the full post-exposure course and RIG. Two booster vaccine regimens are recommended [3,4].

- *Standard IM two-dose regimen*
  Days 0 and 3: one IM dose is injected into the deltoid (Table 13.1).
- *Four-site ID single-day regimen* (see above ID injection information)
  Day 0: four ID injections of 0.1 mL, using a 1 mL syringe, are given in the deltoid and thigh or suprascapular areas (Table 13.2).

This is as immunogenic as the IM regimen [9,10]. The 0.1 mL ID dose is the same for all of the vaccines because half a vial is sufficient to boost an antibody response. If a vial contains 0.5 mL (PVRV), a whole dose is used, without wastage. With 1 mL/vial vaccines (HDCV or PCECV), sharing a vial with precautions is economical if treating two patients per day. When treating one patient, remaining vaccine can be used as ID pre-exposure immunization for relatives or others. It may be simpler and safer in inexperienced hands to give a whole ampoule of any vaccine divided between four ID sites on a single day (as for the four-site regimen below).

Medical kits for expeditions going into remote, high-risk areas could include rabies vaccine as an emergency post-exposure booster. The immunogenicity of these lyophilized vaccines does not decrease significantly at tropical ambient temperatures over 1 month [11]. The dose can be given ID in four sites. If more than one person is exposed at the same time, the vaccine available can be shared. However, to be safe, the appropriate post-exposure vaccination is still recommended on return.

Primary post-exposure vaccination (Tables 13.1 and 13.2)

RIG should be given with every primary post-exposure treatment (see below).

- *Standard IM five-dose (Essen) regimen* (five visits, one month)
  Days 0, 3, 7, 14, and 28: one IM dose is injected IM into the deltoid.

Omitting the last dose, a 2-week regimen (days 0, 3, 7, and 14) has been authorized in the United States, but only for healthy patients and if combined with RIG. Immunogenicity data are not available. The significance of low antibody levels observed after four doses had been given in a travel clinic is unknown [12].

- *IM four-dose (Zagreb, 2-1-1) regimen* (three visits, three weeks)
  Day 0: two IM doses are injected into the deltoids
  Days 7 and 21: one IM dose.

This has been used in some countries for many years.

- *ID four-site regimen* (three visits, one month, economical). This is the original eight-site ID regimen adapted for use with all vaccines.
  Day 0: 4 ID injections – using a 1 mL syringe, the entire contents of the vial (see *Note* below) are divided between four sites: the deltoids and either the thighs or suprascapular areas
  Day 7: two ID injections are given in the deltoid areas (0.1/0.2 mL)
  Day 28: one ID injection is given in a deltoid area (0.1/0.2 mL).

Note: The dose per ID site depends on the volume per vial. For PVRV (0.5 mL/vial) the ID dose is 0.1 mL/site. PCECV and HDCV (1.0 mL/vial) are less concentrated, so the equivalent ID dose is 0.2 mL/site. If injecting 0.2 mL ID proves difficult, the needle is withdrawn and the remainder is injected into an adjacent area.

The WHO did not recommend this regimen because the 0.2 mL ID dose does not comply with the stipulation for a universal ID dose of 0.1 mL, a prerequisite for endorsement[13].

- This regimen is the most economical [14]and is as immunogenic as the "gold standard" five-dose IM Essen regimen [3,15].
- If no vials are shared, three vials are used, which is cheaper than any IM regimen.
- Using a whole vial of vaccine without wastage on day 0 is practical in small clinics, and gives the best chance of survival to patients who default.
- Accidental subcutaneous injection should not impair the immunogenicity because half of the dose is immunogenic in trial conditions [16].
- Any vaccine remaining on day 7 or 28 can be used as pre-exposure ID immunization for relatives or others with strict aseptic precautions (see above).
- *ID two-site regimen* (four visits, one month)
  Days 0, 3, 7, and 28: two ID injections of 0.1 mL in the deltoid areas.

This regimen was devised for PVRV (0.5 mL/vial) using 0.1 mL/ID site. For PCECV and HDCV (1.0 mL/vial), the equivalent ID dose of 0.2 mL/ site was used originally. Following a WHO decision, the universal ID dose is now 0.1 mL irrespective of concentration, so half the amount of PCECV is given [17]. As a result, higher potency vaccines are demanded in most of the few Asian countries where it is in use. Vaccine wastage has been estimated at 25% [18].

- *ID four-site regimen* (three visits, one week)
- Days 0, 3, and 7: four ID injections of 0.1 mL/site of any vaccine.

This regimen is being evaluated. It is either more expensive using three vials of PVRV, or it is not suitable for small clinics with PCECV as half vials are given on each occasion. The antibody level is predicted to fall more rapidly after this short course.

Rabies immune globulin

RIG should be given with primary post-exposure treatment as indicated by the severity of risk, but is not needed if the person has been previously vaccinated. It is most important for severe exposure to infection (Table 13.3). Passive immunization neutralizes virus in the wound, providing some protection during the 7–10 days before vaccine-induced immunity appears. Hence RIG is not needed if vaccine has been started >7 days previously. Local analgesia is advisable before injection.

- A dose of human RIG (HRIG), 20 units/kg body weight, should be infiltrated into and around the wound. If this is impossible, for example in a finger, the rest should be given by IM injection far from the vaccination site, preferably the anterolateral thigh, but not the gluteal region.
- Equine RIG (ERIG), 40 IU/kg, is a cheaper alternative used in developing countries.
- The recommended dose of RIG must not be exceeded as this risks impairing the immune response to the vaccine.
- The local and systemic reaction rates to RIG were 0.09% for HRIG and 1.83% for purified ERIG. Serum sickness followed ERIG in 0.73% and after HRIG in 0.007% of patients [19]. Skin testing before ERIG does not predict reactions and is not recommended [4].
- There is a global shortage of RIG, which is not available in several countries. Alternative monoclonal rabies antibody products are undergoing clinical trials.

Table 13.3 Recommended criteria for post-exposure treatment, a modification of WHO recommendations.

Exposure	Source	Treatment
No exposure[a]	Touching animals or licks on intact skin	No treatment
Minor exposureWHO Category II	Nibbling (tooth contact) with uncovered skin, minor scratches, or abrasions without bleeding	Start vaccine immediately
Major exposure WHO Category III	Single or multiple bites, scratches that break the skin, licks on broken skin, licks or saliva on mucosae, or any physical contact with bats	Start vaccine immediately and if not previously immunized, give immunoglobulin (RIG)
	Severe exposure: Bites on the head, neck, hands, or multiple bites are highest risk of infection	Treatment is very urgent and must be complete

For all cases: stop treatment of the patient if the biting dog or cat remains healthy for 10 days, or if animal's brain proves negative for rabies by appropriate tests.
[a]This is WHO Category I, but the term is confusing and best avoided.
Source: WHO 2013 [4]. Reproduced with permission of WHO.

Simplified scheme for economical rabies prophylaxis

The low-dose two-site ID regimen has been recommended by the WHO for 20 years, but poor uptake shows that it is impractical and not trusted.

The simplified economical scheme for pre- and post-exposure regimens (Table 13.2) would be ideal for developing countries where resources are limited. Robust ID vaccine doses may compensate for unfamiliarity with ID injection technique and lack of RIG. The scheme is also suitable to use anywhere with the government authority's approval or if individual doctors will act on evidence of immunogenicity and economy.

References

1 Dobardzic A, Izurieta H, Woo EJ, et al. Safety review of the purified chick embryo cell rabies vaccine: data from the Vaccine Adverse Event Reporting System (VAERS), 1997–2005. *Vaccine* 2007; **25**: 4244–4251.
2 Toovey S. Preventing rabies with the Verorab vaccine: 1985–2005. Twenty years of clinical experience. *Travel Med Infect Dis* 2007; **5**: 327–348.
3 Warrell MJ. Current rabies vaccines and prophylaxis schedules: preventing rabies before and after exposure. *Travel Med Infect Dis* 2012; **10**: 1–15.
4 WHO. *World Health Organization Expert Consultation on Rabies. Second Report.* WHO Technical Report Series 982. Geneva: World Health Organization, 2013.
5 Salisbury D, Ramsay M, Noakes K (eds.) Rabies. In: *Immunisation Against Infectious Disease*, 3rd edn. Norwich: TSO, 2006, pp. 329–345. Updated 2012.

6 Salisbury DM, Begg NT (eds.) *Immunisation Against Infectious Disease*, 2nd edn. *London: HMSO*, 1996, p. 185.

7 Strady A, Lang J, Lienard M, et al. Antibody persistence following preexposure regimens of cell-culture rabies vaccines: 10-year follow-up and proposal for a new booster policy. *J Infect Dis* 1998; **177**: 1290–1295.

8 Centers for Disease Control and Prevention. Human rabies prevention – United States, 2008: recommendations of the Advisory Committee on Immunization Practices. *MMWR Recomm Rep* 2008; **57**(RR-3): 1–28.

9 Khawplod P, Benjavongkulchai M, Limusanno S, et al. Four-site intradermal postexposure boosters in previously rabies vaccinated subjects. *J Travel Med* 2002; **9**: 153–155.

10 Tantawichien T, Benjavongkulchai M, Limsuwan K, et al. Antibody response after a four-site intradermal booster vaccination with cell-culture rabies vaccine. *Clin Infect Dis* 1999; **28**: 1100–1103.

11 Nicholson KG, Burney MI, Ali S, et al. Stability of human diploid-cell-strain rabies vaccine at high ambient temperatures. *Lancet* 1983; **i**: 916–918.

12 Uwanyiligira M, Landry P, Genton B, et al. Rabies postexposure prophylaxis in routine practice in view of the new Centers for Disease Control and Prevention and World Health Organization recommendations. *Clin Infect Dis* 2012; **55**: 201–205.

13 WHO. *Human and Dog Rabies Prevention and Control. Report of the WHO/Bill & Melinda Gates Foundation Consultation, Annecy, France, 7–9 October 2009*. Geneva: World Health Organization, p. 21. http://whqlibdoc.who.int/hq/2010/WHO_HTM_NTD_NZD_2010.1_eng.pdf (accessed 30 January 2015).

14 Hampson K, Cleaveland S, Briggs D. Evaluation of cost-effective strategies for rabies post-exposure vaccination in low-income countries. *PLoS Negl Trop Dis* 2011; **5**(3): e982.

15 Warrell MJ, Riddell A, Yu LM, et al. A simplified 4-site economical intradermal post-exposure rabies vaccine regimen: a randomised controlled comparison with standard methods. *PLoS Negl Trop Dis* 2008; **2**(4): e224.

16 Ambrozaitis A, Laiskonis A, Balciuniene L, et al. Rabies post-exposure prophylaxis vaccination with purified chick embryo cell vaccine (PCECV) and purified Vero cell rabies vaccine (PVRV) in a four-site intradermal schedule (4-0-2-0-1-1): an immunogenic, cost-effective and practical regimen. *Vaccine* 2006; **24**: 4116–4121.

17 Dodet B. Antigen content versus volume of rabies vaccines administered intradermally. *Biologicals* 2011; **39**: 444–445.

18 Gongal G, Wright AE. Human rabies in the WHO southeast Asia region: forward steps for elimination. *Adv Prev Med* 2011; **2011**: 383870.

19 Suwansrinon K, Jaijareonsup W, Wilde H, et al. Sex- and age-related differences in rabies immunoglobulin hypersensitivity. *Trans R Soc Trop Med Hyg* 2007; **101**: 206–208.

CHAPTER 14

Vaccine-preventable diseases

Joseph Torresi[1], Abinash Virk[2], & Jane N. Zuckerman[3]

[1] University of Melbourne, Melbourne, VIC, Australia
[2] Mayo Clinic, Rochester, MN, USA
[3] University College London, London, UK

Principles of vaccine immunology

The development of effective vaccines for infectious diseases has been amongst the most important medical advances resulting in a substantial improvement in human health. The mechanisms underlying vaccine-mediated protection are multifactorial and for many vaccines the correlates of protective immunity have not been completely established. In general, the protective efficacy of vaccines is conferred by the induction of antigen-specific antibodies [1,2]. This has been shown to be true for several bacterial [e.g., pneumococcus, meningococcus, *Haemophilus influenza* B (Hib), diphtheria, tetanus] and viral [(hepatitis B virus (HBV), hepatitis A virus (HAV), yellow fever, human papillomavirus (HPV), rotavirus, measles, mumps, rubella, smallpox, influenza and polio] infections [1,3]. Protection is not only mediated by high-titer antibody but also by the quality of the antibody response as determined by their affinity for a specific epitope and by the overall avidity [1,3]. In contrast to early protective responses, the persistence of antibodies and the development immunologic memory are key components to the effective long-term protective efficacy of vaccines [4]. The development of these antibody responses requires a complex interplay between antigen-presenting cells, B cells and T-helper cells, which are essential to the induction of high-affinity antibodies. In addition to humoral immune responses, the induction of vaccine-associated CD8+ T-cell responses is important in the protective efficacy of vaccines directed against intracellular pathogens such as TB [1,5].

Vaccine-mediated protection

Antibodies that are able to bind to pathogens or to toxins, thereby inactivating them or enhancing their clearance, essentially mediate the protection afforded by vaccines. Antibodies function by binding to active sites of toxins; neutralizing viral binding and entry into cells or preventing viral replication; promoting opsonization of extracellular bacteria and thereby enhancing phagocytosis by macrophages

Essential Travel Medicine, First Edition.
Edited by Jane N. Zuckerman, Gary W. Brunette and Peter A. Leggat.
© 2015 John Wiley & Sons, Ltd. Published 2015 by John Wiley & Sons, Ltd.

or killing by neutrophils; activating the complement cascade; and mediating antibody-dependent cellular cytotoxicity (ADCC) [1].

Cytotoxic CD8$^+$ T cells are also involved in limiting the spread of pathogens by killing infected cells and secreting antiviral cytokines. The maintenance of both B- and CD8$^+$ T-cell response is supported by CD4$^+$ T helper (Th) lymphocytes, which are subdivided into T helper 1 (Th1) and T helper 2 (Th2) subtypes [6], each with a different cytokine profile. Th1 cells characteristically produce IFN-γ, TNF-α/-β, IL-2, and IL-3 and support the activation and differentiation of B cells, CD8$^+$ T cells and macrophages. In contrast, Th2 cells produce IL-4, IL-5, IL-13, IL-6, and IL-10 and support the activation and differentiation of B cells.

For vaccines directed against bacterial capsular polysaccharides (e.g., meningococcus, pneumococcus, and Hib), protection is provided by an immunoglobulin G (IgG) response that is predominantly independent of T-cell help [7,8]. These vaccines are therefore unable to induce a strong memory response [5]. However, by conjugating a bacterial polysaccharide to a protein carrier, it is possible to produce vaccines that are able to recruit antigen-specific CD4$^+$ Th cells, thereby producing more potent immune responses and inducing immunologic memory [9,10]. Similarly, toxoid, protein, inactivated, or live attenuated viral vaccines are also able to produce T-cell-dependent immune responses that induce both higher affinity antibody and immune memory responses [4]. In contrast, BCG is the only vaccine that induces protective T-cell responses in the absence of antibody [11].

Live viral vaccines induce strong CD4$^+$ and CD8$^+$ T-cell responses [4,5,12], although the protective efficacy of both live attenuated vaccines, inactivated and VLP-based viral vaccines (including MMR, yellow fever, Japanese encephalitis, rabies, HAV, HBV, and HPV) is correlated with the induction of neutralizing antibody responses [1,5]. Vaccine-associated CD4$^+$ and CD8$^+$ T-cell responses however, may play an important role in attenuating the severity of viral infections.

Vaccines and activation of innate immune responses

The activation of antigen-presenting cells (APCs), essentially dendritic cells (DCs), is essential for the induction of effective antigen-specific B- and T-cell responses. In natural infections, exposure of immature DCs to pathogens results in maturation of DCs with the expression specific cell surface stimulatory and costimulatory molecules critical to the induction of T- and B-cell responses occurs. Mature DCs also serve a central role in the induction of vaccine responses through their capacity to provide both antigen-specific and costimulatory signals to T cells. DCs interact with pathogens through a series of receptors expressed at the cell surface and that are directed against conserved pathogen patterns. These receptors include Toll-like receptors (TLRs), C-type lectins, and nucleotide oligomerization and binding domain (NOD)-like receptors (NLRs). The engagement of pattern recognition receptors (PRRs) on DCs by pathogens and the subsequent stimulation of DC maturation results in the release of proinflammatory cytokines and chemokines followed by the migration of DCs to the draining lymph nodes [13]. Here DCs interact with CD4$^+$ and CD8$^+$ T cells to drive antigen-specific adaptive immune responses. Designing molecules that are able to bind these cell surface PRRs provides an avenue to developing vaccines that are able to induce strong protective immune responses [14]. The administration of a live viral vaccine results in the activation of DCs at multiple sites followed by their migration to draining lymph nodes and stimulation of T and B cells. In contrast, inactivated vaccines are not associated with microbial replication although they may still bind to pathogen recognition receptors and thereby initiate innate responses but only at the site of their injection. Consequently, inactivated vaccines are generally associated with lower antibody responses.

Vaccine primary and booster antibody responses

Migrating DCs that have been exposed to vaccine antigens activate B cells that are present in the marginal zone of lymph nodes and in the spleen. B cells bind presented antigens with their cell surface immunoglobulins and are activated. The antigen-specific B cells then proliferate and differentiate into antibody-secreting plasma cells that produce low-affinity antibodies. The antigen-loaded DCs also activate Th cells that interact with the antigen-specific B cells and trigger their interaction with follicular dendritic cells (FDCs) in germinal centers (GCs). Here B cells receive additional signals from follicular Th cells, a specific subset of $CD4^+$ T cells, and undergo clonal proliferation, somatic hypermutation in the variable-region segments of immunoglobulin genes, and B-cell receptors (BCRs), immunoglobulin class switching, and affinity maturation. The result is the production of plasma cells that secrete large amounts of high-affinity antigen-specific antibodies [2,3]. In addition, the interaction of B cells with somatically mutated high-affinity BCRs with follicular Th cells results in the development of memory B cells. However, polysaccharide vaccines do not generate the production of somatically mutated high-affinity B cells and BCRs and consequently result in intermediate or low-affinity IgG antibodies and fail to generate memory B cells.

Memory B cells do not produce antibodies; however, an antigen-driven reactivation and differentiation in response to natural infection or to booster immunization results in the rapid production of large amounts of higher affinity antigen-specific antibodies [3]. This reactivation also results in the production of higher affinity memory B cells that can be recalled by lower amounts of antigen and without the involvement of $CD4^+$ Th cells. This underpins the principle of a prime-boost immunization schedule. By allowing a period of time to elapse between the primary and booster doses of a vaccine, the secondary exposure to antigens results in the production of higher affinity antibodies rather than primary responses and that are more likely to be protective.

Adjuvants and the vaccine response

The administration of live attenuated vaccines essentially results in mild asymptomatic infection that leads to the production of long-lived immune responses against the target pathogen. However, for many pathogens and infections it has not been possible to develop live attenuated vaccines (e.g., meningococcal and pneumococcal disease, Hib, pertussis, diphtheria, rabies, HPV, HBV, and HAV). For these infections, vaccines based on whole, inactivated viruses and microorganisms or recombinant proteins have been developed. These vaccines are generally poorly immunogenic and require the addition of additional components, adjuvants, in order to produce strong humoral and cellular immune responses that will provide protection against the target pathogen [14–16]. Adjuvants enhance vaccine-specific T- and B-cell responses, but rather than acting directly on these cells, adjuvants work by stimulating the innate immune system and this subsequently drives specific adaptive immune responses [14,15].

Vaccine adjuvants consist of different classes of compounds, including microbial products (e.g., CpG motifs, MPL), mineral salts (aluminum hydroxide, aluminum phosphate), emulsions (Montanide, QS-21, AS03), PRR adjuvants (e.g., TLR ligands), lipopeptides (e.g., E8-Pam2Cys), microparticles, and liposomes (e.g., ISCOMATRIX) [14–17]. Although there are many adjuvants in various stages of development and in clinical trials, few have been successfully licensed for human vaccines (aluminum hydroxide, aluminum phosphate). However, as our understanding of the critical role that adjuvants play in stimulating innate immunity and the importance of these responses in developing effective adaptive vaccine immune responses increases, the greater will be the interest and drive to license new adjuvants for human vaccines.

Immunization and vaccination

Vaccination is the process of administering a vaccine as a form of prophylaxis or treatment against disease. Immunization is the process by which an individual's acquired immune system is enhanced against certain infectious diseases by natural or artificial means. Immunization can thus provide complete protection against infection from certain diseases or modify the clinical course should an individual become infected, leading to a milder disease with fewer complications. It may be achieved by passive immunization or much more commonly by active immunization.

Passive immunization is defined as the transfer of preformed immunoglobulin (antibodies) to an individual either by injection of donor antibodies or by passive transfer across the placenta from mother to fetus. Although it provides immediate protection against a disease, the levels of antibody are lower than those achieved with vaccination and the duration of protection is limited to a few weeks or months as immunologic memory is not elicited.

Active immunization is defined as the stimulation of an individual's acquired immune system against a particular disease by exposure to natural infection or to a vaccine against the disease. Vaccination is the administration of a vaccine which consists of artificially produced antigens which elicit active immunity to a disease.

Immunization also has a role in protecting populations from infections through herd immunity whereby vaccinated individuals are less likely to be a source of infection to unvaccinated individuals. If vaccination coverage in a population is not maintained, then herd immunity can be lost, leading to the re-emergence of disease in the population.

Live vaccines

Live vaccines include Bacillus Calmette–Guérin (BCG), measles, mumps, and rubella (MMR), oral polio, oral typhoid, varicella, and yellow fever. Live vaccines consist of attenuated microorganisms that with administration mimic natural infection, but with significantly reduced virulence so that they do not cause illness in most circumstances. They do not require adjuvants and are more likely to induce long-lasting or even life-long immunity following administration of a single dose by activating both the cell-mediated and humoral response.

Inactivated vaccines

Inactivated (killed) vaccines are used when live attenuated vaccines are not available or where reversion of an attenuated strain to wild type occurs with relative ease. Inactivated vaccines do not stimulate infection or mimic disease, are generally less immunogenic, and initially induce a predominantly humoral response which provides less efficient immune protection. A primary course of several doses is usually required to induce a sufficient immune response and regular boosters are then often needed to provide long-lasting immunity through the stimulation of both the cell-mediated and humoral immune systems.

Administration of vaccines

It is important to read carefully the manufacturer's Summaries of Product Characteristics (SPCs) for each specific vaccine, which give detailed information on the vaccine's storage, composition, reconstitution and preparation, color and consistency, life span for use once drawn up, administration, side-effects, and contraindications. Different vaccines should not be mixed in the same syringe.

Some vaccines are supplied preprepared and ready for administration. Other vaccines are supplied lyophilized (freeze-dried) and must be reconstituted with the supplied diluant before administration. A 21 G (green) needle is usually recommended for drawing up the diluant and mixing it slowly with the lyophilized vaccine to avoid frothing. Reconstituted vaccine and opened single- or multi-dose vaccine vials must be used within the manufacturer's recommended period (usually within 1 – 4 hrs). Some multi-dose vials maybe used for up to 30 days if immediately stored in a refrigerator after use, unless recommended otherwise by the manufacturer [18–22].

Correct administration of vaccines
Administration of a travel vaccine relies upon the healthcare professional having:
• obtained patient consent
• ensured there are no contraindications to vaccination
• prepared the vaccine correctly
• reconstituted the product where necessary
• used the appropriate needle length for the size of the patient
• selected the correct site and route of administration and demonstrated an appropriate technique.

Post-vaccination management of the site, observation of the patient, and documentation of the process are also vital.

An anaphylaxis management kit containing intramuscular 1:1000 adrenaline should always be available.

Administration technique

It is important in terms of safety, immunogenicity, and protective efficacy, for the recommended dosage of a vaccine to be given by the approved route of administration at the recommended site. Localized reactions are more common when intramuscular vaccines are inadvertently administered subcutaneously, hence most vaccines are given by intramuscular injection. Generally, vaccines with an adjuvant are given intramuscularly to reduce the risk of localized irritation and granuloma formation. Some vaccines are given by subcutaneous or intradermal injection. Patients with bleeding disorders (e.g. hemophilia) should also have intramuscular vaccines given by the deep subcutaneous route to reduce the risk of bleeding.

Intramuscular and subcutaneous injection

Intramuscular and subcutaneous vaccines should be administered into the anterolateral aspect of the thigh of infants and children less than 2 years old, and into the deltoid region of the upper arms in adults and older children to avoid large blood vessels and nerves. Vaccines are not administered into the buttock where there is a risk of damage to the sciatic nerve, particularly at a site other than the upper outer quadrant. There is also an increased likelihood of injecting the vaccine into fatty tissue in the buttocks leading to reduced vaccine efficacy owing to a lack of phagocytic or antigen-presenting cells in fat and increased enzyme denaturation of vaccine antigens. This is well illustrated with hepatitis B vaccines, which are 2 - 4 times more likely to fail to reach a minimum antibody level of 10 mIU/L when injected into the buttock than into the arm.

Intramuscular and subcutaneous vaccines should be administered with a 25 mm needle of either 23 or 25 G. Very small infants may require a smaller 16 mm, 25 G needle and likewise larger adults may require a longer 38 mm, 21 G needle. Intramuscular vaccines are administered by stretching the skin at the site of injection between the thumb and forefinger and then inserting the needle at 90° to the skin into the muscle. Subcutaneous vaccines are given by bunching (pinching) the skin together and then inserting the needle at 45° to the skin and into the subcutaneous tissue. It is not necessary to aspirate the syringe before injecting the vaccine and vaccines are never given intravenously; one should ensure that all of the vaccine has been injected before withdrawing the needle to avoid tracking.

Intradermal injection

Intradermal vaccines should be administered with a 26 G, 10 mm needle. The upper arm should be positioned at 45° to the body by resting their hand on their hip or holding the arm extended in young children. The skin should be stretched between the thumb and forefinger of one hand and then the needle inserted almost parallel to the skin at a very slight angle with the bevel facing upwards about 2 mm into the superficial dermis so that one can see the needle just below the epidermis. The vaccine is then injected against the resistance of the dermis, forming a bleb in the skin and a bleb of 7 mm diameter is approximately equivalent to 0.1 mL of vaccine administered. If there is no resistance during administration, the needle should be removed and reinserted before giving the remainder of the vaccine. The technique of intradermal vaccine administration is specialized, requiring that the healthcare professional receives appropriate training and assessment before such administration is undertaken.

BCG vaccine is always given by intradermal injection over the insertion of the left deltoid muscle, avoiding the tip of the shoulder, which predisposes to keloid scar formation. Some other vaccines may also be given intradermally, with intradermal rabies being one such vaccine, which requires less vaccine antigen per dose and is thus more cost efficient and may be used on occasion. Intradermal vaccination induces a rapid macrophage-dependent T-lymphocyte response via specific epidermal cells and studies with intradermal hepatitis B vaccination have, however, typically shown a relatively poor immune response compared with intramuscular vaccination.

Types of vaccines (Table 14.1)

Vaccine-preventable infectious diseases

1 **Cholera**:
   a. **Epidemiology**: Cholera is an acute gastroenteritis caused by feco-oral transmission of *Vibrio cholerae*, the majority caused by serotypes O1 and O139. Cholera is endemic and epidemic in about 58 developing countries. The most recent outbreak in the Western Hemisphere started in Haiti after Hurricane Sandy in 2010, which spread to the Dominican Republic and other countries. Risk to an average traveler is low except for those visiting friends and family or providing hands-on care in epidemic locations.
   b. **Indications**: Persons traveling into epidemic locations to provide healthcare.
   c. **Type of vaccine**: Two inactivated vaccines are available:
      i. WC-rBS – killed oral O1 with whole-cell with recombinant B subunit of the toxin (Dukoral).
      ii. BivWC – killed oral O1 and O139 (Shanchol or mORCVAX).
   d. **Administration**:
      i. WC-rBS (Dukoral) is licensed for individuals aged ≥ 2 years.
         1. **For individual >6 years of age**: two doses orally at least 1 week (up to 6 weeks) apart with the second dose at least 1 week before entry to risk area. If the interval between first and second doses is longer than 6 weeks, then the primary series should be restarted.
         2. **For children between 2 and 6 years of age**: three doses at 1-week intervals (minimum 1 week and maximum 6 weeks apart). If more than 6 weeks elapse between any of the doses, the primary series should be restarted.
      ii. BivWC (Shanchol) – Two oral doses 14 days apart for individuals aged ≥ 1 year.

e. **Efficacy and need for boosters**:

  i. WC-rBS (Dukoral) –Vaccine efficacy against cholera is about 50–60% in the first 2 years. Protective efficacy is lower (38%) in children aged <5 years. This vaccine also confers short-term 67% protection against travelers' diarrhea caused by enterotoxigenic *Escherichia coli*. A single booster can be given between 2 and 5 years from the last primary series. However, if the primary series was longer than 5 years ago, a repeat primary series is advised.

  ii. BivWC (Shanchol) – One booster dose is recommended after 2 years.

f. **Contraindications**: Hypersensitivity to cholera vaccine previously or to formaldehyde for Dukoral (Crucell Sweden).

g. **Precautions**: Advised to delay if ongoing gastroenteritis. It should be delayed by 8 hours from oral typhoid vaccine.

h. **Minimum time to effectiveness**: 2 weeks.

i. **Adverse effects**: Mild gastrointestinal disturbances.

j. **Storage**: Stored at 2–8 °C (35–46 °F). Should not be frozen. The vaccine can be stored at room temperature (up to 25 °C) for up to 2 weeks on one occasion only. After mixing with the buffer solution, the vaccine should be consumed within 2 hours.

2 **Diphtheria, tetanus, and acellular pertussis (DTaP, Tdap)**:

a. **Epidemiology**: Diphtheria, tetanus, and pertussis are prevalent in all developing and to a lesser extent in developed countries. Diphtheria and pertussis are acquired by close contact with ill persons. Contaminated injuries in unvaccinated persons can lead to tetanus. Patients should have completed their primary series and be up-to-date for recommended boosters. Adults who have not had diphtheria, tetanus, and acellular pertussis vaccine (Tdap) as an adult booster ever should receive that before travel.

b. **Indications**: All international travelers.

c. **Type of vaccine**: Inactivated combination vaccines. DTaP is the pediatric and Tdap the adult formulation.

d. **Administration**:

  i. **Primary series**: Three primary injectable doses given at 8 weeks (minimum 4 weeks) apart.

e. **Efficacy and need for booster**: Efficacy ranges from 59 to 89%. Tetanus/diphtheria (Td) boosters are recommended every 10 years. Tetanus toxoid is advised earlier in case of a contaminated injury if the last dose was 5 years or more previously. Tdap is recommended only as a single adult dose.

f. **Contraindications**: Hypersensitivity to a previous diphtheria, tetanus, and pertussis vaccine or a vaccine component. Encephalopathy attributed to a previous dose of DTP, DTaP, or Tdap.

g. **Precautions**:

  i. History of Guillain–Barré syndrome <6 weeks after a previous dose.

  ii. History of Arthus-type hypersensitivity after a tetanus or diphtheria toxoid-containing vaccine (including MCV4). Defer vaccination for at least 10 years from last tetanus-containing vaccine.

  iii. Moderate to severe acute illness with or without fever.

  iv. Specific precautions for DTaP:

1. Progressive neurologic disorder, including infantile spasms, uncontrolled epilepsy, progressive encephalopathy; defer DTaP until neurologic status clarified and stabilized.
2. Temperature of ≥105 °F (≥40.5 °C) within 48 hours after vaccination with a previous dose of DTP or DTaP.
3. Collapse or shock-like state (i.e., hypotonic hyporesponsive episode) within 48 hours after receiving a previous dose of DTP/DTaP.
4. Seizure ≤3 days after receiving a previous dose of DTP/DTaP.
5. Persistent, inconsolable crying lasting ≥3 hours within 48 hours after receiving a previous dose of DTP/DTaP.

h. **Minimum time to effectiveness**: 4 weeks from first dose.
i. **Adverse effects**: Mild local and systemic adverse events can occur. More serious adverse events [e.g., fever ≥105 °F (≥40.5 °C), persistent crying of ≥3 hours duration, hypotonic hyporesponsive episodes, and seizures] can occur in infants but are rare.
j. **Storage**: Vaccine should be stored at 2–8 °C (35–46 °F). Should not be frozen. Vaccine that has been exposed to freezing should not be used.

3 *Haemophilus influenzae* **type b** (**Hib**):
  a. **Epidemiology**: *Haemophilus influenzae* causes severe invasive bacterial disease including pneumonia and meningitis worldwide. Risk is highest for children; however, adults also can develop severe illness. Risk is increased in asplenic individuals. Travelers can acquire disease from direct exposure to an ill person.
  b. **Indications**: All traveling children over 4 months of age should complete primary series. Asplenic travelers should have at least one dose ever.
  c. **Type of vaccine**: Conjugated inactivated *Haemophilus influenzae* type b (Diphtheria CRM 197 Protein Conjugate) (HbOC), manufactured by Praxis Biologics, Haemophilus b Conjugate Vaccine (Meningococcal Protein Conjugate) (PRP-OMP), manufactured by Merck Sharp and Dohme, and Haemophilus b Conjugate Vaccine (Tetanus Toxoid Conjugate) booster dose manufactured by GlaxoSmithKline.
  d. **Administration**: Primary schedule is three doses given 8 weeks apart. Minimal interval is 4 weeks apart.
  e. **Efficacy and need for boosters**: Efficacy is 93–100%. No boosters are recommended.
  f. **Contraindications**: Severe allergic reaction (e.g., anaphylaxis) after a previous dose or to a vaccine component. Age <6 weeks.
  g. **Precautions**: Moderate to severe acute illness with or without fever
  h. **Minimum time to effectiveness**: 4 weeks from first dose.
  i. **Adverse effects**: Mild adverse effects include fever, local symptoms.
  j. **Storage**: Vaccine should be stored at 2–8 °C (35–46 °F). Should not be frozen.

4 Hepatitis A virus (**HAV**):
  a. **Epidemiology**: Hepatitis A is a food- and water-transmitted viral hepatitis. It is common in all developing countries. Symptoms include fever, diarrhea, and jaundice. Symptoms and risk of mortality increase with age (1.8% in persons >50 years of age) and with underlying chronic liver disease.
  b. **Indications**: All travelers to developing countries, including parents of adoptee children. Persons with chronic liver disease, clotting factor disorders,

men who have sex with men, or those who work with non-human primates. Persons who work at child care centers, food handling, healthcare institutions, schools, institutions for persons with disability or exposed to sewage.

c. **Type of vaccine**: There are two types of hepatitis A vaccines:

   i. Inactivated vaccines: used in most countries. Commercially available as Havrix and Vaqta.

   ii. Live attenuated vaccines: Manufactured and used mainly in China and India.

d. **Administration**: Intramuscular injections given at least 6 months apart for a two-dose regimen. Inactivated HAV vaccines are available in pediatric dose (0.5 mL) for children aged >1 to 15 years and in adult dose (1 mL).

e. **Efficacy and need for boosters**: Inactivated and attenuated HAV have efficacy reaching 86–95%. The second dose of the inactivated vaccines should ideally be given 6–12 months after the first but studies have shown that it can be boosted up to more than 8 years after the first dose. Re-starting the primary series is never indicated. Immunity from vaccination is expected to last for 25–30 years.

f. **Contraindications**: Severe allergic reaction (e.g., anaphylaxis) after a previous dose or to a vaccine component.

g. **Precautions**: Pregnancy and lactation are precautions.

h. **Minimum time to effectiveness**: 2–4 weeks from vaccination.

i. **Adverse effects**: Most common adverse effects are fever, injection-site reactions, rash, and headache.

j. **Storage**: Hepatitis A vaccines should be stored and shipped in the refrigerator at 2–8 °C (35–46 °F). The vaccine should not be frozen.

5 **Hepatitis B virus (HBV)**:

a. **Epidemiology**: HBV can cause chronic liver disease that can further place the patients at risk for hepatocellular carcinoma. An estimated 350 million people are living with chronic hepatitis B worldwide (1). HBV is prevalent worldwide particularly in Asian and African countries. Risk of transmission to a traveler is from blood or body fluid exposure from sexual or non-sexual contact. Non-sexual contact includes needlestick exposures via parenteral drug abuse or healthcare exposures.

b. **Indications**: Individuals at higher risk for acquiring hepatitis B include frequent or prolonged travelers to countries with high prevalence of HBV, travelers engaged in high-risk activities such as healthcare or other work that may expose them to blood/body fluids (policemen, firefighters, jail wardens, etc.), sexual exposure, or medical tourism abroad.

c. **Type of vaccine**: Recombinant DNA technology, produced in yeast.

d. **Administration**: A three-dose primary HBV series is given as intramuscular injections at 0, 1, and 6 months. Accelerated (0, 1, 2, and 12 months) and hyper-accelerated (0, 7, and 21 days and 12 months) schedules are effective after the first three doses and are available for persons at high risk and leaving imminently.

e. **Efficacy and need for boosters**: Vaccine efficacy is about 95% or higher after three doses. About 10% of vaccinees are non-responders. If there is documentation of hepatitis B surface antibody response, then no boosters are needed. However, testing is not recommended for most travelers. For the highest risk group, such as surgeons, serologies should be done to document vaccine response. Boosters may be needed in someone who is seronegative.

f. **Contraindications**: Hypersensitivity to a previous dose or component.

g. **Precautions**: Moderate to severe acute illness with or without fever.

h. **Minimum time to effectiveness**: Protective antibody response is induced in approximately 30–55% of healthy adults 4 weeks after the first dose, 75% after the second dose, and >90% after the third dose. The vaccine response is lowered by age, nicotine dependence, obesity, and immunosuppression.

i. **Adverse effects**: No serious adverse effects have been causally linked with hepatitis B vaccination.

j. **Storage**: Refrigerated at 2–8 °C (36–46 °F) and should not be frozen. Discard if the product has been frozen.

6 Combination hepatitis A and B vaccination

a. **Epidemiology**: As described above for HAV and HBV.

b. **Indications**: Persons at risk for both should be considered for this vaccination if available in the clinic.

c. **Type of vaccine**: Combination of inactivated hepatitis A (Havrix) and recombinant DNA hepatitis B vaccine (Engerix).

d. **Administration**: A three-dose primary series is given as intramuscular injections at 0, 1, and 6 months. An accelerated schedule of 0, 1, 2, and 12 months or a hyper-accelerated schedule of 0, 7, 21, and 12 months is available for those traveling imminently.

e. **Efficacy and need for boosters**: Vaccine efficacy is about 98% or higher 1 month after completing three doses for the combined hepatitis A and B vaccines.

f. **Contraindications**: Hypersensitivity to a previous dose or component.

g. **Precautions**: Moderate or severe illness. Pregnancy and lactation are precautions.

h. **Adverse effects**: No serious adverse effects.

i. **Minimum time to effectiveness**:

j. **Storage**: Refrigerated at 2–8°C (36–46 °F) and should not be frozen. Discard if the product has been frozen.

7 Human papillomavirus (HPV):

a. **Epidemiology**: Genital HPV is the most common cause of cervical cancers worldwide. Approximately 11.4% of women worldwide are estimated to have cervical HPV infection. HPV infection is acquired by sexual and non-sexual direct contact with an infected person. Risk to travelers is predominantly via sexual exposure.

b. **Indications**: Sexually active young men and women who are <26 years of age irrespective of travel. Children, especially girls, prior to onset of sexually activity.

c. **Type of vaccine**: There are two inactivated vaccines available, HPV4 and HPV2. Both are composed of virus-like particles (VLPs) prepared from recombinant L1 capsid protein of HPV. Quadrivalent HPV4 has two non-oncogenic types 6 and 11, and two oncogenic types 16 and 18, while the bivalent HPV2 is directed against two oncogenic types HPV 16 and 18.

d. **Administration**: HPV vaccine is approved for females aged 9–26 years and males aged 9–21 years. In the United States, HPV vaccines are routinely recommended for 11–12-year-old girls and boys.

e. **Efficacy and need for boosters**: Efficacy against HPV 16- or 18-related cervical intraepithelial neoplasia grade 2 or 3 or adenocarcinoma in situ is over 90%.

f. **Contraindications**: Hypersensitivity to a previous dose or component.

g. **Precautions**: Not recommended for pregnant women. Moderate to severe acute illness with or without fever.

h. **Minimum time to effectiveness**: 4 weeks after completing the course.

i. **Adverse effects**: Fever, injection site pain, fainting.

j. **Storage**: The vaccine should be stored in a refrigerator at 2–8 °C (35–46 °F). The vaccine should not be frozen.

8 **Japanese encephalitis (JE)**: See Chapter 7.

9 **Measles, mumps, and rubella viruses (MMR)**:

a. **Epidemiology**: Despite availability of the MMR vaccine worldwide, measles is one of the leading causes of death among young children globally. Transmission is via contact with respiratory secretions of an ill person.

b. **Indications**: All travelers should be vaccinated against MMR.

c. **Type of vaccine**: Live attenuated viral vaccine. Measles and mumps viruses are propagated in chick embryo cell cultures whereas rubella virus is propagated in human diploid cells.

d. **Administration**: Two doses of the MMR vaccine with the first dose at 12–15 months and revaccination prior to elementary school entry. In the United States, those born before 1957 are considered immune based on the prevalence of diseases at that time. For assessment of immunity, patients should either have proof of vaccination or serologic evidence or be vaccinated if there is no evidence of immunity prior to travel to developing countries.

e. **Efficacy and need for boosters**: Two doses of the vaccine induce 99% protection against MMR. Routine boosters are not recommended.

f. **Contraindications**: Congenital or acquired immunocompromised status, pregnancy, age <9 months. Pregnancy is a contraindication.

g. **Precautions**: Receipt of antibody-containing blood product may impair vaccine response, hence vaccination should be delayed. The duration of delay depends on the type of blood product received. Thrombocytopenia and thrombocytopenic purpura are relative contraindications. Tuberculin skin testing within 4 weeks of receiving MMR may be falsely negative; therefore, tuberculin skin testing or tuberculosis interferon-γ release assay should be delayed by 4 weeks after MMR.

h. **Minimum time to effectiveness**: 4 weeks.

i. **Adverse effects**: MMR vaccine can cause fever, transient rashes, transient lymphadenopathy, or parotitis. There is evidence supporting a causal relationship between MMR vaccination and anaphylaxis, febrile seizures, thrombocytopenic purpura, transient arthralgia, and measles inclusion body encephalitis in persons with demonstrated immunodeficiencies. Evidence refutes the association of MMR vaccination with autism, inflammatory bowel diseases, and type 1 diabetes mellitus.

  j. **Storage**: Vaccine should be stored at −50 to +8 °C (−58 to +46 °F) to maintain potency.

10 **Meningococcal disease**:

  a. **Epidemiology**: *Neisseria meningitidis* infections (meningitis and meningococcemia) occur worldwide. In a number of Sub-Saharan African countries from Senegal to Ethiopia, epidemics occur annually during the dry season (November to June). While serogroups A, B, and C are more common in industrialized countries, serogroups A and W-135 are more common in Africa. Hajj and Umrah pilgrims to Saudi Arabia are also at risk for meningococcal disease due to the congregation of large populations coming from all over the world, especially those coming from the "meningitis belt" of Africa. Saudi Arabia requires proof of vaccination for entry into the country to attend the Hajj and Umrah pilgrimages. Young children, adolescents, immunocompromised persons and asplenic subjects are at higher risk of meningococcal disease. Students traveling for study abroad, especially those who live in dormitories, are at risk for meningococcal disease.

  b. **Indications**: Vaccination is indicated for travelers to high-risk countries in Africa and to Saudi Arabia for Hajj or Umrah pilgrimage. Healthcare workers to risk countries and patients with asplenia should be vaccinated. Students living in a dormitory or study abroad programs should also be vaccinated.

  c. **Type of vaccine**: There are three different types of meningococcal vaccines available worldwide with variable availability of specific vaccines in different geographic locations. The four most common serotypes, A, C, Y, and W-135, are represented in three different combinations in the available vaccines – as A and C, as A, C, and W-135, and as tetravalent. Meningococcal vaccines are either polysaccharide or conjugate polysaccharide vaccines.

  d. **Administration**: Intramuscular injections as a single dose for immunocompetent patients. For asplenics and patients with complement deficiencies, the vaccine is given as a two-dose primary series.

  e. **Efficacy and need for boosters**: Meningococcal vaccines have an efficacy of 85–100% in persons over 2 years of age. Boosters are recommended every 3–5 years for asplenics or complement deficiencies. For immunocompetent patients, revaccination is only needed if traveling back to risk areas.

  f. **Contraindications**: Allergy to a previous dose or a component of the vaccine.

  g. **Precautions**: Moderate or severe illness.

  h. **Minimum time to effectiveness**: Vaccine takes about 2 weeks to become fully effective.

  i. **Adverse effects**: Fever, headache, and syncope can occur with the meningococcal vaccines.

  j. **Storage**: The vaccines should be stored in a refrigerator at 2–8 °C (35–46 °F). The vaccine should not be frozen.

Table 14.1 Vaccines.

Vaccine	Primary course	Boosters	Accelerated schedule	Contraindications/precautions	Possible side-effects
Hepatitis A	**Ages 12 months–18 years** 0.5 mL IM deltoid **≥19 years** 1.0 mL IM deltoid **Usual schedule:** 0 and 6–18 months	None	None	Allergy to aluminum or aluminum hydroxide Age <12 months Moderate/severe illness with or without fever Pregnant Serious reaction to previous dose	Injection site pain, warmth, swelling, headache
Hepatitis B	**Age <19 years** 0.5 mL IM deltoid or anterolateral thigh **Age 11–15 years** 1.0 mL IM deltoid or anterolateral thigh **Adult ≥20 years** 1.0 mL IM deltoid **Usual schedule:** 0, 1, 6 months	None	0, 1, 2, and 12 months 0, 7, 21 days and 12 months	Anaphylaxis to a previous dose of HB vaccine Hypersensitivity to yeast Pregnancy	Injection site pain, fever, headache, itching, nausea; rarely: anaphylaxis or other systemic effect
Twinrix – combined hepatitis A and hepatitis B	**≥18 years** 1.0 mL **Usual schedule:** 0, 1, 6 months	None	Doses at 0, 7, and 21–30 days with a booster dose 12 months after first dose	Anaphylaxis to a previous dose of Twinrix, or a previous dose of monovalent hep A or hep B vaccine. Hypersensitivity to latex, aluminum, aluminum phosphate, aluminum hydroxide, 2-phenoxyethanol, formalin, thimerosal, neomycin or yeast protein Age <18 years Moderate/severe illness with or without fever Pregnancy	Injection site pain, warmth, swelling; headache; fatigue (mild, self-limiting not lasting more than 48 hours)

Haemophilus influenzae type b	**Age 2 months–adult** 0.5 mL IM deltoid or anterolateral thigh **Usual schedule**: 2, 4, 6 months	Single booster dose at 12–18 months of age	Youngest age for 1st dose: 6 weeks	Anaphylaxis to a previous dose of the vaccine Anaphylaxis to any component (tetanus toxoid, ammonium sulfate, formalin) Age <6 weeks Moderate or severe illness with or without fever.	Injection site redness, tenderness or swelling, mild fever, irritability, restless sleep, lethargy, rhinorrhea and possible urticaria, decreased appetite, rarely vomiting, rarely diarrhea, rarely anaphylaxis
Human papillomavirus vaccine (HPV) (Gardasil)	Females and males **Females: >9–26 years** **Males: >9–21 years** 0.5 mL IM deltoid **Usual schedule**: 0, 1–2, 6 months	None	0, 4, 24 weeks Minimum intervals between HPV vaccine doses: • 4 weeks between doses 1–2 • 12 weeks between doses 2–3 • 24 weeks between doses 1–3	Anaphylaxis to a reaction to a previous dose Anaphylaxis to yeast Pregnant	Injection site pain, headache, fever, nausea, dizziness, swelling, erythema, pruritus and bruising. Syncope, therefore need to observe for 15 minutes after vaccination
FluMist Influenza Healthy persons aged 2–49 years Live attenuated viral vaccine	**≥2–49 years** >8 years: single dose 2–8 years: 2 doses 8 weeks apart "Mist" of 0.1 mL in each nostril **Usual schedule**: Once each influenza season	No specific boosters		Anaphylactic reactions to eggs, gentamicin, gelatin, arginine, MSG or previous dose. ASA therapy History of Guillain–Barré syndrome Receipt of antivirals within the last 48 hours Immunocompromised[a] Age <2 years and ≥50 years Other live attenuated viral vaccine within past 28 days Pregnant	

(continued overleaf)

Table 14.1 (*continued*)

Vaccine	Primary course	Boosters	Accelerated schedule	Contraindications/precautions	Possible side-effects
Influenza – inactivated injectable IIV3 – trivalent IIV4 – quadrivalent Injectable	**Ages 6–35 months** 0.25 mL IM anterolateral thigh **3–8 years** 0.5 mL IM anterolateral thigh or deltoid **≥9 years** 0.5 mL IM deltoid **>65 years** IIV3 Fluzone high-dose vaccine can be given **Usual schedule:** **6 months – 8 years:** 2 doses as primary initial series **>8 years:** single dose	None	None	Acute respiratory or other active infections or illness Anaphylaxis to eggs Allergy to gelatin, gentamicin, or thimerosal (presence varies on the specific vaccine type) History of Guillain–Barré syndrome Age <6 months Serious reaction to a previous dose	Injection site pain Fever, malaise, muscle pain Immediate reactions (hives, angioedema, allergic asthma, systemic anaphylaxis) rarely occur
Japanese encephalitis virus IXIARO	**≥2 months to ≤3 years** 0.25 mL IM **≥3 years** 0.5 mL IM **Usual schedule:** 0, 28 days	If primary series received more than 1 year but less than 2 years ago, a single booster dose may be given. If more than 2 years ago: data unavailable to give evidence-based recommendations	None	Anaphylaxis reaction to a previous dose or formaldehyde, bovine serum albumin, host cell DNA or proteins, sodium metabisulfite, and protamine sulfate Less than 28 days prior to departure Pregnant	Injection site pain, redness, or swelling, headache, muscle aches

Rabies – pre-exposure	**Any age** 1.0 mL IM deltoid or anterolateral thigh **Usual schedule**: Days 0, 7, and 21 or 28	None routinely recommended unless extremely high risk	Days 0, 7, and 21 Minimum intervals: • 7 days between doses 1 and 2 • 14 days between doses 2 and 3 • Each minimum interval must be followed	Allergy to processed bovine gelatin, chicken protein, eggs, neomycin, chlortetracycline and amphotericin B Moderate/severe illness with or without fever Pregnant Severe reaction to previous dose	Injection site redness, swelling Localized lymph node swelling Headache, myalgia, malaise, dizziness Rarely: fever, gastrointestinal complaints, swollen lymph nodes, severe headache, sweating, chills, transient numbness/tingling, anaphylaxis, encephalitis, meningitis, temporary paralysis
Meningococcal conjugate – quadrivalent (Menactra)	**≥2–≤55 years** 0.5 mL IM **≥9 months to ≤23 months** 0.5 mL IM **Usual schedule**: Single dose Two doses 8 weeks apart if immunocompromised	**Age <7 years**: every 3 years if continued risk **>7 years**: every 5 years if continued risk	None	Anaphylaxis reaction to a previous dose, diphtheria toxoid or ingredients: formaldehyde or formalin, phosphate buffers (e.g., disodium, monosodium, potassium, and sodium dihydrogen phosphate), and latex (found in vial preparations) History of Guillain–Barré syndrome Age >55 years Pregnant	
Meningococcal MENOMUNE	**≥2 years** 0.5 mL SQ **Usual schedule**: Single dose	Every 3–5 years if at risk	None	Allergy to thimerosal Age <2 years Moderate/severe illness with or without fever Pregnant Severe reaction to previous dose	Injection site pain, redness Transient fever in 2% of children

(continued overleaf)

Table 14.1 (*continued*)

Vaccine	Primary course	Boosters	Accelerated schedule	Contraindications/precautions	Possible side-effects
Measles, mumps, rubella (MMR) Live attenuated viral vaccine	**>12 months – adult** 0.5 mL SQ **Usual schedule**: Primary: 1 dose at 12–15 months with a second dose at age 4–6 years Adults: 2 doses with 4–8 week interval	No additional boosters	None	Active untreated tuberculosis Allergy to a previous dose Allergy to neomycin, gelatin, eggs, egg proteins Blood dyscrasias, leukemia, lymphoma, bone marrow suppression History of seizures History of thrombocytopenia or thrombocytopenic purpura Immunocompromised[a] Age <6 months Other live attenuated viral vaccine within past 28 days Pregnant or planning to become pregnant in next 3 months Receipt of immunoglobins or blood products in past 8 months	Injection site burning, pain, redness Fever Swollen lymph nodes Transient rash (5%) Rarely: transient thrombocytopenia within 2 months, anaphylaxis or other systemic effects
Pneumococcal 13-valent conjugate (PCV-13)	**6 weeks–59 months of age** 0.5 mL IM deltoid or anterolateral thigh (4 doses) **>19 years of age with immunocompromising conditions**		**Primary series in children** **6 weeks–59 months of age**: 3 doses, each minimum of 4–8 weeks apart No accelerated schedule in adults	Anaphylaxis with a previous dose of PCV7, any PCV7 component (CRM-197 carrier protein and aluminum phosphate), latex or diphtheria toxoid Moderate or severe illness with or without fever Pregnant or lactation	Injection site redness, tenderness, or swelling, mild fever, irritability, restless sleep, decreased appetite, rarely vomiting, rarely diarrhea, rarely anaphylaxis

	0.5 mL IM deltoid **Usual schedule:** **6 weeks–59 month of age** Primary: 3 doses minimum of 4–8 weeks apart each. (Typical schedule at ages 2, 4, 6 months) followed by 4th dose at 12–15 months of age **>19 years of age with immuneocompromising conditions** PCV-13 followed 8 weeks later by PPSV23 If PPSV23 received previously, then minimum interval from last PPSV23 is 12 months		
Pneumococcal 23-valent Pneumovax 23 (PPSV23)	**≥2 years** 0.5 mL IM or SQ **Usual schedule:** Single dose	**Children ≥24 months–2 years** with risk factors for severe pneumococcal disease who had PCV13 previously: 1 dose of PPSV23 at 2 years at least ≥8 weeks after last PCV13 **2–64 years with risk factors for severe disease:** aged >10 years, single booster ≥5 years after previous dose and at least ≥8 weeks from PCV13 **≥65 years:** booster dose if a previous dose received ≥5 years and patient was <65 years old at the time	None Allergy to phenol Anaphylaxis to a reaction to previous dose Age <2 years Moderate/severe illness with or without fever Pregnant	Injection site pain, redness, or swelling Rarely: fever/myalgia, or severe systemic effects

(continued overleaf)

Table 14.1 (*continued*)

Vaccine	Primary course	Boosters	Accelerated schedule	Contraindications/precautions	Possible side-effects
Poliovirus-Injectable IPOL	**Dose (all ages)** 0.5 mL SQ **Usual schedule:** **<18 years:** 3 doses at ages 2, 4, 6–18 months **≥18 years:** 3 doses at intervals 0, 2, 8–14 months	**<18 years** 1 dose at 4–6 years of age unless third primary dose was administered after age 4 years **>18 years** If previously completed primary series ≥10 years ago, single, one-time IPV dose to travelers to risk areas	**<18 years** **Primary series** 3 doses 4–8 weeks apart **>18 years** **Primary series:** If 8 weeks until travel: 3 doses 4 weeks apart If 4–8 weeks until travel: 2 doses 4 weeks apart If <4 weeks until travel: first dose with completion of primary series at location or after return	Allergy to a previous dose Allergy to neomycin, polymyxin B or streptomycin Moderate/severe illness with or without fever Pregnant	Injection site pain and fever most common Rarely: anaphylaxis or other systemic effects
Tdap Age ≥7 years Tetanus/diphtheria/ acellular pertussis	**Age ≥7 years** 0.5 mL IM deltoid or anterolateral thigh **Usual schedule:** Single dose at age 11–12 years Single dose for all adults Pregnancy ≥27 weeks gestation	None	None	Allergy to pertussis vaccine History of encephalopathy not due to another cause occurring 7 days following previous DTaP	Injection site pain, fever, irritability; rarely Guillain–Barré syndrome, anaphylaxis

	Usual schedule	Booster		Contraindications	Adverse effects
Td Ages ≥7 years Tetanus/diphtheria	**Age ≥7 years** 0.5 mL IM **Usual schedule:** **Primary series in unimmunized adults and children:** 3 doses at 0, 2, 12 months **Previously completed primary series:** single dose every 10 years	Every 10 years	The 3 primary doses can be accelerated to 0, 2, and 6 months	Allergy to a previous dose (Td, DTP, DTaP, DT) Allergy to thimerosal Age <7 years Moderate/severe illness with or without fever	Injection site redness, swelling, pain, nodule Painful swelling from shoulder to elbow 2–8 hours after injection Uncommon: fever, systemic symptoms, neurologic symptoms, generalized rash/itching, anaphylaxis
DTaP ONLY for children ≤7 years of age	**Age 6 weeks to <7 years** 0.5 mL IM deltoid or anterolateral thigh **Usual schedule:** **Primary:** 3 doses at ages 2, 4, 6 months. Fourth dose of DTaP at age 12–18 months with minimum interval of 6 months from the third primary dose	**Booster:** 1 dose at age 4–6 years	Youngest age for first dose: 6 weeks with the remaining 2 primary doses completed with a minimum of 4 week intervals	Allergy to pertussis vaccine (give DT in this situation to children <7 years old) History of encephalopathy not due to another cause occurring 7 days following previous DTaP	Injection site pain, fever, irritability; rarely Guillain–Barré syndrome, anaphylaxis
Tick-borne encephalitis	**≥18 months–15 years** 0.25 mL IM in the deltoid. **>16 years** 0.5 mL IM deltoid **Usual schedule:** 0, 1–3, and 5–12 months	First booster 3 years after primary series if at continued risk Every 3–5 years after that if continued risk	0, 14 days and 5–12 months	Anaphylaxis to a previous dose of the vaccine Anaphylaxis to aluminum or aluminum hydroxide, sucrose, formaldehyde, neomycin, gentamicin or protamine sulfate	Injection site pain, redness Transient fever, headache, joint or muscle pains

(continued overleaf)

Table 14.1 (*continued*)

Vaccine	Primary course	Boosters	Accelerated schedule	Contraindications/precautions	Possible side-effects
Typhoid Injectable Typhim Vi	**≥2 years–adult** 0.5 mL IM deltoid/vastus lateralis in children **Usual schedule**: Single dose at least 2 weeks prior to exposure	Single IM injection every 2 years with repeated exposure	None	Age <18 months Moderate/severe illness with or without fever Pregnancy Allergy to phenol <2 weeks prior to exposure Age <2 years old Moderate/severe illness with or without fever Pregnant Severe reaction to previous dose	Injection site pain, redness, swelling Occasional fever, flu-like symptoms, headache, tremor, abdominal pains, vomiting, diarrhea, cervical pains
Typhoid – Oral TY21a Live attenuated viral vaccine	**≥6 years–adult** 4 capsules orally every other day on days 0, 2, 4, 6 **Usual schedule**: Capsule taken orally on empty stomach every other day x4 capsules. Vaccine needs to remain refrigerated	Repeat 4-dose series every 5 years with repeated exposure	None	Acute vomiting/diarrhea Antibiotics 24 hours prior initiating or 72 hours after completing doses Immunocompromised[a] Age <6 years Moderate/severe illness with or without fever Pregnant Requires mefloquine within 24 hours of completing typhoid vaccine Severe reaction to previous dose Unable to completed 1 week prior to exposure	Fewer side effects with oral vaccine Rarely: nausea, abdominal pain, cramps, vomiting, fever, headache, rash

| Varicella Varivax Live attenuated viral vaccine | 12 months 0.5 mL SQ deltoid **Usual schedule**: Primary: 2 doses 4–8 weeks apart | None. | Minimum interval between 2 primary doses is 4 weeks | Active, untreated tuberculosis Anaphylaxis to a previous dose of Varivax Anaphylaxis to neomycin or gelatin Anti-varicella antivirals (e.g., acyclovir, famciclovir, or valacyclovir) within 24 hours of vaccination Aspirin therapy Family history of immunodeficiency and living with high-risk persons Immunodeficiency (hematologic and solid tumors; congenital immunodeficiency; long-term immunosuppressive therapy, blood dyscrasias, taking long-term or large doses of corticosteroids) Age <12 months Other live attenuated viral vaccine within past 28 days Pregnancy/lactation Recent administration of immunoglobulin, whole blood, or other blood products | Pain, redness, induration, swelling at injection site, fever Chicken pox-like rash (local or general) in 3–6% of vaccinees |

(continued overleaf)

Table 14.1 (*continued*)

Vaccine	Primary course	Boosters	Accelerated schedule	Contraindications/precautions	Possible side-effects
Shingles (herpes zoster) Zostavax Live attenuated viral vaccine	**≥50 years** 0.65 mL SQ deltoid **Usual schedule:** Single dose	None	None	Active, untreated tuberculosis Anaphy axis to neomycin or gelatin Anti-varicella antivirals (e.g., acyclovir, famciclovir, or valacyclovir) within 24 hours of vaccination Family history of immunodeficiency and living with high-risk persons Immunodeficiency (hematologic and solid tumors; congenital immunodeficiency; long-term immunosuppressive therapy, blood dyscrasias, taking long-term or large doses of corticosteroids) Age <5C years Other live attenuated viral vaccine within past 28 days Pregnancy/lactation Recent administration of immunoglobulin, whole blood, or other blood products	Pain, redness, induration, swelling at injection site, fever Chicken pox-like rash

Vaccine	Dose/Schedule	Booster	Contraindications	Adverse effects
Yellow fever YF-VAX Live attenuated viral vaccine	**≥9 months** 0.5 mL SQ deltoid **Usual schedule**: Single dose	Every 10 years	None	Anaphylaxis to a reaction to previous dose Anaphylaxis to eggs, chicken, gelatin or egg protein Immunocompromised[a] <10 days prior to arrival in endemic county Age <9 months Other live attenuated viral vaccine within past 28 days Pregnant Received other live antigen vaccines within past 4 weeks (MMR, oral typhoid, varicella or OPV) Recent administration of immunoglobulin, whole blood, or other blood products Thymectomy or thymus gland problem (myasthenia gravis, DiGeorge syndrome or thymoma)	Mild: Pain, redness or swelling at injection site, mild headaches, myalgia, low-grade fevers Rarely: Neurotropic adverse effects: 1 per 150,000–250,000 doses. Viscerotropic adverse effects: 1 per 200,000–300,000 doses for otherwise healthy persons, 1 per 40,000–50,000 doses in persons aged 60 years or older

IM, intramuscular; SQ, subcutaneous.

[a]Immunocompromised: HIV/AIDS, leukemia, lymphoma, generalized malignancy, undergoing long-term chemotherapy, radiation therapy, taking large doses of corticosteroids (>2 mg/kg/day or >20 mg per day), status post-organ transplant and on immunosuppression, <3 months since completing immunosuppressive medications.

11 **Pneumococcal disease**:
   a. **Epidemiology**: *Streptococcus pneumoniae* commonly causes respiratory or other organ infections. Risk factors for severe pneumococcal infections include nicotine dependence, immune compromise including older age, diabetes, congenital or acquired immunodeficiency, presence of cochlear implants, and asplenia. Travel itself does not increase the risk, but may be associated with multi-drug-resistant pneumococcal infection.
   b. **Indications**: Individuals with risk factors for severe pneumococcal disease should receive pneumococcal vaccination irrespective of travel. The following persons should receive pneumococcal vaccination: those with iatrogenic or acquired immunodeficiency, asplenia, diabetes, age over 65 years, nicotine dependence, sickle cell disease, cochlear implant and chronic kidney, lung or cardiac disease. Travelers with risk factors should be vaccinated if not already vaccinated.
   c. **Type of vaccine**: Two main types of pneumococcal vaccines are available: 23-valent polysaccharide (PPSV23) and conjugated 7- or 13-valent (PCV7 or PCV13). The conjugated 13-valent is recommended predominantly for severely immunocompromised patients.
   d. **Administration**: Intramuscular injection.
   e. **Efficacy and need for boosters**: Pneumococcal vaccines have an estimated efficacy against invasive pneumococcal disease of 50–80% in immunocompetent hosts and slightly lower in immunocompromised hosts. For immunocompromised patients, a repeat single booster is recommended at 5 years after the initial vaccine.
   f. **Contraindications**: Hypersensitivity to a previous dose or component.
   g. **Precautions**: Acute illness is a relative contraindication for vaccination.
   h. **Minimum time to effectiveness**: 4 weeks.
   i. **Adverse effects**: The primary adverse effect is a local reaction, which is more common with the booster.
   j. **Storage**: The vaccines should be stored in a refrigerator at 2–8 °C (35–46 °F). The vaccine should not be frozen.

12 **Poliomyelitis**:
   a. **Epidemiology**: Poliomyelitis is nearing eradication in the world. Currently only a handful of countries have active transmission of wild strains of poliomyelitis, including Afghanistan, Nigeria, Pakistan, Angola, Chad, and the Democratic Republic of the Congo. There is some risk of polio when millions of worshippers from all over the world congregate in Saudi Arabia for the Hajj or Umrah pilgrimage. Saudi Arabia requires travelers for these pilgrimages to have documentation of recent polio vaccination prior to entry. Transmission is from fecal–oral contamination. The risk to average travelers is extremely low.
   b. **Indications**: Travel to an endemic country.
   c. **Types of vaccine**: The two types of polio vaccines, the oral live attenuated (OPV) and the injectable inactivated vaccine (IPV), are trivalent.
   d. **Administration**: In children, the four-dose IPV series should be administered at ages 2, 4, and 6–18 months and 4–6 years. Those who completed

the primary series and are traveling to an endemic country should receive a one-time booster if the primary series was more than 10 years prior.

e. **Efficacy and need for boosters**: 90–100% of recipients develop protective antibodies after 3–4 doses. Vaccine effectiveness of the IPV is approximately 90%. Other than a one-time adult booster prior to travel to endemic countries, no additional boosters are needed.

f. **Contraindications**: Hypersensitivity to a previous dose or component. Live attenuated oral polio vaccine is contraindicated in immunocompromised patients. Of note, the oral polio vaccine is currently not used in many developed countries.

g. **Precautions**: Pregnancy.

h. **Minimum time to effectiveness**: 8 weeks.

i. **Adverse effects**: Minimal adverse effects from the IPV. The OPV carries a small risk of vaccine-associated poliomyelitis.

j. **Storage**: The IPV should be stored in a refrigerator at 2–8 °C (35–46 °F). The vaccine should not be frozen.

13 **Rabies**: See Chapter 13.

14 **Rotavirus**:

a. **Epidemiology**: Rotavirus is the leading cause of severe gastroenteritis in children aged <5 years worldwide. Rotaviruses are estimated to result in more than 25 million infections and 2 million hospitalizations annually. Approximately half a million deaths are attributed each year to rotavirus infections, predominantly in low-income countries. Rotavirus infections typically peak in the winter in temperate countries but occur year round in the tropics. Risk with travel is predominantly to children less than 5 years of age. Transmission is from fecal–oral contamination.

b. **Indications**: Rotavirus vaccination is routinely recommended to all infants in countries where available and especially prior to travel to developing countries.

c. **Type of vaccine**: Two live, attenuated, oral rotavirus vaccines are available: RotaTeq (RV5) (Merck) and Rotarix (RV1) (GlaxoSmithKline Biologicals).

d. **Administration**: RV5 is administered orally in a three-dose series, with doses at ages 2, 4, and 6 months. RV1 is to be given orally in a two-dose series, with doses given at ages 2 and 4 months. There are strict age limits for starting and completing the series. The first dose should be between 6 weeks and 14 weeks and 6 days of age. All doses should be completed by age 8 months and 0 days. The minimum interval between doses of rotavirus vaccine is 4 weeks. Infants who inadvertently receive the first dose at age 15 weeks and 0 days or older should proceed and complete the series by age 8 months and 0 days.

e. **Efficacy and need for boosters**: Rotavirus vaccine efficacy with the RV5 against severe disease is 98% and against any disease is 85%. Boosters are not recommended.

f. **Contraindications**: Hypersensitivity to a previous dose or component. Immunodeficiency and history of intussusception are contraindications.

g. **Precautions**: These vaccines should be given with caution to children with chronic gastrointestinal disease. Owing to the presence of latex in the vaccine and the potential for latex allergy in spina bifida or bladder exstrophy, these vaccines should be administered with caution in such children.

h. **Minimum time to effectiveness**: 4 weeks.

i. **Adverse effects**: Mild symptoms include irritability, diarrhea, and emesis. Rare risk with intussusception exists within 1 week after the first or second dose. Risk is estimated to be about 1 in 20,000 to 1 in 100,000 US infants who receive rotavirus vaccine.

j. **Storage**: The vaccines should be stored and transported refrigerated at 2–8 °C (35–46 °F). The vaccine should not be frozen.

15 Seasonal influenza:

a. **Epidemiology**: Influenza is the most common vaccine-preventable travel-related illness. It is non-seasonal in the tropics and in the winter months in temperate zones. The monthly incidence is 1.0–2.3% and overall attack rate is 1.2–2.8%. Influenza results in >1% patients requiring medical attention abroad or after return and results in changes in travel plans for 0.2% of the travelers. Influenza is acquired by respiratory droplet exposure. Influenza can be severe in persons at extremes of age and immunocompromised patients.

b. **Indications**: All travelers and non-travelers annually. Influenza vaccination is especially recommended for those at risk for severe influenza such as children aged <5 years, persons with asthma, chronic lung, or heart disease, and immunocompromised subjects. Travel clinics should consider keeping the most recent season's influenza vaccine until its expiration so that it can be offered to travelers to the tropics or to temperate regions on either Hemisphere during their winter.

c. **Type of vaccine**: Currently three main classes of influenza vaccines are available: (1) inactivated injectable vaccines which are egg-based and cell culture-based trivalent inactivated influenza vaccines (IIV3), and egg-based quadrivalent inactivated influenza vaccine (IIV4); (2) the recombinant trivalent recombinant hemagglutinin influenza vaccine (RIV3); and (3) quadrivalent live-attenuated influenza vaccine (LAIV). These vaccines mostly contain two influenza A strains and one or two influenza B strains based on the most recent prevalent strains.

d. **Administration**:

   i. **IIV3 and IIV4**: Single intramuscular injection given once per year to all aged 6 months and over. Age limits and specific doses vary based on specific manufacturer recommendations.

   ii. **RIV4**: Single intramuscular injection given once per year to persons with severe egg allergy aged between 18 and 49 years.

   iii. **LAIV**: Single nasal live attenuated vaccine is given intranasally as a spray once per year for those between the ages of 2 and 49 years.

e. **Efficacy and need for boosters**: Frequent viral reassortment results in emergence of new annual influenza strains for which there is no cross-protection from previous vaccinations. This necessitates a new vaccine each year that contains a new combination of viral antigens. The influenza vaccine efficacy varies greatly depending on age and comorbidities. For otherwise healthy persons, the influenza vaccination affords approximately 60–90% protection. This decreases in individuals with immunosuppression and at extremes of age.

f. **Contraindications**:

    i. **IIV3 and IIV4**: Hypersensitivity to a previous dose or component or anaphylaxis to eggs is a contraindication. Of note, cell culture-based IIVs are not considered egg free since part of their process is in eggs and they contain a small amount of egg protein.

    ii. **RIV4**: Hypersensitivity to a previous dose or component is a contraindication.

    iii. **LAIV**: Contraindicated in immunocompromised patients. Hypersensitivity to a previous dose or component or anaphylaxis to eggs is a contraindication.

g. **Precautions**:

    i. **IIV and LAIV**: Risks should be weighted before vaccination of a person who developed Guillain–Barré syndrome (GBS) within 6 weeks of previous influenza vaccination. Persons with a history of only hives with eggs can receive the inactivated injectable vaccine, but should be observed for 30 minutes for a potential reaction.

    ii. **LAIV**: Anti-influenza antivirals (e.g., amantadine, rimantadine, zanamivir, or oseltamivir) should be avoided for 48 hours before vaccination and for 14 days after vaccination.

h. **Minimum time to effectiveness**: 2 weeks.

i. **Adverse effects**:

    i. **IIV3 and IIV4**: Mild adverse effects include injection site local pain, fever, and headaches. More serious adverse effects include seizures, especially in children who may have also received pneumococcal vaccine (PCV13) at the same time. Rare risk of GBS.

    ii. **LAIV**: Mild symptoms such as runny nose or nasal congestion, sore throat, cough, chills, tiredness/weakness, and headache can occur after nasal vaccine.

j. **Storage**: The inactivated injectable and LAIV vaccines should be stored in a refrigerator at 2–8 °C (35–46 °F). The vaccine should not be frozen. IIV that has been frozen should be discarded.

16 Tick-borne encephalitis (TBE):

a. **Epidemiology**: Tick-transmitted viral encephalitis is prevalent in the wooded parts of Europe, the Russian Federation, northern Japan, and north-eastern China. Risk to the average traveler is minimal. Risk increases with significant outdoor exposure, especially in wooded areas.

b. **Indications**: Persons expecting extensive outdoor exposure during spring or summer in the geographic locations mentioned above. The traveler may need to receive the vaccine in the country of travel owing to limited availability of the vaccine outside risk areas. Generally, this vaccine is not needed for the average traveler. Insect precautions are advised.

c. **Type of vaccine**: Inactivated envelope glycoprotein vaccine from virus grown in chick embryo cell cultures.

d. **Administration**: Vaccine is not available in the United States. Where available, the three-dose vaccine series is given on a schedule of 0, 1–3, and 5–12 months

e. **Efficacy and need for boosters**: Vaccine efficacy is 99% after three doses. Boosters are recommended every 3 years if there is continued risk of exposure.

f. **Contraindications**: Hypersensitivity to a previous dose, vaccine components, or eggs.

g. **Precautions**: Pregnancy and lactation are precautions.

h. **Minimum time to effectiveness**: Within 1 week after the second dose. An accelerated schedule can be accomplished by giving the second dose 2 weeks after the first and the third dose can be given 5–12 months after the second dose.

i. **Adverse effects**: Apart from local injection site adverse effects, patients can develop fevers.

j. **Storage**: TBE vaccine should be stored in a refrigerator at 2–8 °C (35–46 °F). The vaccine should not be frozen. IIV that has been frozen should be discarded.

17 **Typhoid fever caused by *Salmonella enterica* subspecies *typhi***:

a. **Epidemiology**: Typhoid is acquired by consuming contaminated food or water. It is more common in developing countries, especially in south central and southeast Asia. The risk of acquisition is highest from the Indian subcontinent.

b. **Indications**: All travelers to developing countries with higher risk for typhoid.

c. **Type of vaccine**: There are two types of vaccines available: an inactivated injectable and a live attenuated oral bacterial vaccine.

d. **Administration**:

   i. **Oral vaccine**: The oral typhoid comprises of three (Australia and Europe) or four (North America) capsules, taken every other day on an empty stomach.

   ii. **Injectable vaccine**: Intramuscular injection given in the deltoid.

e. **Efficacy and need for boosters**:

   i. **Oral vaccine**: The oral vaccine provides immunogenicity of approximately 70%. Duration of efficacy of the oral typhoid vaccine is 5 years for the four-dose formulation and 3 years for the three-dose formulation.

   ii. **Injectable vaccine**: The injectable vaccine has an efficacy of 60–70% and lasts for 2 years.

f. **Contraindications**:

   i. **Oral vaccine**: The oral live attenuated vaccine is contraindicated in immunocompromised hosts and pregnant women. Hypersensitivity to a previous dose or component.

   ii. **Injectable vaccine**: Hypersensitivity to a previous dose or component. Pregnancy.

g. **Precautions**: The oral typhoid vaccine should be separated by 8 hours from oral cholera vaccine.

h. **Minimum time to effectiveness**: 2 weeks for both vaccines.

   i. **Adverse effects**: Overall both are extremely safe. Fever can occur with either. Rarely, stomach pain, nausea, vomiting, and rash can occur with the oral typhoid.

   j. **Storage**: Both vaccines should be stored in a refrigerator at 2–8 °C (35–46 °F). The vaccine should not be frozen.

18 Varicella:

   a. **Epidemiology**: Chickenpox is prevalent worldwide. In developing countries, the prevalence is higher among older children and adults, unlike in developed countries, where it is mostly seen in children.

   b. **Indications**: All non-immune persons should be vaccinated irrespective of travel.

   c. **Type of vaccine**: Live attenuated viral vaccine.

   d. **Administration**: The two-dose varicella vaccine series given 4 weeks apart.

   e. **Efficacy and need for boosters**: The efficacy of the two-dose primary varicella vaccination series is 98%. No indication for boosters.

   f. **Contraindications**: Pregnancy and immunocompromised status are contraindications. Hypersensitivity to a previous dose or component.

   g. **Precautions**: Recent receipt of antibody-containing blood product may preclude vaccination (the duration of delay depends on the specific type and dose of immunoglobulin received). Anti-varicella antivirals (e.g., acyclovir, famciclovir, or valacyclovir) should be withheld for 24 hours before vaccination and for 14 days after vaccination.

   h. **Minimum time to effectiveness**: 4 weeks.

   i. **Adverse effects**: Fever can occur. Rare reactions include rash, seizures, or pneumonia.

   j. **Storage**: Vaccine should be stored frozen at an average temperature of –15 °C (5 °F) or colder.

19 Yellow fever vaccine: See Chapter 8.

20 Zoster vaccine:

   a. **Epidemiology**: Reactivation of the varicella virus can cause dermatomal or disseminated zoster. The risk of reactivation is highest among elderly and immunocompromised patients. Risk is not related to travel but reactivation could occur during a trip.

   b. **Indications**: Immunocompetent persons over 60 years of age or those between 50 and 60 years old if impending commencement of immunosuppressive medications.

   c. **Type of vaccine**: Live attenuated viral vaccine.

   d. **Administration**: Single herpes zoster intramuscular injection.

   e. **Efficacy and need for boosters**: Zoster vaccine protects approximately 50% of patients from developing dermatomal zoster when they received the vaccine at age 60 years. For those who develop dermatomal zoster, the symptoms are less severe and last a shorter duration. The vaccine is 66.5% efficacious in preventing post-herpetic neuralgia. The protective efficacy of the vaccine decreases when received later in life.

   f. **Contraindications**: Immunocompromised status and pregnancy are contraindications.

g. **Precautions**: Recent receipt of antibody-containing blood product may preclude vaccination (the duration of delay depends on the specific type and dose
of immunoglobulin received). Anti-varicella antivirals (e.g., acyclovir, famciclovir, or valacyclovir) should be withheld for 24 hours before vaccination and
for 14 days after vaccination.

h. **Minimum time to effectiveness**: 2 weeks.

i. **Adverse effects**: Local injection site viral eruption (rare). Headache can
occur rarely.

j. **Storage**: Vaccine should be stored frozen at an average temperature of $-15\,^\circ$C
($5\,^\circ$F) or colder [23–36].

References

1 Plotkin SA. Correlates of protection induced by vaccination. *Clin Vaccine Immunol* 2010; **17**:
   1055–1065.
2 Hangartner L, Zinkernagel RM, Hengartner H. Antiviral antibody responses: the two
   extremes of a wide spectrum. *Nat Rev Immunol* 2006; **6**: 231–243.
3 Baumgarth N. How specific is too specific? B-cell responses to viral infections reveal the
   importance of breadth over depth. *Immunol Rev* 2013; **255**: 82–94.
4 Castellino F, Galli G, Del Giudice G, Rappuoli R. Generating memory with vaccination. *Eur
   J Immunol* 2009; **39**: 2100–2105.
5 Pulendran B, Oh JZ, Nakaya HI, et al. Immunity to viruses: learning from successful human
   vaccines. *Immunol Rev* 2013; **255**: 243–255.
6 Sant AJ, McMichael A. Revealing the role of CD4$^+$ T cells in viral immunity. *J Exp Med* 2012;
   209: 1391–1395.
7 Lee CJ, Lee LH, Lu CS, Wu A. Bacterial polysaccharides as vaccines – immunity and chemical
   characterization. *Adv Exp Med Biol* 2001; **491**: 453–471.
8 Weintraub A. Immunology of bacterial polysaccharide antigens. *Carbohydr Res* 2003; **338**:
   2539–2547.
9 Papaevangelou V, Spyridis N. MenACWY-TT vaccine for active immunization against invasive meningococcal disease. *Expert Rev Vaccines* 2012; **11**: 523–537.
10 Gruber WC, Scott DA, Emini EA. Development and clinical evaluation of Prevnar 13, a
   13-valent pneumococococcal CRM197 conjugate vaccine. *Ann N Y Acad Sci* 2012; **1263**: 15–26.
11 Hanekom WA. The immune response to BCG vaccination of newborns. *Ann N Y Acad Sci*
   2005; **1062**: 69–78.
12 Graham BS. Advances in antiviral vaccine development. *Immunol Rev* 2013; **255**: 230–242.
13 Aoshi T, Koyama S, Kobiyama K, et al. Innate and adaptive immune responses to viral
   infection and vaccination. *Curr Opin Virol* 2011; **1**: 226–232.
14 Coffman RL, Sher A, Seder RA. Vaccine adjuvants: putting innate immunity to work. *Immunity* 2010; **33**: 492–503.
15 Lambrecht BN, Kool M, Willart MA, Hammad H. Mechanism of action of clinically approved
   adjuvants. *Curr Opin Immunol* 2009; **21**: 23–29.
16 Mbow ML, De Gregorio E, Valiante NM, Rappuoli R. New adjuvants for human vaccines.
   Curr Opin Immunol 2010; **22**: 411–416.
17 Brown LE, Jackson DC. Lipid-based self-adjuvanting vaccines. *Curr Drug Deliv* 2005; **2**:
   383–393.
18 World Health Organization. *Immunization Training Resources.* http://www.who.int/
   immunization/documents/MLM_module1.pdf?ua=1 (accessed 1 June 2014).

19 EMC: Electronic Medicines Compendium. *Summary of Product Characteristics.* https://www. medicines.org.uk/emc/ (accessed 1 June 2014).

20 Public Health England. *Immunisation Training Resources for Healthcare Professionals.* http://www.hpa.org.uk/EventsProfessionalTraining/HealthProtectionAcademy/Additional OpportunitiesAndInformation/ImmunisationTrainingResources/ (accessed 1 June 2014).

21 Chiodini J, Cotton C, Genasi F, et al. *UK Guidance on Best Practice in Vaccine Administration.* London: Shire Hall Communications, 2001.

22 Zuckerman JN. The importance of injecting vaccine into muscle. *BMJ* 2001 **322**, 364.

23 World Health Organization. *International Travel and Health* 2014. http://www.who.int/ith/en/ (accessed 1 June 2014).

24 Public Health England. *Immunisation Against Infectious Disease – The Green Book.* https://www. gov.uk/government/collections/immunisation-against-infectious-disease-the-green-book (accessed 1 June 2014).

25 Brunette G (ed.) *CDC Health Information for International Travel 2014*: *The Yellow Book.* New York: Oxford University Press, 2014. http://wwwnc.cdc.gov/travel/page/yellowbook-home -2014 (accessed 1 June 2014).

26 Australian Government Department of Health. *The Australian Immunisation Handbook,* 10th edn., 2013. http://www.immunise.health.gov.au/internet/immunise/publishing.nsf/ Content/Handbook10-home (accessed 1 June 2014).

27 New Zealand Ministry of Health. *New Zealand Immunisation Handbook* 2014. http://www. health.govt.nz/publication/immunisation-handbook-2014 (accessed 1 June 2014).

28 Public Health Agency of Canada. *Canadian Immunization Guide.* http://www.phac-aspc.gc.ca/ publicat/cig-gci/index-eng.php (accessed 1 June 2014).

29 Centers for Disease Control and Prevention. *Morbidity and Mortality Weekly Report (MMWR).* www.cdc.gov/mmwr (accessed 1 June 2014).

30 World Health Organization. *Weekly Epidemiological Record (WHR).* www.who.int/wer/ (accessed 1 June 2014).

31 Centers for Disease Control and Prevention. *Travelers' Health.* http://wwwnc.cdc.gov/travel/. (accessed 1 June 2014).

32 World Health Organization. *Global Alert and Response (GAR).* http://www.who.int/csr/en/ (accessed 1 June 2014).

33 Plotkin SA, Orenstein WA, Offit PA (eds.) *Vaccines,* 6th edn. Philadelphia, PA: WB Saunders, 2013.

34 Zuckerman JN, Jong EC. *Travelers' Vaccines,* 2nd edn. Shelton, CT: People's Medical Publishing House – USA, 2010.

35 Keystone JS, Freedman DO, Kozarsky P, et al. (eds.) *Travel Medicine,* 3rd edn. Philadelphia, PA: Saunders Elsevier, 2013.

36 Zuckerman JN (ed.) *Principles and Practice of Travel Medicine,* 2nd edn. Oxford: Wiley-Blackwell, 2013.

Travelers with underlying medical problems and special needs

CHAPTER 15

Women's health and travel

I. Dale Carroll

The Pregnant Traveler, Spring Lake, MI, USA

Introduction

This chapter gives an overview regarding women who are traveling. More detailed information can be found in reference textbooks in travel medicine and journal articles [1–4].

Pre-travel counseling

Pre-travel counseling for individual women will vary according to their life stage and lifestyle.

The effects of travel may cause menses to cease or become irregular and more symptomatic. Instruction can be given regarding amenorrhea, abnormal uterine bleeding, voluntary delay of menses, and needed supplies. Urinary tract infections are common during travel. Patients should be taught to recognize the symptoms and adopt preventive measures. Similar instructions are needed regarding vaginitis. Safe sex and the recognition of symptoms of sexually transmitted disease should also be discussed.

Advice should include recommendations for both routine and emergency contraception.. Nausea, vomiting, or diarrhea may decrease absorption of oral contraceptives. The risk of venous thromboembolism increases slightly while using oral contraceptives and significantly with pregnancy. Details of appropriate medical kits for both pregnant and non-pregnant women can be found in the literature [1–4].

Long-term travelers and expatriates should have a general health screening prior to travel, including Pap smear and mammogram. Psychologic issues should also be discussed. It is also important to consider the roles of women and men at the traveler's destination.

Essential Travel Medicine, First Edition.
Edited by Jane N. Zuckerman, Gary W. Brunette and Peter A. Leggat.
© 2015 John Wiley & Sons, Ltd. Published 2015 by John Wiley & Sons, Ltd.

Pregnancy

General considerations

Although pregnancy is a normal condition, it produces an altered state of health and requires special consideration. An early ultrasound will help to establish gestational age and identify potential problems. Laboratory data and the medical and obstetric history should be reviewed carefully. The patient should carry a copy of her prenatal record and her physician's contact information.

For the patient's comfort, attention should be paid to airline seating, hotel accommodations, and the intensity of the itinerary. A traveling companion is also recommended. Preparation includes education regarding minor pregnancy discomforts and the early recognition of complications. Finally, one should consider the psychologic impact of a pregnancy complication or loss during the trip.

Complications

Some pregnancy complications may be managed adequately to allow safe travel, particularly when there is advanced obstetric care available at the destination. Bleeding less than a menstrual flow is usually harmless. Rh immunoglobulin, if needed, may not be available in many areas. Premature labor and premature rupture of the fetal membranes are two conditions that require prompt medical attention. Travel would be contraindicated, however, when events could occur in transit that would threaten the lives of both mother and infant, such as major bleeding, active labor, or an ectopic pregnancy. In such cases, it is preferable to bring appropriate help to the patient. Arrangements should be made prior to travel for obstetric care at the destination. Insurance policies must be reviewed to make sure that they cover pregnancy and care of the neonate.

Transportation and environmental risks

Most travel risks exposure to infectious disease. One must also prepare for common discomforts such as edema and abdominal distension. Venous thrombosis prevention includes oral hydration, avoiding immobility, and wearing compression stockings [5].

Airlines restrict travel beyond 32–36 weeks' gestation and cruise lines beyond 28 weeks' gestation. Airport security machines are not considered to be harmful to the fetus. Vehicular accidents with blunt trauma are a common cause of maternal and fetal morbidity. The main health risk associated with sea voyages is the exacerbation of the nausea and vomiting associated with pregnancy. Falls due to movement of the vessel are another.

Air pollution, heat, and humidity may be particularly problematic during pregnancy.

Short exposure to moderate altitudes appears to have no adverse effects on the woman or the fetus, but the pregnant traveler at altitude may experience exaggerated breathlessness and palpitations. Acetazolamide is best avoided. The greatest concern in such travel is the remoteness from medical care.

The pregnant traveler should be discouraged from undertaking unaccustomed vigorous physical activity. Swimming and snorkeling are generally safe, but water-skiing and scuba diving are ill-advised.

Trauma is both more likely and more difficult to triage and treat during pregnancy. In fact, treatment delay in pregnant women has been shown to increase the risk of fetal and maternal death [6].

Infectious diseases

Travelers' diarrhea is more frequent and apt to be more severe in pregnancy, with complications such as dehydration, ketosis, and acidemia. Vigorous oral hydration is the treatment of choice. Loperamide might be considered in severe cases, but bismuth salicylate is contraindicated. Antibiotic use will depend on the severity of disease.

Influenza and pneumococcal vaccines might be regarded as "pre-travel" vaccines. Nasal decongestants should be used sparingly.

Hepatitis A has been reported to increase the risk of placental abruption and premature delivery. Hepatitis E is also a major threat during pregnancy and maternal hepatitis B presents the risk of transmission to the neonate.

Listeria and toxoplasmosis, commonly found in cheeses and meat, may result in abortion or stillbirth. Intestinal helminths rarely warrant treatment during pregnancy but infections from those such as giardia, ameba and cryptosporidia often do.

Female genital schistosomiasis may cause infertility and also facilitate the spread of sexually transmitted disease. Women who are pregnant or postpartum also have an increased risk for severe disease and death from amebiasis. In the case of leishmaniasis, pregnancy seems to reactivate even latent disease and worsen its course, and transplacental infection has been reported.

Malaria and pregnancy

Not only are pregnant women more apt to get malaria, but also the severity of the disease may be much greater than when non-pregnant. It will often be complicated by heavy parasitemia, severe anemia, and profound hypoglycemia, progressing to cerebral malaria and pulmonary edema. Sequestration of parasites in the placenta often results in fetal loss due to abruption, premature labor, and miscarriage. The infant is apt to be of low birth weight and suffer from dehydration, seizures, thrombocytopenia, and splenic rupture [7].

The pregnant traveler should, if possible, avoid travel to *Plasmodium falciparum* -endemic areas. Otherwise she should use all available protective measures, including insecticides and insect repellents.

None of the currently used antimalarials other than tetracycline have any demonstrated teratogenic effect [8]. Primaquine use is not recommended in pregnancy because of the inability to test the infant for G6PD deficiency. Mefloquine, chloroquine–proguanil, pyrimethamine–sulfadoxine, and atovaquone–proguanil have not shown any increase in adverse pregnancy outcomes when used in the first trimester of pregnancy. For prophylaxis, which medication to use should be determined by resistance patterns. A safe but ineffective medication will be worse than no medication at all.

Vaccines

There is reason for caution in the use of vaccines yet it should be remembered that none of the currently available vaccines are known to harm the fetus whereas many of the diseases they prevent are clearly harmful [9]. There has also been recent emphasis on encouraging maternal immunization to protect the newborn against certain childhood diseases. In general, live vaccines should be used during pregnancy only if the risk of exposure to a vaccine-preventable disease outweighs a possible theoretical risk of the vaccine.

Sometimes, the need for the vaccine may be obviated simply by a modification of the itinerary, or, if the vaccine is recommended simply due to local regulations, the patient may be given a waiver. Because pregnancy is a relatively immune-suppressed state, there is concern that vaccination may not produce an adequate immune response. In addition, pregnancy slows intestinal transit and may increase the risk of gastrointestinal adverse events from live bacterial vaccines such as cholera and typhoid.

Medications

It is recommended that practitioners advising pregnant women should use relevant print or web-based references rather than drug classification systems [10,11]. As with vaccination, the use of medications in pregnancy requires consideration of both safety and efficacy. Because of the physiologic changes in pregnancy, many medications are absorbed, distributed, and metabolized differently during pregnancy. Travel-related drugs may also interact with other commonly used medicines, and side-effects may become more pronounced. In addition, most drugs transfer across the placenta and drug transfer increases with gestation.

There are several simple remedies that often are effective in relieving the symptoms of morning sickness and these same remedies may help to prevent motion sickness. Antihistamines such as meclizine and dimenhydrinate appear to have a good safety record and scopolamine has also been used safely in pregnancy, but near term it may cause fetal heart rate abnormalities.

Pregnant women should avoid the use of highly concentrated DEET-containing repellents [12]. Animal studies of the newer agent icaridin have shown no adverse reproductive effects even at toxic levels.

Permethrin is not so much a repellent as a topical insecticide. There are no reports of harm from this agent in human pregnancies.

Breastfeeding while traveling

There are many factors that affect drug transfer into breast milk, such as molecular weight, lipid solubility, and protein binding. Once a drug is in the breast milk, its effect on the infant will be further modulated by the frequency and volume of breastfeeding, bioavailability from the infant's intestine, and a host of other factors. In general, however, it appears that few commonly used medications would pass to the infant in sufficient amount to be either harmful or helpful and the infant will need to be treated medically as a separate patient.

Unlike pregnancy, breastfeeding is not an immune-modulated state, hence there is little reason to expect any alteration in the efficacy of the vaccine in the mother. Whether the antibodies thus produced with be protective to the breastfed infant or, on the other hand, interfere with subsequent immunization of the child will vary depending on the vaccine. Care should be exercised, however, when giving yellow fever vaccine in the first weeks after delivery as encephalitis has been reported in newborns to breastfeeding mothers.

The patient, meanwhile, may be more concerned with the practical and cultural issues involved such as privacy, breast pumping, and milk storage.

It is wise to emphasize the importance of adequate hydration, especially if the patient travels to high altitude or suffers from diarrhea. Cleanliness of the hands, breasts, and all equipment is essential to prevent either mastitis or infant diarrhea. Even the avoidance of mosquito bites when getting up at night to feed may need to be emphasized. As for cultural differences and norms, it may be encouraging to the patient to realize that she may, by successful breastfeeding, serve as a good role model in areas of the world where the practice is being largely abandoned to the detriment of infants.

Conclusion

Travel medicine advisors should be able to address the key travel health issues for women across the life span during the pre-travel assessment. Pre-travel advice should include information on contraception, emergency contraception and prevention of sexually transmitted disease. The woman traveler's itinerary should be carefully evaluated for exposure to any travel or tropical disease that might have long-term consequences.

References

1 Zuckerman J (ed.) Principles and Practice of Travel Medicine, 2nd edn. Oxford: Wiley-Blackwell, 2013.
2 Keystone JS, Freedman DO, Kozarsky PE, et al. (eds.) *Travel Medicine*, 3rd edn. Amsterdam: Elsevier; 2012.
3 Brunette G (ed.) *CDC Health Information for International Travel 2014: The Yellow Book*. New York: Oxford University Press, 2014.
4 Carroll ID, Williams DC. Pre-travel vaccination and medical prophylaxis in the pregnant traveler. *Travel Med Infect Dis* 2008; **6**: 259–275.
5 American College of Obstetricians and Gynecologists. Air travel during pregnancy. ACOG Committee Opinion No. 443. *Obstet Gynecol* 2009; **114**: 954–955.
6 Henderson SO, Mallon WK. Trauma in pregnancy. *Emerg Med Clin North Am* 1998; **16**: 209–228.
7 Desai M, ter Kuile FO, Nosten F, et al. Epidemiology and burden of malaria in pregnancy. *Lancet Infect Dis* 2007; **7**: 93–104.
8 Phillips-Howard PA, Wood D. The safety of antimalarial drugs in pregnancy. *Drug Saf* 1996; **14**: 131–145.

9 American College of Obstetricians and Gynecologists. Immunization During Pregnancy. ACOG Committee Opinion No. 282. *Obstet Gynecol* 2003; **101**: 207–212.

10 Briggs GG, Freeman RK, Yaffe SJ. *Drugs in Pregnancy and Lactation*, 9th edn. Philadelphia, PA: Lippincott Williams & Wilkins, 2012.

11 Reproductive Toxicology Center. *Reprotox*. www.reprotox.org (accessed 1 February 2015).

12 McGready R, Hamilton KA, Simpson JA, et al. Safety of the insect repellent *N,N*-diethyl-*m*-toluamide (DEET) in pregnancy. *Am J Trop Med Hyg* 2001; **65**: 285–289.

CHAPTER 16

Traveling with children

Karl Neumann[1], Andrea P. Summer[2], & Philip R. Fischer[3]

[1] *Weill Medical College of Cornell University, USA*
[2] *Medical University of South Carolina, Charleston, SC, USA*
[3] *Mayo Clinic, Rochester, MN, USA*

Introduction

The ease, speed, and comfort of modern travel enable parents to take ever younger children to ever more exotic destinations. And most parents, by good fortune or good judgment, rarely choose destinations that lie beyond the boundaries of acceptable risk. Although no statistics exist, a recent survey of members of the International Society of Travel Medicine and other surveys of and by travel medicine practitioners show that children "surprisingly" rarely experience serious illnesses or accidents while traveling. Moreover, traveling locally or staying home is not risk free, either.

Family travel is never all fun and games, but for the most part it is a positive experience for all. Most children are great travelers. They are inquisitive and, when motivated, adaptable and inexhaustible. Whether a weekend camping trip at a nearby State park, a week in Paris or the Caribbean, or a safari in Africa, travel provides children with knowledge and experiences that enrich their education, build their self-confidence, promote family cohesiveness, and create memories for tomorrow. The question often arises of whether young children who will not remember trips also benefit from travel – or are just backpacks. Likely, travel is a positive experience for very young children and years later they will enjoy seeing pictures of themselves as part of the family in fun situations, sometimes in faraway places, or perhaps on the lap of a grandparent that they never meet again.

Closely linked with the growth in family travel is a huge increase in helpful, up-to-the-minute, easily accessible information on keeping children healthy and safe for travel. Planning to do so parallels keeping them healthy at home. An upcoming trip presents parents with an opportune time to review their preparedness to deal with children when they become ill, at home or away.

For example, are children's immunizations up-to-date – and will they need additional immunizations for the trip? Do family health/accident insurance policies need adjusting as children grow older, and do the policies cover the family away from home? Is the list of all of the children's health providers current, and are the names in the parent's cell phone? Whenever, and wherever, children become ill, if possible the family health providers should be consulted first.

Essential Travel Medicine, First Edition.
Edited by Jane N. Zuckerman, Gary W. Brunette and Peter A. Leggat.
© 2015 John Wiley & Sons, Ltd. Published 2015 by John Wiley & Sons, Ltd.

Parents should also check their children's medications on hand. These medications should be the basis of a traveling medical kit. Are they outdated? Most illnesses that children acquire when traveling are illnesses that they experience at home – stomach upsets, respiratory infections, and allergies, for example. Carrying medications from home avoids the hassle of buying items with unfamiliar names and doses and, in some developing countries, avoiding items that may be outdated, counterfeited, or improperly stored. The kit should also contain items specific for the trip (antimalarials, for example) and precise instructions on how to administer the medications – including if the child vomits the dose.

Family travel is such an integral part of family life that it should be discussed at all healthcare visits. At sick visits, parents should be asked about recent travel, and at well checkups, about upcoming travel plans. Parents need to be reminded to plan accordingly and to visit travel healthcare professionals, if indicated. Common scenarios calling for such visits include:

- Air travel for infants less than 1 year old who experienced serious perinatal cardiopulmonary events or who were born significantly premature. Such children, even when asymptomatic at home, may have large decreases in their arterial blood oxygen levels at cruising altitudes.
- Ongoing illnesses that may be affected by travel and/or may need prompt treatment (seizure disorders, diabetes, and severe asthma, for example).
- Children going to destinations that require travel-related immunizations, preventive medications, or specific advice regarding poor sanitation, altitude, or insect bite prevention.
- Children returning home with illnesses that primary healthcare providers cannot easily identify.

Pre-trip preparation for traveling children and adolescents

Preventing injury and illness

Appropriate pre-trip preparation can help ensure that young travelers avoid injury and illness while successfully enjoying [1] a wealth of life-enhancing opportunities. Travel health-trained professionals can help insure that their pediatric travelers (1) avoid injury, (2) prevent insect-borne infections, (3) decrease the risk of diarrhea and appropriately manage diarrheal illness when it occurs, and (4) receive immunizations as appropriate to both the traveler and the travel plan [2,3].

Although *all* traveling children should benefit from good pre-travel input, a currently under-met need is for care for children and adolescents traveling to visit friends and relatives (VFR) [4]. The itineraries and healthcare habits of these VFR families leave these children at increased risk of health problems during travel [4,5]. Efforts should continue to ensure that VFR travelers receive good pre-travel care [4,6].

Avoiding injury

Although most travel-associated injuries are not intentional, they are usually the result of missed opportunities for preventive interventions. From the superficial photo-trauma of sunburn to life-threatening motor vehicle accidents, most injuries can be avoided. The most common serious pediatric injuries in travelers are road traffic accidents and drownings [7].

Sunburn

Sunburn is common in traveling children, especially those traveling from cooler northern climates to sunny equatorial regions. In fact, 19% of traveling Dutch children developed significant sunburn [8]. Sadly, blistering sunburn during childhood is a major risk factor for cutaneous malignancy later in life [9]. Outdoor activities around reflective surfaces such as water and snow are particularly risky. Protective clothing and hats may be worn for some outdoor activities, and sunscreen should be applied prior to anticipated sun exposures. Sunscreen with a sun protection factor (SPF) of 30 blocks 96% of potentially damaging rays and can be reapplied after water exposure or heavy sweating; routine reapplication is not otherwise needed [10].

Road traffic accidents

Life-threatening injuries are uncommon among travelers, but motor vehicle accidents account for the majority of deaths in young travelers [11]. Careful attention to travel arrangements can help reduce the risk of crashes and mitigate the extent of injury in the event of a crash. In a study of British volunteers overseas that included adolescent students with a mean duration of service of approximately 1 year, 12% reported being involved in a motor vehicle accident [12]. Related to their small size and reduced visibility, children are at particular risk of pedestrian injuries. Related to the relative contribution of the heads of young children to their total weight, unrestrained young children are also at particular risk of serious injury when propelled within a suddenly stopped vehicle.

Therefore, young children should be well supervised when near roads, and all travelers should be well trained to "look both ways" before stepping into a street. (Looking both ways would have prevented Winston Churchill from a scalp laceration and broken ribs during a 1930s visit to New York. Less worldly-wise children should be especially careful around moving traffic.) This is particularly important when visiting an area where vehicles travel on the "other" side of the road to that in one's home country [13].

All car passengers should be appropriately restrained so as not to be propelled against a hard surface during a sudden stop or crash [14]. For children, back seats are less dangerous than front seats. Rear-facing safety seats are most useful during the first year of life. Forward-facing seats can be used for children from 1 to 5 years of age (when neck control has matured). Booster seats and seat belts can be used after the beginning of the school-age years [14]. Of course, itineraries should be planned with a restrained child in mind! Adequate stops and breaks should be provided to allow all passengers to move around and refresh themselves. As for adult travelers, drivers should be well prepared to drive safely, and night travel in risky areas should be avoided.

Water safety

Drowning is the second highest cause of death in travelers (after motor vehicle accidents) [7]. Approximately eight British children drown in other countries each year (compared with one each year in British municipal pools), with most overseas drownings occurring in hotel pools [15]. Adequate training and, especially, supervision are necessary for children around water. Adolescent travelers will be more independent with less adult supervision and should be counseled about the dangerous risks of combining alcohol ingestion with boating and other aquatic activities.

Safe lodging

Falls and electrical injuries can occur most anywhere in the world. Traveling children are likely at particular risk owing to their curiosity about unfamiliar objects and settings. Adults should "child-proof" new settings to ensure that stairs and balconies and electrical outlets are either safe or out of reach of young children. Children are less intimidating to animals, whether those animals are rabid or not, and should avoid close contact with animals that could bite (whether cute "pets" along streets or interesting monkeys in game reserves).

Adolescents and risk-taking behaviors

Travel affords exposure to new ways of life and to new experiences. However, new-found adolescent "freedom" when mixed with alcohol, drugs, and/or sex (or even non-sterile tattoo ink) can have devastating life-altering consequences for traveling adolescents [16]. Transmissible germs remind us that "what happens in Vegas" does not always "stay in Vegas." And sometimes, "when in Rome," adolescents should *not* try to "do as the Romans."

A pre-travel consultation affords traveling adolescents (and even their parents) the opportunity to gain information about the risks of ingested substances and body fluid exposures. Hearing about the risks of non-sterile body piercing and tattooing [17] might alter subsequent exposure decisions. Raising discussions and fostering risk-decreasing peer pressure can reduce the risk of some dangerous behaviors [18]. Families and group leaders can also suggest or even impose some safe habits, such as the use of seat belts in cars and helmets when on two-wheeled vehicles.

Ready for contingencies

Families traveling with children should carry copies of travel documents to facilitate replacement in the event that original documents are lost or stolen. They should take along medical information (a clear listing of current medications and doses, allergies, and immunizations). Medications (and supplies such as needles and syringes, for patients with some chronic medical conditions) should be safely stored for use during travel. Also, awareness of pediatric care facilities along the route can be helpful should such information become needed.

Preventing insect-borne infections

Awareness of specific details of risk for insect-borne diseases can help target insect bite avoidance measures. For instance, West Nile virus is usually limited to summertime in the United States. Dengue-transmitting mosquitoes can bite indoors and outdoors but are most active during the daytime, whereas malaria-transmitting *Anopheles* bite more during evening and night hours [19]. Chikungunya virus has spread from the

Table 16.1 Malaria chemoprophylaxis for children.

Medication	Timing	Dosing	Comments
Chloroquine	Weekly 1 week pre- to 4 weeks post-exposure	5 mg/kg/dose (max. 250 mg)	
Mefloquine	Weekly 2 weeks pre- to 4 weeks post-exposure	5 mg/kg/dose (max. 250 mg)	Not if active seizures, dysrhythmia, psychiatric concerns; can crush pills, but unpleasant taste
Atovaquone/ proguanil	Daily 1 day pre- to 7 days post-exposure	¼ pill per 10 kg (max. 1 pill)	1 pill contains 250 mg atovaquone and 100 mg proguanil
Doxycycline	Daily 1 day pre- to 28 days post-exposure	2 mg/kg (max. 100 mg)	Not in young children (<8 years of age)

Indian Ocean to many parts of Asia. In fact, traveling children should avoid insect bites day and night, indoors and out, wherever they are traveling.

Once dried for a few hours, permethrin-impregnated clothes and bednets are safe for use in children. DEET (diethyl-*m*-toluamide) is safe at all ages, provided that ingestion and eye contact are avoided; young children should avoid DEET use around the eyes and on the hands. Picaridin is similarly safe at all ages.

Practically, however, not all insect bites can be avoided. Children traveling in malaria-endemic areas should use chemoprophylaxis; the same indications apply as for adults, and weight-based doses may be used.(Table 16.1). Doxycycline should be avoided in young children since it can lead to permanent staining of developing teeth; it is not a problem during and after the adolescent years.

Decreasing and managing diarrhea

Children are at greater risk of getting diarrhea than are their adult traveling companions [20], and about 30% of young travelers are affected [8]. The microbial epidemiology of travelers' diarrhea is similar to that seen in adults.

Prevention of travelers' diarrhea in children follows the same "recently well-cooked food, bottled or boiled drinks, clean hands" guidance as for adults. By their mobility and curiosity, however, children need specific attention to hand hygiene. In a variety of settings, access to and use of alcohol-based hand sanitizer can decrease the risk of infection in children.

Hydration is the key element of management of travelers' diarrhea when it happens in children. Any pure beverage is sufficient when the child is not dehydrated. If there are already hints of dehydration, such as dry eyes, dry mouth, or decreased urine output, however, an "oral rehydration solution" should be used. These solutions contain a small amount of sugar (to power the intestinal sodium channels to facilitate fluid and salt absorption while avoiding osmotic diarrhea) and generous quantities of salt. However, the "low osmolar" solutions are adequate for non-cholera diarrhea.

Table 16.2 Vaccines for traveling children and adolescents.

Illness/vaccine	Usual age	Comments
Hepatitis A	>1 year	6 months
Typhoid, Ty21a, oral	>6 years	
Typhoid, Vi, intramuscular	2 years	
Yellow fever	9 months	Encephalitis risk <4 months of age
Cholera	1 year?	Limited infant data
Escherichia coli	Infancy?	Limited pediatric data
Meningococcus	2 years	A component suitable for 3-month-old infants
		C component suitable for 2-year-old children
Japanese encephalitis	>1 year	12–36-month-old children: ½ adult dose
Rabies	Any age	Underused
Malaria		Pending

Antimotility agents are usually not needed in children (who are less compelled to follow formal schedules away from restrooms than are adults). Also, young children (especially before age 3 years) should avoid loperamide and other antimotility agents since they are at risk of adverse side-effects [21].

Presumptive use of an antibiotic for a traveling child with diarrhea follows the same principles as for adults. Azithromycin (10 mg/kg once daily for up to 3 days) is effective against main pathogens, including some of the quinolone-resistant *Campylobacter*. Quinolones such as levofloxacin may be used, but they carry some risk of adverse effects on connective tissues.

Obtaining appropriate vaccinations

Vaccine-preventable illnesses continue to cause significant morbidity and mortality in children. Although deaths due to infection are rare in pediatric travelers, those that occur would still have been largely avoidable. Details of vaccines [22] specific for traveling children are summarized in Table 16.2.

"Routine" immunization schedules vary between countries due to variations in disease epidemiology and to practical feasibilities of vaccination programs. A pre-travel consultation provides an excellent opportunity to ensure that traveling children are up-to-date with their "routine" vaccines. This is a particular issue for adolescent travelers who might have missed opportunities for new or newly recommended vaccines. Influenza vaccine should be provided to all children of at least 6 months of age who are traveling into an area around the time of seasonal outbreaks.

Hepatitis A poses a risk not only to the traveler but also to future contacts of that traveler. Thus, even though hepatitis A is often asymptomatic in young children, all international travelers over 1 year of age may be vaccinated for hepatitis A. The vaccine is safe in younger children and is often used down to 6 months of age even though there is a possibility that remaining transplacentally-acquired maternal antibodies might block vaccine effectiveness.

Typhoid fever is a risk in most "developing" countries. Vaccines are effective in older children, but no adequately safe and effective vaccine is currently available for use in the first two years of life. Families of young children will concentrate their typhoid prevention efforts on careful food, water, and hand hygiene measures.

Meningococcal disease is a risk in many parts of Africa and Asia. Vaccines are fairly effective even in young children. Children at least 9 months of age can benefit from meningococcal conjugate vaccine, and younger children can be helped by some of the monovalent meningococcal vaccines (when available).

The indications for yellow fever vaccine are the same for adults and children. However, there is a real risk of vaccine-induced yellow fever disease in young children, especially those 4 months of age or younger. Most specialists would defer travel for children less than 9 months of age or else depend on mosquito-avoidance measures. The yellow fever vaccine may be safely used after 9 months of age.

Children are at particular risk of animal bites. Rabies vaccine may be used at any age.

Relatively new Japanese encephalitis virus vaccines are safe and effective in children. Dosing details are noted in Table 16.2.

When additional protection is needed in young travelers who are not already up-to-date with their home country's routine vaccinations, "accelerated" schedules may be used. Table 16.2 provides some details about "early" initiation of vaccines and also about safe and effective "short" time periods between vaccine doses.

Advancing higher?

Of course, there are concerns for traveling children beyond safety, insects, diarrhea, and vaccines. Mostly, those concerns are managed as for adults. For instance, children traveling to high altitude seem to have the same risk of acute mountain sickness as do adults [23]. Preventive management involves slow ascent and, when desired, acetazolamide (2 mg/kg per dose up to 125 mg per dose, with timing as for adults).

Traveling children have life-enhancing experiences and exposures. Attention to these "basic" means of avoiding injury and illness and managing common conditions such as diarrhea can help ensure that health problems do not significantly negate the value of pediatric travel.

International adoption

Since 2004, there has been a steady decline in international adoptions. This reduction has primarily resulted from the implementation of tighter restrictions and more government oversight to battle corruption and child trafficking. Over the past several years, adoptions from Sub-Saharan Africa and especially Ethiopia have increased significantly. These children have often lost one or both parents to HIV/AIDS, tuberculosis, or malaria and are placed in orphanages when extended families are unable to assume their care.[24]. Regardless of country of origin, adopted children today have typically spent a portion if not all of their lives in institutionalized settings and have experienced varying degrees of environmental deprivation, malnutrition, and neglect [25–27]. Since the majority of adopted children were institutionalized in resource-poor and sometimes tropical countries, they are susceptible to a variety of infectious diseases and also extensive nutritional, growth, developmental, and behavioral issues [28–30]. Consequently, all internationally adopted children should be considered to have special medical and developmental–behavioral needs.

Pre-adoption

Physicians may become involved in the adoption process after families receive a referral, which contains information on a specific child for the family to consider for adoption. These prospective parents will often request a physician to review the information and give advice. The amount and quality of medical and family information documented in the referral can vary tremendously. Written medical reports are usually brief, except those from South Korea, which give detailed information that is usually accurate and current. Reports from Russia often contain frightening terms such as perinatal encephalopathy, hypertension–hydrocephalus syndrome, and infringement of cerebral circulation that suggest serious central nervous system pathology, but this is usually not confirmed when the child is evaluated post-adoption [28]. Ultrasound reports may also contain unusual terminology.

Birth countries usually provide photographs and sometimes videotapes of the child, which again may vary in content and quality. These tapes can help identify obvious medical or neurologic conditions [31] and, when they provide close-up views of the child's face, can be used to assess roughly for stigmata of fetal alcohol syndrome. Information on height, weight, and head circumference is almost always provided and can be very useful for tracking trends when multiple measurements are given. Laboratory information varies but usually includes results for HIV, hepatitis B and C, and syphilis screening. Additionally, a complete blood count and urinalysis are often included in records from China. Information on the child's development may be documented in the form of a checklist, but often the information is sparse or cryptic, making it difficult to interpret.

Ideally, pre-adoption medical evaluations should be performed by clinicians who have expertise in international adoption medicine. The clinician's role in this process is to provide a risk assessment based on the information provided and help the family anticipate the child's medical and developmental needs. The clinician should also prepare the family for the possibility of unsuspected infections or medical diagnoses that may not be included in the child's records [30].

Pre-adoption travel preparation of families and caregivers

Before parents travel to complete the adoption process and bring their child home, they should be encouraged to seek pre-travel consultation. The consultation should include the usual recommendations addressing all preventive measures, with a strong emphasis on routine and travel-specific vaccine preventable diseases. All caregivers and family members should be current on routine immunizations. Many adults have only received one dose of measles, mumps, rubella (MMR) vaccine and consequently should receive a booster dose, as several cases of measles have been confirmed in adoptees from China.[32]. Booster doses of tetanus, diphtheria, and acellular pertussis should also be provided to those who are not current.

Additionally, all caregivers and family members should receive both hepatitis A and B vaccines. Many countries in Asia and Africa have a higher prevalence of vertical transmission of hepatitis B, which may leave some children chronically infected. Recent prevalence of hepatitis B infection among adoptees has been found to be from 1–7% [28,33,34]. Since horizontal transmission can occur within households, family members and caregivers should be protected through vaccination [35,36]. Over the past several years, as more adoptions have taken place in Sub-Saharan Africa, acute infections with hepatitis A have led to multiple community outbreaks that have included contacts of the adoptee who have never traveled [37]. As a result, in 2009 the Advisory Committee on Immunization Practices recommended routine hepatitis A vaccination for family members and caregivers of children adopted from countries with intermediate or high hepatitis A endemicity [38].

Other vaccination recommendations for the traveling parents are country specific and must take into account the following factors: duration and season of travel, accommodations, anticipated contact with the local populace, and rural versus urban location. Many parents spend less than 2 weeks in the country finalizing the adoption, whereas others may be required to stay for several weeks.

Parents will undoubtedly have questions about the trip home with their new child. To facilitate travel, an umbrella stroller or front/back carrier back may be useful depending on the age of the child. Bulkhead seating and small age-appropriate toys to keep the child comfortable and entertained during the long trip home can also be helpful. In addition to a basic first aid kit, scabies and lice treatment is often prescribed. Motion sickness aids such as dimenhydrinate or diphenhydramine may also be recommended. Advice regarding proper use of rehydration solution for vomiting or diarrheal illness should be emphasized. Any questions regarding feeding practices and special formula recommendations for severely malnourished and neglected children should be referred to a provider knowledgeable in international adoption.

Post-adoption evaluation

All internationally adopted children undergo a medical evaluation in their country of origin just prior to departure. These examinations are usually cursory and the process is often focused more on legal requirements for the issue of an immigrant visa. Screening for tuberculosis with PPD (purified protein derivative) or QuantiFERON testing is an important component of this screening evaluation for children 2 years and older. After children have arrived home with their adoptive family, a comprehensive assessment is strongly recommended. The post-adoption evaluation is often performed in a multidisciplinary setting with medical and developmental–behavioral specialists included in the process. Assessing the child's nutritional status and testing for infectious screening are a major part of the medical evaluation, the details of which will be included here.

Growth

The effects of institutionalization on growth can be profound. The prevalence of underweight, short stature, and reduced head circumference is high among children who have spent time in institutionalized settings. The longer the period of institutionalization, the more severely growth appears to be affected [39–41]. Children living in abusive or neglectful environments have been shown to experience growth delay even when adequate caloric intake is provided [42]. Growth delay of this nature is termed psychosocial short stature or dwarfism.

An additional characteristic of children with psychosocial short stature is that once placed in a nurturing environment, they undergo notable improvement in growth velocity. Since the severity of growth delay tends to correlate with the duration of institutionalization, children adopted during infancy demonstrate better catch-up growth than children adopted at an older age [43]. Catch-up growth for head circumference is typically modest and incomplete, but in the majority of studies head circumference has only been assessed through 72 months of age [44–46].

In addition to growth delay, micronutrient deficiencies are also often identified in international adoptees. The most common deficiencies are iron and vitamin D [41,47]. Even rickets has been reported, although rarely [26].

Post-arrival screening for immigrants, refugees, and adoptees
Infectious diseases
Recommendations for infectious diseases screening for newly arriving children generally include tuberculosis, hepatitis B and C, HIV, syphilis, and intestinal parasites [48,49]. In addition, a malaria smear and also serologic testing for *Trypanosoma cruzi* and lymphatic filariasis should be considered in children from endemic countries. Testing for hepatitis A has more recently been emphasized in international adoptees owing to reports of hepatitis A infection among adoptees and their contacts, as mentioned previously [37,50]. If an acute hepatitis A infection is identified, all family members and close contacts, including babysitters, should be immunized if not done prior to adoption.

Stool examination for ova and parasites should be obtained. Multiple stool specimens increase the likelihood of pathogen identification and are recommended for high-risk individuals regardless of symptoms [51–53]. In addition, antigen-specific testing for *Giardia intestinalis* and *Cryptosporidium* species should be carried out on all adoptees.

Children who are found to have an eosinophilia (absolute eosinophil count >450 cells/mm^3) and negative stool specimens require additional evaluation. The first step is usually serologic testing for *Strongyloides* and *Toxocara*. Adoptees with eosinophilia from Sub-Saharan Africa, South-East Asia and certain parts of Latin America should also be screened for *Schistosoma* species. If serology for these pathogens is negative, further parasitic testing should be tailored to the country of origin. Additional causes of eosinophilia such as allergy, medications, and malignancy should be considered in those for whom no parasitic cause is identified.

Hematologic
A complete blood count with differential and red blood cell indices should be obtained. An elevated eosinophil count should increase suspicion for parasitic diseases. Serum iron studies may be indicated if a microcytic anemia is found. In addition, hemoglobin electrophoresis should be carried out if thalassemia or sickle cell disease is suspected. Finally, glucose-6-phosphate dehydrogenase (G6PD)

deficiency screening is frequently obtained on children from the Mediterranean, Asia, and Africa.

Biochemistry

A urinalysis should be considered for children from areas endemic for urinary schisto-somiasis and also for any children with suspected renal disease. Thyroid function tests are often obtained for children with poor growth. Liver enzymes should be obtained on children with jaundice or concerns for systemic illness. Lead levels are gener-ally recommended for immigrant children and especially refugees due to a higher probability of lead exposure in less developed countries [54,55].

Immunizations

Immunizations should be administered according to local recommendations. Records of immunizations from the child's country of origin may be accepted if the month, day, and year are documented for each vaccine and the spacing between vaccines is concordant with the schedule for the country of resettlement. International adoptees are an exception, because data suggest that immunization records for children who have resided in orphanages are not predictive of protective immunity [56,57]. There are two approaches to immunizations for international adoptees: (1) re-immunize completely or (2) obtain titers for documented vaccines and repeat any immunizations for titers that are not protective. Many immigrant children will not have received immunizations such as *Haemophilus influenza*, *Pneumococcus*, and hepatitis B owing to lack of availability in their country of origin. These vaccines will need to be administered according to the recommended catch-up schedule for the country of resettlement.

Care for children following travel to the tropics

Children who have returned from a long-term trip or who have had extensive contact with the local populace should be evaluated for tuberculosis by PPD or QuantiFERON testing. Ill returning children, especially those with fever, require immediate evalu-ation to rule out life-threatening illnesses such as malaria, typhoid, and meningo-coccemia. Once life-threatening illnesses have been eliminated, both travel-related infections and illnesses common in the patient's country of origin should be con-sidered. Laboratory evaluation should be narrowed by taking a comprehensive his-tory and considering potential exposures and sequence of symptoms in conjunction with typical incubation periods for potential pathogens. Children found to have an eosinophilia should be evaluated similarly to immigrant children as described in a previous section.

References

1 Fischer PR, Sohail MR. Children and airplanes: are we having fun yet? *Minn Med* 2011; **94**: 33–35.

2 Stauffer W, Christenson JC, Fischer PR. Preparing children for international travel. *Travel Med Infect Dis* 2008; **6**: 101–113.

3 Summer AP, Fischer PR. Travel with infants and children. *Clin Fam Pract* 2005; **7**: 729–743.

4 Han P, Yanni E, Jentes ES, et al. Health challenges of young travelers visiting friends and relatives compared with those traveling for other purposes. *Pediatr Infect Dis J* 2012; **31**: 915–919.

5 Hagmann S, Benavides V, Neugebauer R, Purswani M. Travel health care for immigrant children visiting friends and relatives abroad: retrospective analysis of a hospital-based travel health service in a US urban underserved area. *J Travel Med* 2009; **16**: 407–412.

6 Valerio L, Roure S, Sabrià M, et al. Epidemiologic and biogeographic analysis of 542 VFR traveling children in Catalonia (Spain). A rising new population with specific needs. *J Travel Med* 2011; **18**: 304–309.

7 Galvin S, Robertson R, Hargarten S. Injuries occurring in medical students during international medical rotations: a strategy toward maximizing safety. *Fam Med* 2012; **44**: 404–407.

8 van Rijn SF, Driessen G, Overbosch D, van Genderen PJ. Travel-related morbidity in children: a prospective observational study. *J Travel Med* 2012; **19**: 144–149.

9 Gloster HM, Brodland DG. The epidemiology of skin cancer. *Derm Surg* 1996; **22**: 217–226.

10 Diffey BL. When should sunscreen be reapplied? *J Am Acad Dermatol* 2001; **45**: 882–885.

11 Leggat PA, Fischer PR. Accidents and repatriation. *Travel Med Infect Dis* 2006; **4**: 135–146.

12 Bhatta P, Simkhada P, van Teijlingen E, Maybin S. A questionnaire study of Voluntary Service Overseas (VSO) volunteers: health risk and problems encountered. *J Travel Med* 2009; **16**: 332–337.

13 Baldwin A, Harris T, Davies G. Look right! A retrospective study of pedestrian accidents involving overseas visitors to London. *Emerg Med J* 2008; **25**: 843–846.

14 Durbin DR, Committee on Injury, Violence, and Poison Prevention. Child passenger safety. *Pediatrics* 2011; **127**: e1050–e1066.

15 Cornall P, Howie S, Mughal A, et al. Drowning of British children abroad. *Child Care Health Dev* 2005; **31**: 611–613.

16 Neld LS. Health implications of adolescent travel. *Pediatr Ann* 2011; **40**: 358–361.

17 Quaranta A, Napoli C, Fasano F, et al. Body piercing and tattoos: a survey on young adults' knowledge of the risks and practices in body art. *BMC Public Health* 2011; **11**: 774.

18 Patrick ME, Morgan N, Maggs JL, Lefkowitz ES. "I got your back": friends' understandings regarding college student spring break behavior. *J Youth Adolesc* 2011; **40**: 108–120.

19 Wilder-Smith A. Dengue infections in travellers. *Paediatr Int Child Health* 2012; **32**(Suppl 1): 28–32.

20 Pitzinger B, Steffen R, Tschopp A. Incidence and clinical features of traveler's diarrhea in infants and children. *Pediatr Infect Dis J* 1991; **10**: 719–723.

21 Li ST, Grossman DC, Cummings P. Loperamide therapy for acute diarrhea in children: systematic review and meta-analysis. *PLoS Med* 2007; **4**(3): e98.

22 Greenwood CS, Greenwood NP, Fischer PR. Immunization issues in pediatric travelers. *Expert Rev Vaccines* 2008; **7**: 651–661.

23 Yaron M, Waldman N, Niermeyer S, et al. The diagnosis of acute mountain sickness in preverbal children. *Arch Pediatr Adolesc Med* 1998; **152**: 683–687.

24 Miller LC, Tseng B, Tirella LG, et al. Health of children adopted from Ethiopia. *Matern Child Health J* 2008; **12**: 599–605.

25 Juffer F, van Ijzendoorn MH. Behavior problems and mental health referrals of international adoptees: a meta-analysis. *JAMA* 2005; **293**: 2501–2515.

26 Reeves GD, Bachrach S, Carpenter TO, Mackenzie WG. Vitamin D-deficiency rickets in adopted children from the former Soviet Union: an uncommon problem with unusual clinical and biochemical features. *Pediatrics* 2000; **106**: 1484–1488.

27 Miller LC, Kiernan MT, Mathers MI, Klein-Gitelman M. Developmental and nutritional status of internationally adopted children. *Arch Pediatr Adolesc Med* 1995; **149**: 40–44.

28 Albers LH, Johnson DE, Hostetter MK, et al. Health of children adopted from the former Soviet Union and Eastern Europe. Comparison with preadoptive medical records. *JAMA* 1997; **278**: 922–924.

29 Miller LC. International adoption: infectious diseases issues. *Clin Infect Dis* 2005; **40**: 286–293.

30 Hostetter MK, Iverson S, Dole K, Johnson D. Unsuspected infectious diseases and other medical diagnoses in the evaluation of internationally adopted children. *Pediatrics* 1989; **83**: 559–564.

31 Boone JL, Hostetter MK, Weitzman CC. The predictive accuracy of pre-adoption video review in adoptees from Russian and Eastern European orphanages. *Clin Pediatr (Phila)* 2003; **42**: 585–590.

32 Update: measles among adoptees from China – April 14 2004. *MMWR Morb Mortal Wkly Rep* 2004; **53**: 309.

33 Hostetter MK, Iverson S, Thomas W, et al. Medical evaluation of internationally adopted children. *N Engl J Med* 1991; **325**: 479–485.

34 Stadler LP, Mezoff AG, Staat MA. Hepatitis B virus screening for internationally adopted children. *Pediatrics* 2008; **122**: 1223–1228.

35 Sokal EM, Van Collie O, Buts JP. Horizontal transmission of hepatitis B from children to adoptive parents. *Arch Dis Child* 1995; **72**: 191.

36 Davis LG, Weber DJ, Lemon SM. Horizontal transmission of hepatitis B virus. *Lancet* 1989; **i**: 889–893.

37 Fischer GE, Teshale EH, Miller C, et al. Hepatitis A among international adoptees and their contacts. *Clin Infect Dis* 2008; **47**: 812–814.

38 Updated recommendations from the Advisory Committee on Immunization Practices (ACIP) for use of hepatitis A vaccine in close contacts of newly arriving international adoptees. *MMWR Morb Mortal Wkly Rep* 2009; **58**: 1006–1007.

39 Johnson DE, Miller LC, Iverson S, et al. The health of children adopted from Romania. *JAMA* 1992; **268**: 3446–3451.

40 Miller LC. Initial assessment of growth, development, and the effects of institutionalization in internationally adopted children. *Pediatr Ann* 2000; **29**: 224–232.

41 Miller LC Hendrie NW. Health of children adopted from China. *Pediatrics* 2000; **105**: E76.

42 Widdowson EM. Mental contentment and physical growth. *Lancet* 1951; **i**: 1316–1318.

43 Van Ijzendoorn MH, Bakermans-Kranenburg MJ, Juffer F. Plasticity of growth in height, weight, and head circumference: meta-analytic evidence of massive catch-up after international adoption. *J Dev Behav Pediatr* 2007; **28**: 334–343.

44 Benoit TC, Jocelyn LJ, Moddemann DM, Embree JE. Romanian adoption. *The Manitoba experience. Arch Pediatr Adolesc Med* 1996; **150**: 1278–1282.

45 Landgren M, Andersson Gronlund M, Elfstrand PO, et al. Health before and after adoption from Eastern Europe. *Acta Paediatr* 2006; **95**: 720–725.

46 Rutter M. Developmental catch-up, and deficit, following adoption after severe global early privation. English and Romanian Adoptees (ERA) Study Team. *J Child Psychol Psychiatry* 1998; **39**: 465–476.

47 Gustafson KL, Eckerle JK, Howard CR, et al. Prevalence of vitamin D deficiency in international adoptees within the first 6 months after adoption. *Clin Pediatr (Phila)* 2013; **52**: 1149–1153.

48 AAP. *Red Book.* 2012 Report of the Committee on Infectious Diseases. Elk Grove Village, IL: American Academy of Pediatrics, 2012.

49 Swinkels H, Pottie K, Tugwell P, et al. Development of guidelines for recently arrived immigrants and refugees to Canada: Delphi consensus on selecting preventable and treatable conditions. *CMAJ* 2011; **183**: E928–E932.

50 Abdulla RY, Rice MA, Donauer S, et al. Hepatitis A in internationally adopted children: screening for acute and previous infections. *Pediatrics* 2010; **126**: e1039–e1044.

51 Staat MA, Rice MA, Donauer S, et al. Intestinal parasite screening in internationally adopted children: importance of multiple stool specimens. *Pediatrics* 2011; **128**: e613–e622.

52 Nazer H, Greer W, Donelly K, et al. The need for three stool specimens in routine laboratory examinations for intestinal parasites. *Br J Clin Pract* 1993; **47**: 76–78.

53 Thomson RB, Jr.,, Haas RA, Thompson JH, Jr., Intestinal parasites: the necessity of examining multiple stool specimens. *Mayo Clin Proc* 1984; **59**: 641–642.

54 Raymond JS, Kennedy C, Brown MJ. Blood lead level analysis among refugee children resettled in New Hampshire and Rhode Island. *Public Health Nurs* 2013; **30**: 70–79.

55 Eisenberg KW, van Wijngaarden E, Fisher SG, et al. Blood lead levels of refugee children resettled in Massachusetts 2000 to 2007. *Am J Public Health* 2011; **101**: 48–54.

56 Verla-Tebit E, Zhu X, Holsinger E, et al. Predictive value of immunization records and risk factors for immunization failure in internationally adopted children. *Arch Pediatr Adolesc Med* 2009; **163**: 473–479.

57 van Schaik R, Wolfs TF, Geelen SP. Improved general health of international adoptees, but immunization status still insufficient. *Eur J Pediatr* 2009; **168**: 1101–1106.

CHAPTER 17

Travelers with underlying medical conditions

Anne E. McCarthy & Kathryn N. Suh
University of Ottawa, Ottawa, Canada

Introduction

Increasingly, individuals with significant underlying medical conditions are traveling the world, as documented from a recent study of Boston area travel clinics where 18% of over 15,000 travelers were considered high risk due to immunosuppression or medical comorbidities; 86% were traveling to areas of malaria risk and 23% to countries endemic for yellow fever. The authors concluded that these complex travelers have increased requirements for counseling [1]. These travelers may be at increased risk of adverse outcomes during or after travel [1,2]. A recent study of Dutch travelers showed that those with underlying health conditions, especially those with immune compromise, were at increased risk of travel-related gastrointestinal illness in particular. Of concern, less than 20% had protection against hepatitis B and almost 3% required hospitalization during their travel [3]. Preparing travelers with pre-existing medical conditions requires consideration of not only the standard travel-related risks and prevention strategies outlined in this text, but also whether the travel itself, the diseases encountered, and the drugs used for prevention/treatment will impact their underlying disease or routine medications [4].

There are few absolute contraindications to travel, although airlines may refuse to transport individuals with unstable or acute medical conditions. All travelers with significant medical conditions should ensure that their underlying disease is stable before they travel and check with their routine care provider, well in advance of departure, to discuss any potential concerns related to the planned travel. Travel often includes exertion and therefore travelers should optimize cardiovascular and muscular fitness prior to departure.

Providers should consider supplying the traveler with an emergency medical contact at home, a telephone number or email address, and also advice about where best to seek specialty care at the destination. Travelers should carry an adequate supply of all medications, including routinely used non-prescription medication and medical supplies, in their hand luggage, to avoid loss. Medication should be carried in the original, labeled container. Replacement or replenishment of drugs at the destination may not be easy, since the composition and potency of drugs may vary with different

Essential Travel Medicine, First Edition.
Edited by Jane N. Zuckerman, Gary W. Brunette and Peter A. Leggat.
© 2015 John Wiley & Sons, Ltd. Published 2015 by John Wiley & Sons, Ltd.

manufacturers, and some drugs may not be available. Counterfeit medications are also common in some countries. Travelers should request from their pharmacy an itemized list of all medications, including dosing instructions and generic names, in case there is a need for documentation or replacement. In addition, travelers should carry a provider letter outlining the name and contact information of their primary provider, and also the underlying diagnosis(es), treatment requirements, allergies, and the need to carry medications and other medical supplies, in case documentation is requested or medical attention is required during travel. In addition, they should have copies of important documents such as a recent EKG, for those with significant cardiac disease, and a list of the make, model, and lot number of implanted devices (e.g., pacemakers, defibrillators, and prosthetic cardiac valves or joints) and date of insertion. Copies of other significant and relevant laboratory results should also be carried. It is prudent to carry the name and telephone number/email address of a family member or friend to contact in the event of an emergency. In addition, plans for possible access to medical expertise during travel and at the destination should be made prior to departure. Possible resources for travelers include their primary care provider for the underlying condition, organizations and associations related to the underlying disease, their insurance provider, and organizations such as the International Association for Medical Assistance for Travelers (IAMAT; www.iamat.org), which provides access to an international network of doctors and clinics around the world. The Joint Commission International (www.jointcommissioninternational.org) provides accreditation to international healthcare facilities.

If required, special consideration in transit such as meals and in-flight oxygen should be arranged with the carrier at least 48 hours prior to departure. When selecting seats, any special needs should be considered. In addition, requests for extra assistance or a wheelchair should be arranged at the time of booking. Travelers should allow adequate time for travel through the terminal and for check-in. When crossing multiple time zones, dosing of medications should be gradually altered over days; modification of insulin dosing is discussed below in the section on diabetes.

Health insurance coverage is particularly important for those with underlying medical conditions. Travelers should verify the extent of medical coverage that their provider offers, ensuring that any supplemental insurance cover, if required, is purchased prior to departure. Insurance should be sufficient to cover the costs of emergency medical care, and also evacuation and repatriation. For many out-of-country medical services the traveler may be required to pay at the time the service is provided, with subsequent reimbursement from the insurance company.

In this chapter, we concentrate on those travelers with immune compromise, diabetes, and cardiopulmonary disease.

Immunocompromised

There are many reasons why travelers may have compromised immune systems, whether due to the specific underlying disease or due to the treatment. These travelers need to consider the potential risk or limitation of prevention and treatment strategies and also possible increased risk of illness at travel destinations [5,6]. In general, the vaccine recommendations are similar to those for all travelers. However, certain vaccines, in particular live vaccines, may be contraindicated. In addition, the degree of immunosuppression may decrease vaccine efficacy [7–10]. The US Centers for Disease Control and Prevention (CDC) provide a very useful table of vaccines for those with immunodeficiency, including contraindications and effectiveness [11].

An additional consideration in immunocompromised travelers may be the provision of self-treatment for anticipated infections, such as treatment for skin and soft tissue infections, since mild infections may quickly progress in this population. In addition, instructions should be provided on when to seek medical attention [12].

This section specifically addresses travelers with immunocompromise due to human immunodeficiency virus (HIV), and those with iatrogenic immunocompromise due to systemic steroid therapy, biologics, or antirejection therapy.

Human immunodeficiency virus infection

The advent of highly active antiretroviral therapy (HAART) has remarkably changed the natural history of HIV, allowing the potential for extensive travel [13,14]. Despite this, there are certain factors for travel medicine providers to consider for these travelers before, during, and after the voyage [15]. Of note, there may be imposed travel restrictions for those with HIV infection in some countries, such as those in Eastern Europe and the Middle East. Some countries may request HIV testing for foreigners as a requirement of entry, and deny entry to those testing positive. Although this often applies to those planning longer stays, travelers should check with individual embassies or consulates to inquire about the need for HIV testing. Identification of a physician knowledgeable in HIV is ideal prior to travel. A list of organizations involved in the care and support of those with HIV across the world is available at www.aidsmap.com/e-atlas.

Pre travel preparation must take into consideration the degree of immune deficiency related to HIV infection, particularly when assessing vaccine recommendations. Those with severe immunocompromise (CD4 counts less than 200/mm^3) should avoid live attenuated viral and bacterial vaccines, owing to the risk of vaccine-associated illness. In addition, these individuals will have an attenuated response to inactivated vaccines. Ideally, vaccines should be administered 3 months after immune reconstitution with antiretroviral therapy. Some authorities [4] recommend readministering any vaccines given during the time of severe immunocompromise. HIV-infected travelers with CD4 counts between 200 and 500/mm^3 have limited immune deficits and may have a less robust vaccine response, but in general vaccine responses should be protective. Yellow fever vaccine can be considered in this group after a careful assessment of the risks and benefits of the vaccine based on the planned travel itinerary. In general, HIV-infected individuals with CD4 counts above 500/mm^3 are not considered significantly immunocompromised, and can be prepared as any other traveler would be. Travel preparation is a good time to ensure that routine vaccines, including pneumococcal, influenza, and hepatitis B vaccines, are up-to-date. For the latter, it is prudent to confirm serological immune response.

HIV infection may increase the risk for more severe illness with a number of food- and water-transmitted diseases, including *Salmonella*, *Cryptosporidium parvum*,

Microsporidia, and *Cyclospora* [16]. Attention to food and water precautions is critical. *Cryptosporidium* is resistant to both iodine and chlorine, so bottled, boiled, or filtered (pore size <1 μm) water should be used and extra care should be taken to avoid swallowing contaminated water during swimming or recreational water activities. Prophylaxis for travelers' diarrhea is not routinely recommended; however, self-treatment is advised, as for all travelers, with attention to potential medication interactions.

Malaria prevention is important in travelers with HIV infection, as in all travelers. However, there are additional considerations for malaria drugs used for prevention. The website www.hiv-druginteractions.org addresses potential interactions between drugs used for malaria chemoprophylaxis and those used in HAART regimens. In general, mefloquine is the most likely drug to have interactions, whereas doxycycline and chloroquine are less likely. The protease inhibitors are the most likely antiretroviral drugs to be associated with antimalarial drug interactions, with less likely interactions using nucleoside reverse transcription inhibitors and integrase inhibitors. The optimization of prevention strategies is key since the drugs often used for treatment of malaria, the artemesinins and quinine, may as well have interactions with HAART [17].

Respiratory infections may be a concern with immunocompromised HIV-infected travelers [18]. These include infections with pneumococcus, influenza, and tuberculosis (TB), and care should be taken to avoid exposure. Travelers should be up-to-date for both pneumococcal and influenza vaccines and, owing to concern about influenza vaccine efficacy, it may be prudent to consider a prescription of self-treatment for influenza with high-risk travel, such as cruises. Travelers with HIV infection should be educated about the risk of exposure to endemic mycoses, such as histoplasmosis, penicilliosis, and coccidioidomycosis, which may result in severe or disseminated disease [19]. Spelunking (caving) with exposure to bat-infested caves should be avoided.

Insect avoidance measures are important for more than malaria in immunocompromised individuals, including those with HIV, owing to the risk of more severe illness with visceral leishmaniasis [20] from sand-fly bites and Chagas disease from reduviid bug exposure [21].

Travelers taking steroids and/or immune-modulating drugs

Increasingly, individuals are treated with systemic steroids and immune-modulating drugs for inflammatory diseases and post-transplantation. While the advent of biologics and their use in autoimmune diseases have remarkably improved the lives of many affected [22], they have also increased the opportunity for exotic travel in this immunosuppressed population [1–3,23,24]. All of these drugs are associated with increased risk of infectious diseases that need to be carefully considered when carrying out a pre-travel assessment [5,25].

It is imperative to assess the degree of immunosuppression, since this will affect the safety of live vaccines and the efficacy of all vaccines, and provide an indication of the risk of travel-related and other infections. There is little or no immunosuppression associated with the following: <20 mg prednisone or equivalent daily; inhaled or topical steroids; >1 month since high-dose steroid therapy (≥20 mg daily for 2 weeks); >2 years after bone marrow or human stem-cell transplant (with no graft-versus-host disease); and autoimmune disease not on treatment. Severe immune deficiency is associated with the following: active leukemia or lymphoma; high-dose steroids (>2 mg/kg body weight or >20 mg daily for 2 weeks); alkylating agents (e.g., cyclosporine); antimetabolites (e.g., azathioprine); post-transplant on immune-modulating drugs; tumor necrosis factor blocking drugs; and other biologics.

Those with minimal immunosuppression can be vaccinated as recommended for regular travelers. For those with severe immunodeficiency, live vaccines including yellow fever vaccine are contraindicated. If the travel itinerary cannot be altered, then extra attention to insect precautions is required to prevent infection with yellow fever, as this may be more severe with immunocompromise. Inactivated vaccines are safe; however, there may be an attenuated immune response. Protective serologic response should be confirmed for hepatitis B vaccine and also rabies vaccine, if administered. Travel provides an ideal time to ensure that influenza and pneumococcal vaccines are up-to-date. Owing to the anticipated immunosuppression with immune-modulating drugs, it may be prudent to inquire about future travel plans prior to severe immunosuppression, and to administer vaccines while the immune system is still intact, providing more safety for live vaccine administration and improved response to all vaccines.

Malaria chemoprophylaxis is important where indicated, as for all travelers. Of note, there may be interaction of antimalarials with antirejection drugs. A prudent plan is a trial of therapy for at least a few doses prior to travel, monitoring and adjusting antirejection medication levels closely, in conjunction with the transplant care team. Similar monitoring is required as the traveler finishes the malaria chemoprophylaxis.

Travelers' diarrhea posses a particular risk since immunosuppressed individuals may be at increased risk for severe disease with some pathogens, including complications such as bacteremia. In addition, diarrhea may interfere with medication absorption, putting individuals at risk for disease exacerbation or low drug levels. There is also danger related to dehydration that may lead to concentration of and toxicity from antirejection drugs. Diligent adherence to food and water precautions is key, and also a detailed treatment plan, including antibiotics for self-treatment. Prophylaxis for travelers' diarrhea may be considered for the high-risk, short-term traveler.

Individuals taking tumor necrosis factor-blocking drugs are known to be at increased risk of infections, including TB, invasive fungal infections, skin and soft tissue infections, listeriosis, and pneumonia [26]. These travelers need to avoid high-risk activities. In addition, TB testing should be carried out after return. Consideration should be given to providing presumptive therapy for skin/soft tissue and pulmonary infections, with strict instructions about when to seek medical care.

Diabetes

Diabetic travelers need to optimize their diabetic control and understanding of their condition prior to travel. In addition, they need to consider potential complications in transit and at their destination. Travel involves exertion and stress, both of which may change requirements for hypoglycemic therapy. In addition, crossing multiple time zones may require adjustment of hypoglycemic therapy, both oral and injectable (see below). More frequent blood glucose monitoring is the best way to avoid the serious consequences of hypoglycemia and to determine insulin needs.

Individuals traveling with diabetes are common, representing 12% of those with medical comorbidities in a recent study [1]. During travel they may have problems related to their diabetes. One in 10 diabetics using insulin experiences problems while traveling, mostly due to hypoglycemia [27]. Patient education may help to reduce the incidence of problems in diabetic travelers. Preparation is key. Diabetics should carry an adequate supply of everything required for diabetes care on their person during travel, including an additional supply of medications and also food, glucose tablets, and glucagon, if appropriate, in case of unforeseen transportation delays. Ideally, insulin should be stored in a refrigerator; however, it is stable at room temperature for up to 1 month. Extremely high temperatures should be avoided. Those taking insulin should be reminded that insulin absorption increases in hot climates and that travel to altitude may interfere with glucometer and insulin pump function.

Travelers can get assistance from organizations such as the American Diabetes Association (ADA) (www.diabetes.org) and their airline carrier to confirm policies regarding carrying diabetes medication and supplies. Those traveling with diabetes should know how to use the local language at their destination to communicate that they have diabetes and how to request sugar or orange juice should they experience an episode of hypoglycemia. Diabetic individuals should carry a diabetes alert card, available in several languages from the ADA, and wear a medical bracelet. The International Diabetes Federation (www.idf.org) provides a list of regional and country email addresses should the traveler require specialist care abroad.

Travelers with diabetes are not at increased risk of many travel related illness [12], such as travelers' diarrhea; however, they may be at increased risk of complications. Diabetics should utilize oral rehydration solutions to maintain hydration, and should be reassured that solutions with glucose or rice can be safely used [28]. Malaria prevention advice is no different for diabetics than it is for non-diabetic individuals. Immunization is also not remarkably different for these patients. However, given the possibility of need for hospitalization abroad, ideally the hepatitis B vaccine series should be completed prior to travel, with serologic confirmation of response. In addition, immunizations should include annual influenza vaccine and up-to-date pneumococcal vaccine. Tuberculosis testing should be considered for those at added TB risk, such as those doing medical work in endemic regions.

Routine concerns for diabetic care, including skin and soft tissue infections, should be anticipated and prevented. Careful instructions regarding diligent foot care and management of early ulcers are essential, in addition to providing an antibiotic to cover staphylococci and group B streptococci, with care to provide coverage for methicillin-resistant *Staphylococcus aureus* (MRSA). Other infections experienced by diabetic individuals, such as urinary tract infections in women, should have a plan of management and a prescription for standby medication to be used as directed, in the hope of averting more severe infection and need for hospitalization. When diabetic travelers visit areas endemic for melioidosis, such as South-East Asia and northern Australia, they should be advised about avoidance of this soil-derived infection, which is more severe in diabetics [29]. *Burkholderia pseudomallei* is particularly prevalent in rice paddies during the rainy season and infections seem to be acquired by several routes, including inoculation and inhalation.

During travel, diabetic control remains important and individualized advice by the primary diabetic care specialist is best. Although tight control is stressed for all diabetics, it is prudent to accept higher values during travel, when there may be a risk of hypoglycemic episodes while crossing multiple time zones or during an intercurrent travel-related illness. Travelers taking oral hypoglycemics do not require additional doses, but should adjust their medication according to local time, taking care not to miss meals. For those taking insulin, no adjustment in dosage is required for those traveling north–south or those crossing fewer than six time zones. Those crossing six or more time zones do need to adjust insulin dosage; for example, those flying eastwards will require less insulin. Sane et al. provided a simplified approach, recommending a decrease in the daily dose of insulin by 2–4% for each hour of time shift with eastward flights, and increasing the same amount for each hour of time shift for westward flights [30].

Diabetics traveling to high (>3000 m) and extreme (>5000 m) altitudes may experience additional challenges. A review by Brubaker outlined the research on altitude risk for type 1 diabetics [31]. Symptoms of altitude illness, for example, acute mountain sickness with headache, dizziness and nausea, are difficult to differentiate from those of hypoglycemia. In addition, altitude induces anorexia, which may increase the risk of episodes of hypoglycemia. High-altitude retinal hemorrhage is a risk in some diabetics, and a dilated-pupil ophthalmologic examination and /or fluorescein angiogram are recommended before considering trips involving exposure to high altitude. Glycemic control is altered by altitude, and the stress related to the exertion and altitude complicate good control, requiring frequent glucose monitoring and insulin adjustment. However, glucometers are unreliable at altitude, and may give significant false readings [31,32]. In addition, the traveler must ensure special care of diabetic supplies since insulin pumps may not function properly and insulin may freeze at the low temperatures associated with ascent to high altitude [31].

Cardiovascular and respiratory disease

Cardiovascular disease

Cardiovascular disease is common and can lead to problems during flight, in transit, and at the destination. Therefore, travelers with underlying cardiac disease should undergo a pre-travel examination to optimize cardiovascular status and define preventive measures, including any in-flight oxygen requirements. Prior to departure, the traveler should obtain names of specialist physicians in the cities to be visited in case complications arise. The current medication profile and the specific underlying cardiac disease should be reviewed in detail prior to the prescription of any preventive or treatment medication for travel. Fitness to fly needs to be evaluated and the British Cardiovascular Society has published a comprehensive review of the existing evidence related to fitness to fly for those with underlying cardiovascular disease [33]. A summary of the recommendations is presented in Table 17.1. Those

Table 17.1 Travel restrictions for individuals with underlying cardiovascular conditions.

Condition	Flight restrictions	Comments
Stable angina	None	Make sure to take all medications, and bring all PRN cardiac meds
Acute coronary syndrome	Very low risk – 72 hours Medium risk – 10 days High risk – defer until stable	Very low risk – uncomplicated, <65 years, successful reperfusion, first event, ejection fraction (EF) >45%
		Medium risk– EF >40%, no symptoms of heart failure, no inducible ischemia or arrhythmia, no further investigations planned
		High risk – EF <40%, signs/symptoms of heart failure, those pending further investigations/intervention such as implantable device or revascularization
Heart failure	Acute heart failure – 6 weeks Chronic – no restriction, see comment	Chronic heart failure NYHA class III–IV – consider in-flight oxygen and airport assistance
Arrhythmia	Paroxysmal supraventricular tachycardia, atrial fibrillation, atrial flutter – no restrictions Persistent atrial fibrillation – stabilize on anticoagulants and rate control Ventricular arrhythmia – control before flight or do not fly	
Cardiac catheterization	Uncomplicated – 24 hours	
Elective percutaneous coronary intervention (PCI)	Uncomplicated – 48 hours	
Pacemaker or implantable cardiovascular device insertion	Uncomplicated – 48 hours	
Ablation	Uncomplicated – 24 hours	High risk of deep venous thrombosis/venous thromboembolism for 1 week
Open chest surgery	Uncomplicated – 10 days	Will need to consider ground assistance since limited exertion for 6 weeks post-operatively

Source: Adapted from Smith et al. 2010 [33].

with implanted cardiac devices need to ensure proper functioning prior to travel, with battery replacement as needed, since routine checks or maintenance may not be readily available in destination countries. Portable security magnets may inter-fere with the functioning of an implantable defibrillator and hand searches should be requested. As with all significant medical conditions, a physician's letter should be provided and carried along with a copy of a recent EKG in case medical attention is required while abroad.

High altitudes, usually defined as >2500 m, induce compensatory responses, including increased heart rate and cardiac contractility, which in turn lead to an increase in myocardial workload and cardiac output, with maximal effects during the first few days of exposure [34,35]. A recent consensus statement outlined an evidenced-based approach for travel medicine providers [36]. In general, most individuals with underlying cardiovascular disease can tolerate altitude exposure but do require an individual assessment, based on their disease status, including a plan for management of symptoms related to the underlying disease. This includes gradual ascent above 2000 m above sea level, increasing sleep altitude by <300 m per day. Absolute contraindications to high-altitude exposure include unstable angina or symptoms with mild to moderate exertion, decompensated congestive heart failure or myocardial infarction in the past 6 months, uncontrolled tachyarrhythmias, poorly controlled hypertension, marked pulmonary hypertension, severe valvular heart disease, cyanotic or severe acyanotic congenital heart disease, and defibrillator implantation or intervention in the past 6 months.

The drugs used for the prevention and treatment of altitude illness can have an effect on underlying cardiovascular disease and medications [37]. Acetazolamide metabolism may be impaired by long-term low-dose aspirin and the acetazolamide may increase central nervous system penetration of aspirin, leading to toxicity. The diuretic effects of acetazolamide may augment other diuretic drugs and increase the risk of abnormal electrolytes and dehydration, with additional risks if patients are concurrently taking digoxin. Calcium channel blockers such as nifedipine should be safe in stable coronary artery disease and can be used with caution in those taking other antihypertensive agents; however, short-release formulations should be avoided. Phosphodiesterase inhibitors such as sildenafil and tadalafil, used for the prevention of high-altitude pulmonary edema, reduce pulmonary artery pressure by increasing nitric oxide concentrations in the pulmonary vasculature. They should be avoided in those taking nitrates owing to the risk of profound hypotension. Salmeterol, a long-acting inhaled β-agonist, may interact with β-blockers, if taken together.

Travelers with cardiovascular diseases should have routine travel vaccinations as usual. Malaria prevention and treatment require some special considerations. Mefloquine is not recommended for people with cardiac conduction abnormalities, such as atrioventricular blocks. Coadministration of mefloquine with antiarrhythmic agents, some β-adrenergic blocking agents, and calcium channel blockers may contribute to prolongation of the QTc interval. Drug interactions have to be considered when prescribing mefloquine with warfarin. Standby treatment with artemether/lumefantrine is contraindicated in those with pre-existing cardiac disease associated with a prolonged QTc interval.

Respiratory disease

Travel may impact those with pulmonary disease. Pulmonary function should be optimized prior to travel and during flight by using bronchodilators and/or corticosteroids, if indicated. In flight, adequate hydration will facilitate the clearance of pulmonary secretions. Tracheostomies should not be expected to pose significant problems; however, the traveler should bring any equipment required for care. If there are significant abnormalities, carrying a copy of recent pulmonary function tests and chest X-ray may be advisable.

The air quality at many destinations may put some individuals at risk, hence these travelers should bring not only their routinely used medications, but all PRN puffers and other therapies. Pre-travel preparation should include consideration of providing a standby prescription for a tapering dose of steroids and/or antibiotic therapy for disease exacerbation, with clear guidance on when to initiate these, and when to seek medical attention. The only absolute contraindications to flying for these patients are pneumothorax, bronchogenic cyst, and severe pulmonary hypertension [38].

If oxygen is required, the airline will need to be contacted at least 48 hours prior to scheduled departure. A prescription for oxygen (indicating the flow rate or FiO_2, and specifying continuous versus intermittent oxygen) is required, as is a physician's letter outlining the individual's fitness to travel. In-flight oxygen and equipment will be supplied by the carrier, at a cost to the traveler, usually based on flight segments and/or the number of oxygen canisters required. Although airline attendants can provide basic assistance, such as help with changing canisters, they should not be expected to assist if mechanical problems arise. If oxygen is required during stopovers or at the final destination(s), this has to be arranged separately and well in advance; the traveler's regular oxygen vendor should be able to assist.

Commercial aircraft fly with a cabin pressure at the equivalent of 1500–2500 m (5000–8000 feet) above sea level. This pressure can have adverse effects on those with otitis or sinusitis. In pressurized aircraft cabins, there is a decrease in barometric pressure leading to a decrease in atmospheric oxygen, reflected by a decrease in PaO_2 and in the percentage of oxygen saturated hemoglobin (SaO_2), leading to 15.1% (2500 m) and 17.1% (1500 m) saturation of oxygen [38]. The reduction in atmospheric oxygen during flight may be an additional stress for those with cardiopulmonary disease, necessitating an in-flight assessment for supplemental oxygen [39–41]. The minimum desired PaO_2 during flight is 50 mmHg, and supplemental oxygen should be used if the predicted PaO_2 will be below this level. The hypoxia–altitude simulation test (HAST) is considered to be the best predictor of resting PaO_2 at altitude [42]. A simpler method is the standardized and validated 6 minute walking test, assessing tolerance and oxygen saturation [39]. The very simple 50 m walking test is very practical, but is not standardized. The inspired oxygen concentration (FiO_2) required during flight can be estimated using several methods. For travelers who do not require supplemental oxygen on land, an FiO_2 of 30% (2 L/min) should be adequate. The HAST nomogram can be used, with baseline PaO_2 measured using supplemental oxygen.

References

1 Hochberg NS, Barnett ED, Chen LH, et al. International travel by persons with medical comorbidities: understanding risks and providing advice. *Mayo Clin Proc* 2013; **88**: 1231–1240.

2 LaRocque RC, Rao SR, Lee J, et al. Global TravEpiNet: a national consortium of clinics providing care to international travelers – analysis of demographic characteristics, travel destinations, and pretravel healthcare of high-risk US international travelers, 2009–2011. *Clin Infect Dis* 2012; **54**: 455–462.

3 Wieten RW, Leenstra T, Goorhuis A, et al. Health risks of travelers with medical conditions – a retrospective analysis. *J Travel Med* 2012; **19**: 104–110.

4 Brunette G (ed.) *CDC Health Information for International Travel 2014: The Yellow Book*. New York: Oxford University Press, 2014.

5 Askling HH, Dalm VA. The medically immunocompromised adult traveler and pre-travel counseling: status quo 2014. *Travel Med Infect Dis* 2014; **12**: 219–228.

6 McCarthy AE, Mileno MD. Prevention and treatment of travel-related infections in compromised hosts. *Curr Opin Infect Dis* 2006; **19**: 450–455.

7 Agarwal N, Ollington K, Kaneshiro M, et al. Are immunosuppressive medications associated with decreased responses to routine immunizations? A systematic review. *Vaccine* 2012; **30**: 1413–1424.

8 Rendi-Wagner P, Kundi M, Stemberger H, et al. Antibody response to three recombinant hepatitis B vaccines: comparative evaluation of multicenter travel-clinic based experience. *Vaccine* 2001; **19**: 2055–2060.

9 Rubin LG, Levin MJ, Ljungman P, et al. 2013 IDSA clinical practice guideline for vaccination of the immunocompromised host. *Clin Infect Dis* 2014; **58**: 309–318.

10 van den Bijllaardt W, Siers HM, Timmerman-Kok C, et al. Seroprotection after hepatitis a vaccination in patients with drug-induced immunosuppression. *J Travel Med* 2013; **20**: 278–282.

11 Atkinson W, Wolfe S, Hamborsky J (eds.) *Epidemiology and Prevention of Vaccine-Preventable Diseases*, 12th edn. Washington, DC: Public Health Foundation, 2012.

12 Baaten GG, Geskus RB, Kint JA, et al. Symptoms of infectious diseases in immunocompromised travelers: a prospective study with matched controls. *J Travel Med* 2011; **18**: 318–326.

13 Kemper CA, Linett A, Kane C, Deresinski SC. Travels with HIV: the compliance and health of HIV-infected adults who travel. *Int J STD AIDS* 1997; **8**: 44–49.

14 Salit IE, Sano M, Boggild AK, Kain KC. Travel patterns and risk behaviour of HIV-positive people travelling internationally. *CMAJ* 2005; **172**: 884–888.

15 Franco-Paredes C, Hidron A, Tellez I, et al. HIV infection and travel: pretravel recommendations and health-related risks. *Top HIV Med* 2009; **17**: 2–11.

16 Zacharof A. AIDS-related diarrhea – pathogenesis, evaluation and treatment. *Ann Gastroenterol* 2001; **14**: 22–26.

17 Fehintola FA, Akinyinka OO, Adewole IF, et al. Drug interactions in the treatment and chemoprophylaxis of malaria in HIV infected individuals in sub Saharan Africa. *Curr Drug Metab* 2011; **12**: 51–56.

18 Adenis A, Nacher M, Hanf M, et al. Tuberculosis and histoplasmosis among human immunodeficiency virus-infected patients: a comparative study. *Am J Trop Med Hyg* 2014; **90**: 216–223.

19 Adenis AA, Aznar C, Couppie P. Histoplasmosis in HIV-infected patients: a review of new developments and remaining gaps. *Curr Trop Med Rep* 2014; **1**: 119–128.

20 Diro E, Lynen L, Ritmeijer K, et al. Visceral leishmaniasis and HIV coinfection in East Africa. *PLoS Negl Trop Dis* 2014; **8**(6): e2869.

21 Bern C, Kjos S, Yabsley MJ, Montgomery SP. *Trypanosoma cruzi* and Chagas' disease in the United States. *Clin Microbiol Rev* 2011; **24**: 655–681.

22 Furst DE, Keystone EC, So AK, et al. Updated consensus statement on biological agents for the treatment of rheumatic diseases, 2012. *Ann Rheum Dis 2013*; **72**(Suppl 2): ii2–ii34.

23 Roukens AH, van Dissel JT, de Fijter JW, Visser LG. Health preparations and travel-related morbidity of kidney transplant recipients traveling to developing countries. *Clin Transplant* 2007; **21**: 567–570.

24 Uslan DZ, Patel R, Virk A. International travel and exposure risks in solid-organ transplant recipients. *Transplantation* 2008; **86**: 407–412.

25 Visser LG. The immunosuppressed traveler. *Infect Dis Clin North Am* 2012; **26**: 609–624.

26 Rychly DJ, DiPiro JT. Infections associated with tumor necrosis factor-alpha antagonists. *Pharmacotherapy* 2005; **25**: 1181–1192.

27 Burnett JC. Long- and short-haul travel by air: issues for people with diabetes on insulin. *J Travel Med* 2006; **13**: 255–260.

28 Haider R, Khan AKA, Roy SK, et al. Management of acute diarrhoea in diabetic patients using oral rehydration solutions containing glucose, rice or glycine. *BMJ* 1994; **308**: 624–626.

29 Woods DE, Jones AL, Hill PJ. Interaction of insulin with *Pseudomonas pseudomallei*. *Infect Immun* 1993; **61**: 4045–4050.

30 Sane T, Koivisto VA, Nikkanen P, Pelkonen R. Adjustment of insulin doses of diabetic patients during long distance flights. *BMJ* 1990; **301**: 421–422.

31 Brubaker PL. Adventure travel and type 1 diabetes: the complicating effects of high altitude. *Diabetes Care* 2005; **10**: 2563–2572.

32 Moore K, Vizzard N, Coleman C, et al. Extreme altitude mountaineering and type 1 diabetes; the Diabetes Federation of Ireland Kilimanjaro Expedition. *Diabet Med* 2001; **18**: 749 755.

33 Smith D, Toff W, Joy M, et al. Fitness to fly for passengers with cardiovascular disease. *Heart* 2010; **96**(Suppl 2): ii1–ii16.

34 Naeije R. Physiological adaptation of the cardiovascular system to high altitude. *Prog Cardiovasc Dis* 2010; **52**: 456–466.

35 Rimoldi SF, Sartori C, Seiler C, et al. High-altitude exposure in patients with cardiovascular disease: risk assessment and practical recommendations. *Prog Cardiovasc Dis* 2010; **52**: 512–524.

36 Donegani E, Hillebrandt D, Windsor J, et al. Pre-existing cardiovascular conditions and high altitude travel. Consensus statement of the Medical Commission of the Union Internationale des Associations d'Alpinisme (UIAA MedCom) Travel Medicine and Infectious Disease. *Travel Med Infect Dis* 2014; **12**: 237–252.

37 Luks AM, Swenson ER. Medication and dosage considerations in the prophylaxis and treatment of high-altitude illness. *Chest* 2008; **133**: 744–755.

38 Tzani P, Pisi G, Aiello M, et al. Flying with respiratory disease. *Respiration* 2010; **80**: 161–170.

39 ATS Committee on Proficiency Standards for Clinical Pulmonary Function Laboratories. American Thoracic Society Statement: guidelines for the six-minute walk test. *Am J Respir Crit Care Med* 2002; **166**: 111–117.

40 British Thoracic Society Standards of Care Committee. Managing passengers with respiratory disease planning air travel: British Thoracic Society recommendations. *Thorax* 2002; **57**: 289–304.

41 Aerospace Medical Association, Air Transport Medicine Committee. Medical guidelines for air travel, ed 2. *Aviat Space Environ Med* 2003; **74**: A1–A19.

42 Gong H, Tashkin DP, Lee EY, Simkons MS. Hypoxia–altitude simulation test. Evaluation of patients with chronic airway obstruction. *Am Rev Respir Dis* 1984; **130**: 980–986.

CHAPTER 18

The older traveler and traveling with disability

Kathryn N. Suh & Anne E. McCarthy

University of Ottawa, Ottawa, Canada

Introduction

International travel is now widely accessible to most individuals, regardless of age, medical condition, or disability. Older persons and those with pre-existing conditions account for an increasing number of the almost 1.1 billion travelers who cross international boundaries each year; this number is expected to reach 1.8 billion by 2030 [1].

Only 1–3% of deaths in travelers are attributable to infectious diseases; most are due to natural causes and trauma [2–5]. It is therefore especially important that prevention of non-infectious travel-related illnesses and injury be a focus of the pre-travel assessment for the older or disabled traveler.

General advice for the older or disabled traveler

A general medical check-up should be performed to assess fitness for travel, far enough in advance to allow for investigation and treatment of any undiagnosed conditions that might alter travel plans. A conditioning program started before travel can increase cardiovascular fitness and muscular strength and identify potential limitations or problems. Exercise stress testing for older asymptomatic individuals may be considered if planning remote or lengthy treks [6].

A summary of significant past medical problems, allergies, and the name and telephone number of their physician(s) and an emergency contact should be carried by the traveler. Travelers should consider purchasing supplemental health insurance to cover the costs of emergency medical care, evacuation and repatriation costs, and any costs related to loss, theft, or damage of mobility and visual and hearing aids. Insurance carriers generally will not cover pre-existing health problems and will not insure those over 85 years of age. For many out-of-country medical services, the traveler will be required to pay at the time the service is provided, with subsequent reimbursement from the insurance company.

Essential Travel Medicine, First Edition.
Edited by Jane N. Zuckerman, Gary W. Brunette and Peter A. Leggat.
© 2015 John Wiley & Sons, Ltd. Published 2015 by John Wiley & Sons, Ltd.

Adequate time for travel to the terminal, for check-in, to reach departure areas, and for making connections should be ensured. Specific needs such as wheelchairs or extra assistance should be arranged with the carrier at the time of booking, at least 48 hours prior to departure, and again at the time of check-in.

The older traveler

Travel-related illness in the older traveler

Older travelers are more likely to die from underlying medical conditions but are also at risk of dying due to injury because they have slowed reaction times, auditory or visual impairment, poor coordination, or medication side-effects that may make them more vulnerable to accidents and crime. The older traveler also has additional risks related to physiologic changes of aging. Specific travel recommendations (e.g., malaria chemoprophylaxis, vaccines) and the possibility of adverse medication effects may also be affected by the traveler's age.

The healthy elderly will often have greater difficulty acclimatizing during travel, take longer to adjust to extremes in temperature or humidity and changes in altitude, and be more prone to motion sickness, jet lag, insomnia, and constipation. Non-prescription medications including analgesics, antiemetics, antacids, decongestants, and laxatives may be useful during travel but may cause uncomfortable and potentially serious side-effects in the elderly. Their use should be carefully reviewed prior to travel. Denture adhesive may be difficult to find in foreign destinations. Prescription medications, enough to last the entire trip plus an extra several days' worth, should be carried with the traveler in carry-on luggage at all times, along with a duplicate set of medications (and a prescription for each) in a separate location. Medications should be kept in their original labeled bottles.

Accidents and injury

Injury accounted for 25% of deaths in US travelers between 1975 and 1984 [2] and 38% in Canadians in 1995 [3]. Trauma-related deaths in travelers are more common in males, and in the young and elderly [2]. Motor vehicle accidents, drowning, and violent deaths are the most common causes of accidental death overall, but causes vary by region visited [7]. Most (80%) travelers who die from trauma do so before reaching a hospital; even if transport to a hospital occurs, evacuation is often required because of inadequate medical facilities.

Altitude sickness

The effect of age on acute mountain sickness (AMS) has been disputed. Some studies [8,9] have suggested that advanced age is protective, whereas others have found no association between age and AMS [10]. A reasonable level of fitness and adequate acclimatization will minimize the risk of AMS in the elderly. With a 5-day acclimatization period, the healthy older individual can tolerate altitudes of 2500 m well; hypoxemia, sympathetic activation, pulmonary hypertension, and reduced plasma volume do contribute to reduced exercise capacity, however [11]. Acetazolamide and dexamethasone are effective when used for prevention of AMS, but side-effects must be carefully considered when used in the older traveler.

Hyperthermia and hypothermia

The elderly are more susceptible to the effects of heat and cold. Peripheral vasodilation is impaired with advanced age and perspiration is diminished, reducing the body's cooling mechanisms in hot climates. In the cold, heat-generating mechanisms (i.e., shivering) are diminished. The thirst response may also be reduced in the elderly, leading to dehydration. Proper clothing is essential in both extremes of temperature. Acclimatization to heat or cold may take several days.

Jet lag

Jet lag is more common and may be more severe or prolonged in the elderly. It can be minimized by dividing long trips into segments with multiple stopovers, and adapting to the current time of day upon reaching the destination. Exposure to bright outdoor light may help readjust the circadian rhythm. Benzodiazepines may relieve sleep disturbances, but can result in daytime sleepiness, drowsiness, impaired memory, and fatigue, all of which may be more pronounced in older travelers. Zolpidem, a short-acting imidazopyridine hypnotic used for short-term treatment of insomnia, is effective in the treatment of jet lag [12], but adverse effects such as confusion, ataxia and falls, and gastrointestinal side-effects (cramps, nausea, vomiting, diarrhea) are increased in the elderly; the initial dosage should be halved (5 mg before bedtime) in the older individual. Melatonin may reduce jet lag and improve sleep quality [13] and its use is supported by the American Academy of Sleep Medicine [14]. Doses between 0.5 and 5 mg are effective [15], although most studies have excluded subjects over 65 years of age.

Motion sickness

Adults over 50 years of age are less susceptible to motion sickness, possibly related to age-related decline in vestibular function. Dimenhydrinate, diphenhydramine and related antihistamines, and scopolamine may cause more adverse effects in the older traveler. Scopolamine carries a greater risk of side-effects (drowsiness, dry mouth, blurry vision) than other agents, and may precipitate narrow-angle glaucoma, urinary retention (particularly in older men with prostatic hypertrophy), intestinal ileus, and heatstroke in warmer climates. Dimenhydrinate and diphenhydramine can also cause exaggerated or prolonged drowsiness, confusion, or ataxia in the elderly.

Thromboembolic disease

Observational studies suggest that venous thromboembolism (VTE) occurs in up to 12% of travelers [16], and the risk appears to be increased two- to fourfold compared with the population at large [16–18]. Most deep vein thromboses (DVTs) reported in studies have been asymptomatic; their clinical significance and natural history are unclear [16]. Age alone is not clearly a risk factor for travel-related VTE. Compression stockings, aspirin, and subcutaneous heparin are not generally recommended for VTE prophylaxis in older travelers, but compression stockings or anticoagulants may be indicated for high-risk patients [19].

Travel-related infections
Malaria

Adults ≥65 years of age accounted for 5% of all reported cases of malaria in the United States in 2011 [20]. The assumption that older travelers are at lower risk of acquiring malaria and do not require prophylaxis because their activities are less "risky" can lead to fatal outcomes. Illness may be more severe in the elderly, and mortality from malaria increases with age [21,22]. Chemoprophylaxis is always indicated, and may be better tolerated in the elderly than in younger age groups. Contraindications should be reviewed prior to prescribing antimalarial medications. Atovaquone–proguanil is generally well tolerated when used for prophylaxis, but only small numbers of travelers aged ≥65 years have been included in clinical trials. There is no increased toxicity from N,N-diethyl-3-methylbenzamide (diethyl-m-toluamide; DEET) in the elderly.

Sexually transmitted infections (STIs)

STIs account for less than 1% of reported illnesses among travelers [23,24]. The availability of therapy for erectile dysfunction may increase the likelihood of having unprotected sex and acquiring STIs in older travelers, particularly men. Appropriate counseling regarding the risks of sexual activity and the need for barrier precautions are important, regardless of the age of travelers.

Travelers' diarrhea (TD)

Older travelers are not necessarily at higher risk of TD. However, complications including dehydration and electrolyte imbalance are more poorly tolerated in the elderly. Evidence supporting routine antimicrobial chemoprophylaxis in the elderly is lacking, and possible adverse outcomes include antibiotic-associated diarrhea, *Clostridium difficile* infection, and increased antibiotic resistance. Rifaximin, a non-absorbable derivative of rifampin, has few side-effects and may be an attractive option for TD prophylaxis [25]. Antimotility agents (loperamide, diphenoxylate hydrochloride–atropine) may provide symptomatic relief of TD in the absence of bloody diarrhea, but may cause constipation, paralytic ileus, and central nervous system depression (especially with diphenoxylate, which is a narcotic), and contribute to hyperthermia.

Travel vaccines in the elderly

Vaccine-induced antibody responses may take longer to develop in the elderly and may be less robust. Therefore, the older traveler should seek travel advice early, preferably at least 8 weeks before travel. Data regarding the immunogenicity and efficacy of many travel vaccines in the elderly are scarce. Recommendations for travel immunizations are generally the same as for younger adults, with exceptions noted below.

Older travelers who have lived or traveled in endemic regions, or who have a prior history of jaundice, have a higher prevalence of hepatitis A antibody; screening prior to immunization may be cost-effective in this population. Hepatitis B vaccine may provide protection should unexpected medical care be required in endemic regions.

Immunization for TD may be considered for older travelers who might tolerate TD poorly, despite modest vaccine efficacy at best [26].

Yellow fever (YF) is rare in travelers, but the risk of severe disease from YF increases with age. While vaccine adverse events, serious side-effects, hospitalization, and death attributable to YF vaccine are rare, observational studies suggest that rates of these events increase with advancing age [27–30]. For example, based on passive reporting in the United States, serious systemic adverse events occurred 5.9 times more often for those aged 60–69 years and 10.7 times more often for >70-year-olds compared with 19–29-year-olds [27], and the rates of both viscerotropic and neurotropic reactions were to 2–6-fold higher, respectively [28]. To put this increased risk into perspective, however, viscerotropic and neurotropic reactions would occur in 2.3 per 100,000 vaccinees >70 years of age, and serious adverse effects including death in 12.6 per 100,000 [27]. These increased risk estimates have been questioned given the lack of standardized case definitions and other methodologic issues used in studies, but an association between increasing age and YF vaccine-related side-effects seems clear [31]. In practical terms, the risks of acquiring YF and of YF vaccine-related adverse events must both be carefully considered prior to immunization. It may be reasonable not to immunize (and to "medically exempt") elderly travelers who are at very little risk for YF, even if the vaccine is required by international regulations.

The disabled traveler

Travelers with physical disability

Legislation protects the traveler with special needs against unfair treatment. The Air Carrier Access Act [32] in the United States, the Canada Transportation Act [33] in Canada, the Code of Practice for Access to Air Travel for Disabled People [34] in the United Kingdom, and Regulation (EC) 1107/2006 of the European Parliament [35] were enacted to allow travelers with disabilities to travel safely and without discrimination on commercial aircraft. Similar legislation also exists to ensure that travelers with disabilities have improved accessibility to rail and ferry transport. Some very small vessels or aircraft may be unable to accommodate the traveler with severe physical limitations, however.

Specific needs for physically challenged travelers should be identified and requested well in advance of travel. If a carrier cannot provide the degree of assistance that it feels the traveler requires, it may request that the individual travel with an attendant. An attendant may also be required for safety reasons, if safety of the traveler or other passengers may be compromised; in such cases, the attendant is only required to help in the event of an emergency and is not obliged to provide personal assistance to the traveler.

Disabled travelers should inform transportation carriers, hotels, and tour guides/companies of their disability and identify specific needs or requests at the time of booking travel. Some useful online resources for disabled travelers are listed in Table 18.1.

Table 18.1 Selected online resources for disabled travelers.

Organization[a]	Website[b]
General information	
Access-Able Travel Source	www.access-able.com
Canadian Transportation Agency	www.cta-otc.gc.ca
Society for Accessible Travel and Hospitality (SATH)	www.sath.org
United States Department of Transportation Federal Aviation Agency	www.faa.gov/passengers/prepare_fly/#disabilities
Physically disabled travelers	
Accessible Journeys	www.disabilitytravel.com
Mobility International USA	www.miusa.org
Moss Rehab	http://www.mossrehab.com/disability-resources
The Opening Door	www.travelguides.org
Hearing-impaired travelers	
Action on Hearing Loss	www.actionhearingloss.uk
National Association of the Deaf	www.nad.org
Visually impaired travelers	
American Council of the Blind	www.acb.org
Canadian National Institute for the Blind	www.cnib.ca
Royal National Institute for the Blind	www.rnib.org.uk
Guide Dogs	
Guide Dogs for the Blind	www.guidedogs.com

[a]Organizations listed are not endorsed by the author.
[b]Websites were verified at the time of writing.

Air travel and the physically disabled traveler

A useful source of information for air travelers with disabilities is *New Horizons*, produced by the US Department of Transportation [36].

Mobility aids (canes, crutches, walkers) should be stored onboard at no cost. When a traveler requests assistance from an airline, the airline is obliged to provide access to the aircraft door (preferably by a level entry bridge; if a ramp is not available, a mechanical lift or "boarding chair" may be required), an aisle wheelchair, and a seat with removable armrests. Aircraft with <30 seats are generally exempt from these requirements. Wide-body aircraft with two aisles are required to have a fully accessible lavatory, and any aircraft with >60 seats needs to have an on-board wheelchair. Airline personnel should assist with pushing a wheelchair, including to the area by the lavatory. They should also help with carry-on baggage, and opening and identifying food, but are not required to transfer passengers, to assist with eating or administering medications, or to provide help in washrooms. Washrooms may be too small to accommodate an attendant, if one is required.

Airlines will transport wheelchairs and scooters at no extra cost to the traveler. An alternative may be to rent a wheelchair or scooter at the destination. A small repair kit and voltage adaptor, if required, should be carried. Prior to departure, proper functioning of the device should be ensured. The device and any removable parts should be labeled with proper identification prior to travel. Manual wheelchairs may be stored in the aircraft cabin if space permits, and should not be counted as carry-on baggage. Newer aircraft (those delivered after 1992 in the United States, or after May 2010 for other airlines) must be able to accommodate one folding wheelchair in the cabin, usually on a first-come, first-served basis. Gate checking the device is an alternative. Removable parts (seat cushions, baskets, etc.) should be removed before checking the item. Removal of batteries may also be required. If the wheelchair requires disassembly, it should be returned to the traveler fully reassembled; attaching instructions for disassembly and disconnection of batteries (and reassembly and reconnection) may be helpful. Mobility aids should be returned to the traveler either at (or as close as possible to) the aircraft door or at the baggage claim area, as specified by the traveler.

The traveler should not be required to sign any waiver of liability, except when pre-existing damage to the device is present. Damage during flight is the airline's responsibility, and the carrier is obliged to provide a suitable replacement at no cost to the traveler until the damaged item is repaired or replaced. Coverage for loss may vary, depending on the country of travel, and whether travel is domestic or international. Liability for loss during international travel is stipulated by the Warsaw Convention [37], in which assistive devices are not distinguished from other baggage, hence compensation may not cover replacement costs.

Cruising with a wheelchair or scooter

Newer cruise ships are fitted with features such as wheelchair-accessible washrooms and roll-in showers. Cruise ships can dock if the pier is large enough and in sufficiently deep water to allow this, in which case both traveler and wheelchair can be brought onshore. If the water is too shallow to permit a cruise ship to dock, travelers may need to transfer to a smaller ship to come ashore (tendering); most cruise lines will assist the wheelchair traveler with this process.

The hearing-impaired traveler

Deaf and hearing-impaired travelers may have difficulty hearing announcements and using telephones. Hearing impairment may also subject the traveler to potential safety risks, particularly in emergency settings where verbal or overhead instructions are provided, or where alarms are sounded. Hearing-impaired travelers should ask that information in overhead announcements be provided to them individually. Hotel staff should be made aware of a traveler's hearing impairment. Some hotels will provide visual aids as alerts of alarms or telephone calls. If these are unavailable, knowledge that a traveler is hearing impaired is essential in the event of an emergency. Teletypewriter (TTY) telephones [synonymous with telecommunications devices for the deaf (TDDs), text telephones, and minicoms] allow hearing-impaired (and speech-impaired) persons to use the telephone by typing instead of talking and can be requested, if available, when making reservations. Travelers who use hearing aids should carry extra batteries.

The visually impaired traveler

Extra eyeglasses should be carried during travel. Contact lens wearers should pack all required solutions. For those with significant visual impairment, a white cane may alert others of their disability, and written directions and specific addresses are helpful, especially if the traveler will rely on public transportation or taxis.

Service animals are specifically trained to help an individual with a disability, usually but not always visual impairment. As of 15 March 2011, dogs are the only animals that are recognized as service animals in the United States [38]. Foreign air carriers may not accept animals other than dogs. Certification is generally not required for service dogs to work, but proof of certification may be required for travel. Service dogs should not be barred entry to areas where pets are disallowed. In the United States, the Americans with Disabilities Act stipulates that service animals be permitted to accompany their owners in all areas where the public is allowed, including taxis, public buses, airplanes, restaurants, hotels, and other public facilities [38]. Restrictions may apply if safety concerns take precedence, such as sitting in the emergency exit row of an airplane or in operating rooms. A service animal may be barred if its behavior poses a safety risk to others.

The dog and its harness may be subjected to detailed inspection for security reasons. Restrictions or requirements for transporting a service dog both into and out of a given country (including upon return), including the need for quarantine, should be clarified by contacting the embassy or consulate of that country. Required immunizations and routine treatments should be up-to-date. A certificate of health and a record of immunizations should be obtained; some countries will require that these documents be certified.

A vest or harness that identifies the dog as a service animal can make others aware that the dog is not a pet. A secure collar with tags identifying the owner, with address and telephone number, and date of the most recent rabies immunization can be crucial. A non-metallic collar and harness will not set off security alarms. The dog should not be fed immediately before travel; additional food should be carried if needed en route, and folding dog bowls are useful for this purpose. The dog should not be sedated before travel and should be exercised and have voided prior to boarding. If the dog needs to void between connecting flights, it may need to be taken outside of and then brought back into the secure area of the terminal. The traveler should remember to pack whatever essentials the dog might need while away from home. Finally, the traveler may consider purchasing health insurance for the dog prior to travel. Some policies will include or offer coverage for veterinary services required during travel, but conditions and limitations should be clarified prior to purchase.

Conclusion

Many older individuals, and those with disabilities, are able to travel. Severe limitations may preclude travel but, in general, age and disability are not insurmountable barriers to traveling. Although some aspects of a trip may be limited, proper advanced planning can ensure that the elderly or disabled traveler enjoys a fulfilling, rewarding, and healthy travel experience.

References

1 United Nations World Tourism Organization. *UNWTO Tourist Highlights*, 2014 *Edition*. http://mkt.unwto.org/publication/unwto-tourism-highlights-2014-edition (accessed 12 June 2014).

2 Hargarten SW, Baker TD, Guptill K. Overseas fatalities of United States citizen travelers: an analysis of death related to international travel. *Ann Emerg Med* 1991; **20**: 622–626.

3 MacPherson DW, Guerillot F, Streiner DL, et al. Death and dying abroad: the Canadian experience. *J Travel Med* 2000; **7**: 227–233.

4 Leggatt PA, Wilks J. Overseas visitor deaths in Australia, 2001 to 2003. *J Travel Med* 2009; **16**: 243–247.

5 Redman CA, MacLennan A, Walker E. Causes of death abroad: analysis of data on bodies returned for cremation to Scotland. *J Travel Med* 2011; **18**: 96–101.

6 Backer H.. Medical limitations to wilderness travel. *Emerg Med Clin North Am* 1997; **15**: 17–41.

7 Tonellato DJ, Guse CE, Hargarten SW. Injury deaths of US citizens abroad: new data source, old travel problem. *J Travel Med* 2009; **16**: 304–310.

8 Hackett PH, Rennie D, Levine HD. The incidence, importance, and prophylaxis of acute mountain sickness. *Lancet* 1976; **ii**: 1149–1155.

9 Honigman B, Theis MK, Koziol-McLain J, et al. Acute mountain sickness in a general tourist population at moderate altitudes. *Ann Intern Med* 1993; **118**: 587–592.

10 Stokes S, Kalson NS, Earl M, et al. Age is no barrier to success at very high altitudes. *Age Aging* 2010; **39**: 262–265.

11 Levine BD, Zuckerman JH, deFilippi CR. Effect of high-altitude exposure in the elderly. The Tenth Mountain Division Study. *Circulation* 1997; **96**: 1224–1232.

12 Suhner A, Schlagenhauf P, Hofer I., et al. Effectiveness and tolerability of melatonin and zolpidem for the alleviation of jet lag. *Aviat Space Environ Med* 2001; **72**: 638–646.

13 Herxheimer A. Jet lag. *Clin Evid (Online)* 2014; **4**: 2303.

14 Morgenthaler TI, Lee-Chiong T, Alessi C, et al. Practice parameters for the clinical evaluation and treatment of circadian rhythm sleep disorders. An American Academy of Sleep Medicine report. *Sleep* 2007; **30**: 1445–1459.

15 Suhner A, Schlagenhauf P, Johnson R, et al. Comparative study to determine the optimal melatonin dosage form for the alleviation of jet lag. *Chronobiol Int* 1998; **15**: 655–666.

16 Philbrick JT, Shumate R, Siadaty MS, Becker DM. Air travel and venous thromboembolism: a systematic review. *J Gen Intern Med* 2007; **22**: 107–114.

17 Kuipers S, Schreijer AJM, Cannegieter SC, et al. Travel and venous thrombosis: a systematic review. *J Intern Med* 2007; **262**: 615–634.

18 Pérez-Rodríguez E, Jiménez D, Díaz G, et al. Incidence of air travel-related pulmonary embolism at the Madrid-Barajas airport. *Arch Intern Med* 2003; **163**: 2766–2770.

19 Watson HG, Baglin TP. Guidelines on travel-related venous thrombosis. *Br J Haematol* 2011; **152**: 31–34.

20 Centers for Disease Control and Prevention. Malaria surveillance – United States, 2011. *MMWR Morb Mortal Wkly Rep 2013*; **62**(SS-5): 1–17.

21 Greenberg AE, Lobel HO. Mortality from *Plasmodium falciparum* malaria in travelers from the United States, 1959–1987. *Ann Intern Med* 1990; **113**: 326–327.

22 Legros F, Bouchaud O, Ancelle T, et al. Risk factors for imported fatal *Plasmodium falciparum* malaria, France, 1996–2003. *Emerg Infect Dis* 2007; **13**: 883–888.

23 Chen LH, Wilson ME, Davis X, et al. Illness in long-term travelers visiting GeoSentinel clinics. *Emerg Infect Dis* 2009; **15**: 1773–1782.

24 Field V, Gautret P, Schlagenhauf P, et al. Travel and migration associated infectious diseases morbidity in Europe, 2008. *BMC Infect Dis* 2010; **10**: 330.

25 Hu Y, Ren J, Zhan M, et al. Efficacy of rifaximin in prevention of travelers' diarrhea: a meta-analysis of randomized, double-blind, placebo-controlled trials. *J Travel Med* 2012; **19**: 352–356.

26 Ahmed T, Bhuiyan TR, Zaman K, et al. Vaccines for preventing enterotoxigenic *Escherichia coli* (ETEC) diarrhoea. *Cochrane Database Syst Rev* 2013; (**7**): CD009029.

27 Khromava AY, Eidex RB, Weld LH, et al. Yellow fever vaccine: an updated assessment of advanced age as a risk factor for serious adverse events. *Vaccine* 2005; **23**: 3256–3263.

28 Lindsey NP, Schoreder BA, Miller ER, et al. Adverse event reports following yellow fever vaccination. *Vaccine* 2008; **26**: 6077–6082.

29 Monath TP, Cetron MS, McCarthy K, et al, Yellow fever 17D vaccine safety and immunogenicity in the elderly. *Hum Vaccin* 2005; **1**: 207–214.

30 Lawrence GL, Burgess MA, Kass RB. Age-related risk of adverse events following yellow fever vaccination in Australia. *Commun Dis Intell* 2004; **28**: 244–248 [Erratum appears in *Commun Dis Intell* 2004; **28**: 348–352].

31 Rafferty E, Duclos P, YActayo S, Schuster M. Risk of yellow fever vaccine-associated viscerotropic disease amont he elderly: a systematic review. *Vaccine* 2013; **31**: 5798–5805.

32 United States Department of Transportation. *14CFR Part 382. Nondiscrimination on the Basis of Disability in Air Travel (Air Carrier Access Act). July 2003; and Rule in Effect Beginning May 13, 2009,* 2009 http://airconsumer.ost.dot.gov/rules/rules.htm (accessed 4 July 2014).

33 Canadian Transportation Agency. *Summary of Regulations Covering the Accessibility of air Travel,* 2010. http://www.otc-cta.gc.ca/eng/publication/summary-regulations-covering-accessibility-air-travel (accessed 4 July 2014).

34 United Kingdom Department for Transport. *Access to Air Travel for Disabled Persons and Persons with Reduced Mobility – Code of Practice,* 2008. http:/www.dft.gov.uk/transportforyou/access/aviationshipping/accesstoairtravelfordisabled.pdf (accessed 4 July 2014).

35 European Commission. *Regulation (EC) 1107/2006 of the European Parliament and of the Council of 5 July 2006 Concerning the Rights of Disabled Persons and Persons with Reduced Mobility when Travelling by Air.* http://eur-lex.europa.eu/legal-content/EN/ALL/?uri=CELEX:32006R1107 (accessed 4 July 2014).

36 United States Department of Transportation. *New Horizons. Information for the Air Traveler with a Disability,* 2009. http://airconsumer.dot.gov/%5Cpublications%5CHorizons2009Final.pdf (accessed 4 July 2014).

37 *Warsaw Convention (Amended at the Hague, 1955, and by Protocol No. 4 of Montreal, 1975).* http://www.mcgill.ca/files/iasl/warsaw1929.pdf (accessed 4 July 2014).

38 United States Department of Justice Civil Rights Division, Disability Rights Section. *ADA 2010 Revised Requirements: Service Animals,* 2010. http://www.ada.gov/service_animals_2010.htm (accessed 4 July 2014).

CHAPTER 19

Visiting friends and relatives

Karin Leder[1,2] & Sarah L. McGuinness[2]

[1] Monash University, Melbourne, VIC, Australia
[2] Melbourne Hospital, Parkville, VIC, Australia

Introduction

It is increasingly recognized that reason for travel significantly impacts on disease risks and health outcomes for travelers. One traveler subgroup now recognized to be at high risk for many travel-related diseases is travelers visiting friends and relatives, commonly known as VFRs.

Who are VFRs?

The term VFR does not refer to all individuals traveling for the purpose of seeing loved ones, but instead refers to a distinct and more limited subpopulation. Although exact definitions have varied, the most common use of the VFR term implies a health-risk gradient between the current place of residence and the place being visited, and refers to those individuals originally from a developing country who have moved to live in an industrialized country who subsequently return to their home region for the purpose of visiting friends and relatives [1,2]. VFRs include immigrants, asylum seekers, refugees, and international students. The term additionally includes accompanying family members who may have been born locally, specifically spouses, children, and grandchildren (second- and third-generation VFRs). Different terms for VFRs that have sometimes been used include foreign-born travelers and migrant travelers [3,4].

Why are VFRs an important traveler subgroup?

With increasing global population movement and migration, VFRs are comprising an increasing and substantial proportion of all international travelers, currently estimated at 25–40% [5].

Essential Travel Medicine, First Edition.
Edited by Jane N. Zuckerman, Gary W. Brunette and Peter A. Leggat.
© 2015 John Wiley & Sons, Ltd. Published 2015 by John Wiley & Sons, Ltd.

Why are VFRs at increased risk of disease?

VFRs are often at greater risk of contracting travel-related illnesses than individuals traveling for other purposes [3,6,7], in part because a lower proportion of VFRs
attend for pre-travel advice [6–8]. A major barrier to optimal pre-travel preparation
is the perception among many VFRs that the trip poses minimal risk since they are
"only going home," and the commonly held but erroneous belief that they have
pre-existing immunity to all infections to which they might be exposed during their
trip. Language, cultural, and financial barriers also contribute to low pre-travel visit
rates, as do last-minute decisions to travel (e.g., following the death or birth of a family
member). For those VFRs who do seek pre-travel advice, decreased acceptance of or
compliance with preventive interventions is common. These issues are compounded
by behavioral characteristics that increase exposure risks during the trip. VFRs often
live like local residents, commonly staying in local homes in rural areas. It may be culturally inappropriate for them to refuse home-cooked food prepared by family and
friends, thereby exposing them to potentially contaminated meals. Moreover, they
often travel for long periods, at extremes of age, and while pregnant.

Which diseases are of particular importance among VFRs?

Prospective studies of absolute risk of illness among VFRs compared with other
travelers are lacking, so most of the evidence regarding differential illness risks for
VFRs comes from studies that examine unwell travelers following return from their
trips. Reports of travel-associated illnesses that are more common among VFRs
therefore reflect a mixture of illnesses that (i) have higher absolute acquisition
risks among VFRs, (ii) are more serious, more prolonged, or more frightening to
VFRs, thereby prompting presentation to a healthcare professional, or (iii) are
more common among immigrant groups regardless of recent travel, but which are
diagnosed when a VFR presents for medical care for some other reason following
a trip. Differentiating between these factors to determine why a disproportionate
burden of disease is seen among VFRs is not always possible.

Some health problems for which there is evidence for higher absolute risks among
VFRs include:
- *Malaria:* Increased risk is presumably related to the frequency of travel to rural/
  remote destinations, sleeping in non-air-conditioned rooms without screens, low
  use of mosquito repellants, and low use of malaria prophylaxis. Many global studies
  show that VFRs comprise about 70% of malaria notifications [9]. Given that VFRs
  comprise approximately one-third of all travelers, they are clearly over-represented
  among notified cases. Even if malaria prophylaxis has been prescribed, VFRs are
  often non-compliant, and may prefer to leave their medication supply with their
  family members in the endemic region [10].
- *Enteric fever:* Risk is presumably related both to low immunization rates against
  Salmonella typhi and to high exposure risks. A number of studies suggest that over
  80% of all notified enteric fever cases occur among VFRs, especially among VFRs

to the Indian subcontinent, leading to a 3–8-fold greater risk of infection for VFRs than for other travelers [9].

- *Hepatitis A:* Individuals who have grown up in areas with poor sanitation may have had prior exposure to hepatitis A virus (HAV), thus providing them with life-long immunity. However, accompanying children who were born in the developed country of residence will be non-immune. This underpins the observation of an estimated eightfold risk of HAV among VFRs, predominantly attributable to pediatric VFRs [9].
- *Vaccine-preventable diseases:* These include diseases such as measles and polio, and are related to incomplete, or lack of, childhood vaccination.
- *Influenza:* This presumably relates to close contact with locals and low levels of immunization.
- *Sexually transmitted infections:* Risks again relate to close contact with locals, and also possibly to prolonged travel duration [6,11].
- *"Immigrant" diseases:* These include tuberculosis, human immunodeficiency virus (HIV), hepatitis B, strongyloides, and other infections that can have long latency. In many cases, the diagnosis may be made after a recent trip home if another intercurrent illness prompts the individual to seek medical care, but the relevant infection may have been acquired prior to immigration rather than during the recent VFR trip.

A number of other causes of travel-related morbidity are often described as being important for VFRs, although definitive evidence for an incremental risk among VFRs compared with other travelers is lacking. Examples include:

- *Travelers' diarrhea (TD):* TD is the commonest health problem among all travelers, so it is important for VFRs. VFRs may believe that they are not susceptible to TD owing to prior exposures when living in their country of origin, but most if not all causes of TD are at best associated with partial immunity which wanes over time (often months). Intuitively, behavioral factors would suggest that VFRs should be at a high risk of TD if they eat local foods, but there is some evidence that VFRs are comparatively less likely to present to a healthcare provider with TD following return from a trip than other types of travelers [6]. However, this may be because of a higher threshold for seeking post-travel care with diarrhea among VFRs rather than being due to a true differential illness risk.
- *Dengue:* Long-term immunity to dengue serotypes to which the individual has previously been exposed might decrease their risks of acquiring dengue. On the other hand, diminished adherence to vector precautions and the possible increased risks of complications from infection with a new serotype might make VFRs more likely to present with severe dengue infections.
- *Meningococcus:* Meningococcal infection may intuitively be considered to be more common among VFRs who (i) may have missed out on childhood vaccination, (ii) are less likely to have received vaccination during a pre-travel visit, and (iii) have close contact with locals, thereby potentiating transmission of infections via the respiratory route. However, there are no specific data for incremental risks among VFRs.
- *Rabies:* The contact that VFRs have with local environments might theoretically put them at high risk of exposure to animals, plus long travel durations and repeated

travel may cumulatively increase potential risks. However, in practice, it is unlikely that there is a significant overall difference in rabies risk *per se* among VFR travelers.

- *Accidents:* Trauma and motor vehicle accidents are common among all types of travelers. Cultural factors affecting, for example, use of helmets or seatbelts during transport may put VFRs at higher risk of accidents. However, there currently are no specific data in this regard.

Engaging VFRs

Many pre-travel health services are equipped to deal predominantly with tourist and business travelers. For over a decade, the observed high travel risks among VFRs have prompted researchers, travel health professionals, and public health personnel to suggest that better engagement of VFRs with pre-travel services, improved understanding of their cultural needs, better availability of interpreter services, and better methods for disseminating travel risk messages to VFRs are needed. Despite this, few successful methods have been described, and none have been proven to improve travel outcomes for VFRs. Suggested interventions to engage VFRs have included [12–15]:

- production of multilingual and culturally appropriate educational materials to convey simple travel health messages;
- reducing costs of vaccinations and medications (including malaria chemoprophylaxis);
- educating primary care providers (PCPs) about VFR travel risks, including targeting of PCPs from ethnically diverse backgrounds from whom VFRs may be more likely to seek care;
- opportunistically providing pre-travel advice when individuals present to healthcare providers for other reasons;
- establishing community-based educational activities;
- highlighting the particular vulnerability of children during travel;
- using the media to disseminate travel-risk messages.

Pre-travel advice for VFRs

Recommendations for VFRs do not fundamentally differ from those for other travelers, yet prioritization of interventions – which may often be essential from a practical perspective to minimize costs – often need careful consideration. For example, malaria chemoprophylaxis may be a high priority if there is a risk of life-threatening falciparum malaria at the intended destination. VFRs from malaria-endemic areas may need to be specifically informed that any partial prior immunity to malaria that they had will have started to wane within about 6–12 months. Additionally, the importance of seeking medical attention during or after the trip should a fever develop must be emphasized.

Specific vaccine priorities vary according to the destination and traveler characteristics. Although VFRs may present because they need a required vaccine such as yellow fever, travel immunization recommendations for VFRs almost always extend beyond required vaccines. For example, typhoid vaccine for VFRs to the Indian subcontinent is a high priority. Hepatitis A, especially for pediatric travelers who were born after migration from the endemic area, is often advised, but immunity among individuals born in the endemic area should not be assumed, so screening plus vaccination for these individuals is also recommended. Catch-up immunization for childhood vaccines may be important, not just for the impending trip, but to decrease local risks of hepatitis B, measles/mumps/rubella, meningococcus, tetanus, varicella, and other diseases. Behavioral advice regarding food and water precautions, frequent handwashing and hygiene behavior, avoidance of animal and insect bites, safe-sex messages, and safety advice should also all be provided.

VFRs may find it relatively easy to access health services if needed during their trip as the families they are visiting are likely to know local healthcare providers and language is unlikely to be a barrier. This might make VFRs think that buying presumptive self-treatment (e.g., for TD) or malaria chemoprophylaxis to take with them is unnecessary, and that cheaper medicines can be obtained while traveling if needed. However, the availability and quality of local services may be suboptimal and in some regions counterfeit drugs are common, so relying on drugs acquired during the trip is generally inadvisable.

References

1 Brunette G (ed.) *CDC Health Information for International Travel 2012: The Yellow Book*. New York: Oxford University Press, 2012, Chapter 8. http://wwwnc.cdc.gov/travel/ (accessed 27 June 2013).

2 WHO. *International Travel and Health* 2012. Geneva: World Health Organization, 2012, Chapter 9. http://www.who.int/topics/travel/en/ (accessed 27 June, 2013).

3 Angell SY, Cetron MS. Health disparities among travelers visiting friends and relatives abroad. *Ann Intern Med* 2005; **142**: 67–72.

4 Matteelli A, Carvalho AC, Bigoni S. Visiting relatives and friends (VFR), pregnant, and other vulnerable travelers. *Infect Dis Clin North Am* 2012; **26**: 625–635.

5 United Nations World Tourism Organization. *UNWTO Tourist Highlights, 2011 Edition*, 2011. http://mkt.unwto.org/sites/all/files/docpdf/unwtohighlights11enlr_1.pdf (accessed 28 June 2013).

6 Leder K, Tong S, Weld L, et al. Illness in travelers visiting friends and relatives: a review of the GeoSentinel Surveillance Network. *Clin Infect Dis* 2006; **43**: 1185–1193.

7 Bacaner N, Stauffer B, Boulware DR, et al. Travel medicine considerations for North American immigrants visiting friends and relatives. *JAMA* 2004; **291**: 2856–2864.

8 Leder K, Torresi J, Libman MD, et al. GeoSentinel surveillance of illness in returned travelers, 2007–2011. *Ann Intern Med* 2013; **158**: 456–468.

9 Health Protection Agency. *Foreign Travel-Associated Illness: a Focus on Those Visiting Friends and Relatives*. London: Health Protection Agency, 2008.

10 Pistone T, Guibert P, Gay F, et al. Malaria risk perception, knowledge and prophylaxis practices among travellers of African ethnicity living in Paris and visiting their country of origin in sub-Saharan Africa. *Trans R Soc Trop Med Hyg* 2007; **101**: 990–995.

11 Ansart S, Hochedez P, Perez L, et al. Sexually transmitted diseases diagnosed among travelers returning from the tropics. *J Travel Med* 2009; **16**: 79–83.

12 Angell SY, Behrens RH. Risk assessment and disease prevention in travelers visiting friends and relatives. *Infect Dis Clin North Am* 2005; **19**: 49–65.

13 Hagmann S, Reddy N, Neugebauer R, et al. Identifying future VFR travelers among immigrant families in the Bronx, New York. *J Travel Med* 2010; **17**: 193–196.

14 Navarro M, Navaza B, Guionnet A, Lopez-Velez R. A multidisciplinary approach to engage VFR migrants in Madrid, Spain. *Travel Med Infect Dis* 2012; **10**: 152–156.

15 Leder K, Lau S, Leggat P. Innovative community-based initiatives to engage VFR travelers. *Travel Med Infect Dis* 2011; **9**: 258–261.

CHAPTER 20

Migrants, refugees, and travel medicine

Louis Loutan
University Hospital of Geneva, Geneva, Switzerland

Introduction

Migrants can be considered as members of the group that comprise long-term travelers, but healthcare practitioners need to recognize specific differences. Travelers are free to move anywhere and have unlimited access to services, restricted only by the availability of financial resources. Migrants, however, are bound by regulations and rules beyond their control. They are also likely to have experienced long and often painful administrative procedures and often are waiting for decisions that are pending and that create major uncertainties about their future. From a public health perspective, they are all mobile populations and contribute to the overall impact of global mobility. They share some common factors related to travel and exposure to new environments and risks. However, migrants and travelers are very different in terms of access to health and care determined by their status, conditions of travel and living, duration of residence, and overall personal experiences. It is important to remember that most migrants are healthy and benefit from the "healthy migrant effect," i.e., those moving and ready to leave their country are healthy and dynamic. Migration is not an easy decision; it tends to select the fittest. However, the conditions that may prevail in the migration process can increase vulnerability and be detrimental to health.

The migration process and health

Migrant populations are very heterogeneous in origin in terms of experienced exposures to risk factors, conditions of living in the host country, and their access to healthcare services. Without doubt these many factors will influence their health status, and one way of looking at the health of migrants is to consider it in relation to the very process of migration itself [1].

The pre-departure phase is characterized by the influences of the environment upon health in which an individual or a group of migrants has lived. This refers to a broad spectrum of factors including exposure to endemic diseases such as malaria,

Essential Travel Medicine, First Edition.
Edited by Jane N. Zuckerman, Gary W. Brunette and Peter A. Leggat.
© 2015 John Wiley & Sons, Ltd. Published 2015 by John Wiley & Sons, Ltd.

tuberculosis, intestinal parasites, and viral hepatitis. Nutritional factors such as sufficient intake of micronutrients, vitamins, and proteins will shape the nutritional status and normal growth of children. Social and economic factors such as poverty, illiteracy, unemployment, occupational hazards, poor housing, and unhygienic living conditions are among key factors shaping the future health status of migrants, as is exposure to insecurity, war, violence, torture, and other human rights violations. Religion and cultural background are, of course, of key importance in influencing health beliefs and behaviors. Finally, experiences encountered following contact with the medical services in the country of origin and with other traditional and lay medical providers will also influence a migrant's expectations and rapport with medical services in the country of settlement.

The journey itself may be very short and uneventful, but for many refugees and migrants the journey may be a long process, characterized by uncertainty, deprivation, insecurity, abuse, trauma, and sometimes life-threatening events. This may be particularly the case with illegal migrants smuggled into a new country, and for women.

The resettlement phase may differ greatly according to the legal status of a particular person or community. The level of education, professional skills, and language and communication skills will influence the capacity of migrants to adjust to their new cultural, professional, and social environment, and to interact and integrate progressively into the new society. Living conditions such as overcrowding or isolation may accelerate the transmission of diseases such as tuberculosis and varicella, or they may have an important psychological impact. Restrictive policies aimed at discouraging newcomers to seek asylum may have also a deleterious effect on the mental health of asylum seekers or migrants [2]. Access to health services may be restricted. Nonetheless, arriving in the receiving country may also be a relief and provide an opportunity to start a new life.

When taking the successive steps of the migratory process into account, it is possible to build a clear view of the potential exposures and risk factors that may influence the present health condition of a specific person or community. This can help healthcare providers to connect the present complaint or illness to previous events related to the migration process that the person has undergone.

From medical screening to access to care

At a time of worldwide mobility of millions of travelers, mandatory medical screening continues to be implemented for immigrants and refugees prior to or at the time of entry into the receiving country. It is aimed mainly at identifying communicable diseases such as tuberculosis, hepatitis B, syphilis, and HIV and other health conditions that may cause a financial burden to the receiving country. Preventive measures such as vaccinations are often implemented at this time. With mobile populations becoming a larger component of societies, infectious diseases with long periods of latency or those with subclinical or chronic stable infectious periods pose problems that are not solved by screening at the time of entry. Chronic infectious diseases such as tuberculosis, hepatitis B and C, and schistosomiasis, and infectious diseases with a long latency, such as vivax malaria, will often only be recognized after many months or years of residing in the host country.

Health and diseases in migrants: a practitioner's perspective

Healthcare providers and travel medicine professionals may frequently see migrants or refugees of various origins both for treatment and for preventive measures such as immunization. They need to be able to recognize diseases that are unusual and more "exotic" and they should develop a cultural competence to provide effective care.

Infectious diseases

Coming from regions where many cosmopolitan or tropical communicable diseases are more prevalent, a significant proportion of migrants may have been in contact with or infected with or indeed be a carrier of some specific infectious disease. This is particularly the case with tuberculosis [3]. Pulmonary symptoms lasting more than 2 weeks, fatigue, and weight loss should always raise the possibility of underlying tuberculosis (TB). In migrants and refugees coming from countries where TB is endemic, a significant proportion of cases are extra-pulmonary. Cases of tuberculosis with a history of incomplete treatment are likely to be at a higher risk of developing drug resistance.

Hepatitis B and C are of concern as they can cause chronic infection with serious long-term complications. The prevalence in migrants varies according to the level of endemicity of their country of origin.

Asymptomatic infection with HIV is a consideration with migrants coming from regions where HIV/AIDS is endemic. Voluntary screening, counseling, and information on the disease and its prevention should be encouraged in potentially at-risk groups.

Healthcare practitioners should always consider malaria as a cause of fever in a migrant or refugee who originated from a tropical country, as for *Plasmodium vivax, P. ovale and P. malariae* the latent phase can last for several months and even years after infection.

Intestinal infection due to protozoa and helminths is a very common finding in arriving migrants. Clinical presentation is often non-specific, but the presence of eosinophilia should suggest screening for infection with helminths, particularly *Strongyloides sterchoralis* and schistosomiasis, which can be present for decades. Recently, American trypanosomiasis (Chagas disease) has attracted attention in migrants coming from Latin American countries, where it is endemic, and which can be the cause of serious cardiac complications.

It is worth remembering that a substantial proportion of migrants may not have benefited from organized immunization programs, so healthcare practitioners should always check and provide the complementary immunizations needed.

Non-infectious diseases

Chronic non-infectious diseases are on the rise in migrant populations. As a result of lifestyle changes, the incidence of cardiovascular diseases in populations of immigrants to Canada or the United States tends to adjust with time to those observed in the local population.

Epidemiologic data on migrants should be integrated in a dynamic way as their migratory journey evolves. High blood pressure can be fairly prevalent in black African migrants and diabetes is frequently seen in migrants from South Asia and Pacific islands. Healthcare practitioners should also look at the short- and long-term effects of protein and vitamin deficiencies leading to osteomalacia and bone deformation, iron deficiency, and anemia. Anemia can also be a consequence of genetic traits such as G6PD deficiency or thalassemia. Both are fairly frequent in ethnic minorities in the United Kingdom: 3–10% in Indians, 10–14% in Afro-Caribbeans, and 20–25% in West Africans. Oral health is an often a forgotten problem of particular concern in children, who may show a high proportion of dental caries with long-term consequences.

This very short overview of chronic non-communicable diseases should raise healthcare practitioners' awareness of this commonly overlooked dimension of migrant health. Measures of prevention, counseling and providing sound health promotion advice, and early disease detection and treatment can make a significant difference to the health of migrants.

Mental health and violence

Healthcare practitioners should be aware of possible previous exposure to violence, war, torture, or other trauma and its long-term impact on health. Recognizing physical and psychologic symptoms related to rape, various forms of physical abuse, post-traumatic stress disorder, and depression, including how these may be expressed in a specific society or ethnic group, are of prime importance. Very often victims of organized violence will not present to healthcare practitioners as such, but will present with common non-specific symptoms such as headache, fatigue, and general pain. It is only when trust, confidence, and empathy are established, when the patient feels that the physician or the nurse is open to listening, that they will talk about their traumatic experiences and then allow for the therapeutic process to start.

Acquiring cultural competence

As medical providers and travel medicine practitioners are caring increasingly for patients of diverse sociocultural backgrounds, it is essential to acquire cultural competence. Patient satisfaction and compliance with medical recommendations and treatment are closely related to the effectiveness of communication and the quality of the patient–doctor relationship. Physicians need to understand how each patient's sociocultural background affects their health beliefs and behavior. Much

Table 20.1 A few questions to elicit the patient's explanatory model.

1. What do you (or other people) think has caused your problem?
2. Why do you think it started when it did?
3. What do you think your sickness does to you?
4. How severe is your sickness? Will it have a short or long course?
5. What kind of treatment do you think you should receive?
6. What are the most important results you hope to receive from this treatment?
7. What are the chief problems your sickness has caused for you?
8. What do you fear most about your sickness?

Source: Adapted from Kleinman et al. 1978 [4].

work has already been done in proposing ways for healthcare practitioners to recognize cultural differences and to understand better how patients perceive and experience their health condition or illness.

Acknowledgment and discussion of differences and similarities between the patient's and the healthcare practitioner's understanding lead to a negotiation process that will help in reaching a satisfactory solution [4]. A set of questions helping the clinician to elicit the patient model is given in Table 20.1. Language barriers may be such that working with interpreters and bilingual cultural mediators may be a necessity to provide effective communication between the practitioner and the patient to improve satisfaction and outcome.

To develop cultural competence, medical providers need to integrate health-related beliefs and cultural values, disease incidence and prevalence, and treatment efficacy.

Caring for patients: a patient-based approach

Healthcare practitioners should know about these characteristics and be aware of the epidemiology and clinical manifestations of diseases with which they may not be familiar. More important is the set of core values that should guide their practice.

Communication difficulties, uncertainties about the real needs of the patient, the administrative and financial constraints related to the status of the migrant, and previous traumatic experience that may impair the patient–doctor relationship are all factors that may lead to misunderstanding and frustration on the part of the healthcare practitioner and the patient. This often reflects inherent differences in cultural values and expectations. It may translate into mistrust, or lack of understanding and compassion. As Green and Betancourt stated: "at the heart of any meaningful and successful medical encounter (especially across cultures) there are three core values: empathy, curiosity and respect" [5]. Of course, this triad applies to all patients, not just migrants, but it is crucial to respect it in cross-cultural practice where differences may be more profound and may have a negative influence on the patient–doctor relationship. Learning, understanding, and responding to the patient's feelings and needs are essential. A patient-based approach is at the center of any medical encounter. Taking the time to learn from the patients themselves about their cultures and their belief allows an understanding of their needs and avoids the risk of stereotyping.

References

1 Gushulak B, MacPherson D. *Migration Medicine and Health. Principles and Practice*. Hamilton, ON: BC Decker, 2006.
2 Robjant K, Hassan R, Katona C. Mental health implications of detaining asylum seekers: systematic review. *Br J Psychiatry* 2009; **194**: 306–312.
3 Centers for Disease Control and Prevention. Trends in tuberculosis – United States, 2013. *MMWR Morb Mortal Wkly Rep 2014*; **63**: 229–233. http://www.cdc.gov/mmwr/preview/mmwrhtml/mm6311a2.htm (accessed 2 February 2015).
4 Kleinman A, Eisenberg L, Good B. Culture, illness, and care. Clinical lessons from anthropologic and cross-cultural research. *Ann Intern Med* 1978; **82**: 251–258.
5 Green AR, Betancourt JR. Cultural competence: a patient-based approach to caring for immigrants. In: Walker PF, Barnett ED (eds.) *Immigrant Medicine*. Philadelphia, PA: Saunders-Elsevier, 2007, pp. 83–97.

CHAPTER 21

Study-abroad programs: student health and safety issues

Gary Rhodes[1] & Gary W. Brunette[2]

[1] *University of California at Los Angeles, Los Angeles, CA, USA*
[2] *Centers for Disease Control and Prevention, Atlanta, GA, USA*

Special risks faced by students who study and travel abroad

International travel and study can be a life-changing experience for students, who gain an opportunity to understand better peoples and cultures outside their home country and stand to learn much about themselves and others. People who study abroad face the same risks as all other travelers, but may have an additional layer of risks according to their activities and behaviors.

The most recent data from the Institute of International Education show that annually 283,332 American students study outside the United States for some part of their degree [1], and 46,571 Americans study for full degrees at foreign universities [2]. Recent data have shown an increase in the volume of international study and also an increase in travel to non-traditional study venues that are associated with a variety of health and safety challenges.

In the United States and other developed countries, colleges and universities follow minimum local, state, and national government health and safety standards. An example is the enforcement of minimum fire codes in campus buildings and dormitories. In the United States, the Clery Act requires institutions to provide an annual report of safety incidents and regular updates on safety conditions on and around campus. Additionally, communication systems can provide immediate information by telephone, text, and email about any safety issue that would be of concern for the campus community. These standards and systems for campuses may not exist in other countries.

Many US and European campuses have a student health center and mental health support services easily available for students, with staff and physicians who have formal training. This support may not be available on campuses in other countries, or there may be language barriers for students who wish to access it.

Although most students easily manage the physical and mental health challenges and the realities of campus life in their home countries, they are in familiar surroundings; their daily lives follow a familiar schedule, they understand the language

Essential Travel Medicine, First Edition.
Edited by Jane N. Zuckerman, Gary W. Brunette and Peter A. Leggat.
© 2015 John Wiley & Sons, Ltd. Published 2015 by John Wiley & Sons, Ltd.

fluently, and they are at ease with the culture. Students who travel to a foreign campus may experience difficulties adjusting to their new environment and may pay less attention to their physical well-being. They may also not be aware of psychological stressors, may not recognize mental health problems, and may not receive counseling for stress management or effectively manage mental health medications.

American social norms can be protective on US campuses. As tobacco use and driving under the influence of alcohol or drugs are increasingly recognized as destructive, students in the United States may feel peer pressure not to engage in these behaviors. These social norms may not be the same in more permissive countries, and students may feel free to engage in destructive behavior. Conversely, studying in less permissive countries may actually be protective against risky behavior.

Special challenges for international travel

One of the key challenges for supporting students traveling internationally is that the methods of program development and implementation vary for different programs, institutions, and locations, and the type of program (study, volunteer, internship, community services, research, etc.). No governing institution reviews and approves health and safety policies and procedures for study-abroad programs. As a result, students should review the health policies and procedures for their program and be actively engaged in their health and safety before, during, and after their international experience. The following list of health and safety issues is a place to start when advising students about what issues they might face [3]:

• alcohol and drug use and abuse
• conflict between students or between students and program faculty/staff
• crime and violence
• crisis management
• emergency communication
• environmental challenges and disaster response
• faculty and staff leaders with limited knowledge and skills to support effective decision-making for health and safety
• fire safety
• kidnapping and terrorism
• legal issues abroad
• medical and physical health response
• mental health support
• political instability challenges and response
• responding to discrimination abroad
• responding to guidance by the US Centers for Disease Control and Prevention
• responding to guidance by the US Department of State
• laboratory hazards
• sexual harassment and assault
• supporting students with special needs and disabilities
• transportation safety
• tropical diseases and special health issues in the developing world

- water safety
- other health and safety challenges based on the local environment.

Less than 4% of all students who study abroad as a part of their US degree program do so for more than a semester. Therefore, on top of the challenges listed above, students may pack their time abroad with many non-academic activities so that they can experience as much as possible in a relatively short period of time. As a result, students abroad may take health risks that they would not otherwise take.

One of the challenges is students who are looking for the excitement of high-risk activities to make their overseas experience as memorable as possible. For example, this has resulted in the arrest of university students who took part in political unrest and protests abroad. To reduce costs of travel during their free time, students may also make poor transportation decisions (such as driving at night on unsafe roads, traveling in open buses, using unauthorized taxis, etc.). Students have become injured or died abroad from high-risk activities such as diving into water while intoxicated. There have also been study-abroad students who drowned in the ocean because they were weak swimmers or did not understand local rip currents.

Risk management to support student health and safety abroad

The following actions can guide students and parents in the decision-making process for choosing an international travel program:

- **Risk assessments** – Before making decisions about travel abroad, students should review the health and safety issues for the particular location and program abroad. Faculty and staff can help implement risk assessments. However, program leaders may not have the expertise to do a comprehensive health and safety risk assessment. Country-specific information from governmental organizations such as, in the United States., the US Department of State and the US Centers for Disease Control and Prevention can be helpful. In the United Kingdom, for example, the British Council provides similar comprehensive information alongside the National Travel Health Network and Centre, which is supported by Public Health England. However, reliable information from local authorities is critical. Using other international travel experts/companies such as International SOS and iJet can also be useful to understand local conditions better.
- **Risk management** – Once the risks are understood, students and parents must make an informed decision about whether they are comfortable taking the risks. If students still want to participate in the program, they can learn how best to manage the risks. This can include understanding local transportation safety issues, learning the local language and customs, and learning how to swim.
- **Pre-departure travel health consultation** – Students should have a comprehensive medical examination before international travel. Suggested elements of a pre-travel consultation should include ensuring that [4]:
  - The student is up-to-date on all their routine vaccines and has received any additional vaccines that may be needed for the particular destination.
  - The student has all medications that may be recommended.

- The student is aware of health advice and guidelines, such as
  - country- and region-specific health information
  - food and water safety
  - insect bite precautions
  - gender-specific health information.
- **Students' special needs** – It is important to understand any potential special needs and support which students may require. Certain study-abroad programs may not sufficiently support physical or mental health needs. An important and useful resource in the United States. to support special-needs students during study abroad is Mobility International USA, which is funded by the US Department of State (www.miusa.org). Similar resources may be available in other countries.
- **Orientation of faculty/staff/program leaders** – It is critical that faculty and staff leading programs be trained to manage situations they may encounter overseas. They should be actively involved in all stages of the process, including learning about the risks associated with a particular destination or program, developing an appropriate itinerary with comprehensive support, and in decision-making during the program. Examples of incidents that have occurred and highlight inadequate training in risk management include the following:
  - A student complains to the faculty leader of sexual harassment from a host family father. The student is not removed from the host family and is later sexually assaulted.
  - A group vehicle driven by a faculty leader goes over the side of a hill, resulting in the death of a student.
  - A faculty leader permits travel in an area known for risk of bandits. The group bus is forced to the side of the road where students are robbed and some are sexually assaulted.
  - A student becomes ill in a country where they are not fluent in the language. The student is taken to a medical facility and left there without supervision by a faculty member. The student is given the wrong medical procedure and is sexually assaulted while under anesthesia.
- **Orientation before leaving** – Students must be provided with a comprehensive and realistic orientation of the areas they will be visiting and the expected health and safety issues and challenges for the participants in the program. It is also important to highlight both available resources and those resources that will not be available [5]. Students should be familiar with the medical and mental health support system in the country.
- **Medical care** – To manage physical and mental health needs effectively, students and parents should ensure that critical support is available and accessible at the destination and that special support can be provided in a crisis.
- **Medical and evacuation insurance** – All study-abroad students should have adequate access to 24-hour emergency assistance and have comprehensive health insurance which covers all medical care and procedures and the cost of emergency evacuation, if needed.
- **Emergency response drills** – To support the ability of students to respond to potential emergencies abroad, programs must possess and practice emergency

response procedures. Depending on program length, activities, and students' needs, health and safety orientations should be ongoing.

- **Support services** – Students should be aware of all available support services for issues that they may face. They should be made aware of which services they would expect at their home campus that may not be available for students in some locations.
- **Emergency communication** – Students should be able to communicate with their home program at all times in the event they need support. They should have a full list of emergency contacts and have access to communications. A cell-phone and email are often sufficient. In areas where cell-phone coverage is not supported, a group satellite telephone may be necessary to support continuous communication.
- **Crime and safety records** – Institutions should keep and disseminate information about health and safety incidents to inform planning and program implementation. In the United States and for study-abroad programs, the Clery Act has mandated adequate record keeping on college and university campuses in order to inform parents and students about potential health and safety risks [6].
- **Emergency action plan** – Faculty and staff should be trained to take on leadership roles in avoiding and managing emergency situations abroad. They must participate in developing an emergency action plan to manage crises and they should train students how to respond to crises.
- **Evaluation and feedback** – Faculty, staff, and students should be able to evaluate all aspects of the program and provide feedback to improve health and safety support.

Conclusion

Many health and safety challenges exist with international travel for students. Understanding potential risks, limiting identified risks, and then implementing policies and procedures to manage risks and avoid potential health and safety challenges can result in programs that support student health and safety needs. By managing these processes effectively, students can take part in international study and travel, and have a safe and healthy experience abroad that can provide international learning and understanding not available in their home country.

References

1 Institute of International Education. *Open Doors Data: U.S. Study Abroad.* New York: Institute of International Education, 2013. http://www.iie.org/Research-and-Publications/Open-Doors/Data/US-Study-Abroad (accessed 3 December 2013).
2 Belyavina R, Li J, Bhandari R. *New Frontiers: U.S. Students Pursuing Degrees Abroad.* New York: Institute of International Education, 2013.
3 Center for Global Education. SAFETI audit checklist: analyzing risks and capabilities. *SAFETI Clearinghouse: Safety Abroad First – Education Travel Information.* Los Angeles, CA: Center for

Global Education, UCLA. http://globaled.us/safeti/crisis_and_management/analyze_risk_ and_capabilities.asp (accessed 9 December 2013).

4 Rhodes G, Romana I, Ebner J. Study abroad and other international student travel. In: Brunette G (ed.) *CDC Health Information for International Travel 2014: The Yellow Book*. New York: Oxford University Press, 2014, pp. 598–601.

5 Office of Postsecondary Education. *The Handbook for Campus Safety and Security Reporting*. Washington, DC: Department of Education, 2011.

6 Interorganizational Task Force on Safety and Responsibility in Study Abroad. *Responsible Study Abroad: Good Practices for Health & Safety*, 2002. https://www.nafsa.org/uploadedFiles/ responsible_study_abroad.pdf (accessed 3 December 2013).

CHAPTER 22

Humanitarian aid workers, disaster relief workers, and missionaries

Brian D. Gushulak & Douglas W. MacPherson

Migration Health Consultants, Inc., Qualicum Beach, BC, Canada

Introduction

Humanitarian aid workers, disaster relief workers, and missionaries represent a diffuse group of international travelers. They share significant similarities in terms of travel health risk. They can be distinguished from other groups of travelers by their risk profiles. The focus of this chapter is on operational field workers in these activities. Depending on the size and complexity of the organization involved, not all of them may be "in the field" and, as a consequence, not all workers in the humanitarian sector share the same risk profiles. For the purpose of this chapter, the term "workers" will be used, recognizing that within and between groups that there are significant differences to be considered. This chapter does not reiterate the general assessment and interventions discussed for other international travelers.

Historical overview

Historically, humanitarian, relief, or missionary actions involved the provision of direct assistance to those in need in the immediate community. Early hospitals and care-giving institutions were often associated with temples or religious orders. As society developed, assistance and missionary activities were extended to those at greater distance. Many of these early organized activities were associated with conflict; such as the origin of the Red Cross in relation to the Battle of Solferino in 1859 [1]. Others manifested themselves in compassion for human suffering and/or evangelicalism as exploration and colonization expanded the understanding of the world [2].

Modern humanitarian service can be seen as an extension and institutionalization of these early altruistic actions.

Essential Travel Medicine, First Edition.
Edited by Jane N. Zuckerman, Gary W. Brunette and Peter A. Leggat.
© 2015 John Wiley & Sons, Ltd. Published 2015 by John Wiley & Sons, Ltd.

Current perspectives - the scope of need

At the present time, providing assistance and missionary services to those in need takes place across the planet. The United Nations estimated the number of people in need of humanitarian assistance in 2011 at 62 million individuals [3]. Humanitarian aid, disaster relief, and missionary workers deliver service in situations that result from both natural and man-made events (Table 22.1). When these situations occur, they generate immediate response activities that result in the mobilization of workers to locations of acute need. The duration of the response varies and many other workers travel to assist in long-standing situations.

The level of assistance ranges from individuals or small organizations operating alone, to non-governmental organizations (NGOs), government agencies and

Table 22.1 Characteristics of humanitarian/missionary responses.

Nature of event
- Natural
  - Weather related
    - Storms
    - Floods
    - Droughts
    - Extreme heat/cold
  - Geological
    - Earthquakes
    - Volcanic activity
    - Landslides
- Man made
  - Social equity, equality, and political disparities
  - Conflict
    - Military
    - Social
  - Accidents
  - Forced population displacement
  - Poverty/deprivation
  - Food insecurity

Characteristics of events
- Duration
  - Acute
  - Recurrent
  - Concurrent events: disaster + civil unrest + outbreaks
  - Post-event/transitional
  - Chronic
- Location
  - Urban/rural
  - Coastal/mountainous
  - Arid/flood prone
  - Locations affected by extreme weather

departments, and finally large and structured international agencies and organizations. The service network is large and very diverse. There are estimated to be more than 250 international NGOs involved in humanitarian activity [4]. For some, assisting in humanitarian or disaster relief operations is a periodic activity involving temporary absence from their normal place of work and residence. For others, humanitarian help and assistance are their vocation involving extended periods of time, or their entire life's work, devoted to assisting those in need.

The person

Estimates of the numbers of humanitarian, disaster, and faith-based workers are imprecise. In 2010, there were an estimated 275,000 active humanitarian workers. It is believed that this number is growing by approximately 4% annually [5]. The number of foreign missionaries may be even greater, with estimates in excess of 400,000 individuals [6].

The nature of humanitarian and disaster response activity ensures that many workers are young, healthy, and altruistic. Their engagement in the response activity may be part of an organizational plan or an individual commitment. Their training, preparedness, experience, and field exposures are variable and their response to the work environment may be unpredictable [7]. Risk-taking behaviors, alcohol or substance abuse, and event-related stress are common in this group.

Practice point:

- A detailed profile of the worker and their personal health history will assist in risk assessment. The greatest impacts tend to be physical fatigue, mental burn-out, shifting social practice norms, and acquired risk-taking behaviors [8].

In addition to younger workers, many involved in humanitarian and missionary activities are an older age cohort who use work leave time or early retirement to become involved in field work. Despite their greater life experience, they may also bring the physical, mental, and health consequences of their age. The expectations and needs of those with pre-existing medical conditions can impact on field preparedness and adaptivity.

Practice point:

- The pre-departure evaluation should include a thorough review of the worker's health in terms of need and availability of medications, required investigations, or follow up for pre-existing conditions. This review should be undertaken in the context of capacity of the health and medical infrastructure available in the field.

The place and prevalence gaps

Many events requiring an international humanitarian response occur in resource-limited environments. The magnitude of the impact of the event itself maybe compounded by chronic social, economic, and political disparity which exceeds local response capacities. Some humanitarian emergencies and disasters become increasingly complex events owing to cascading levels of destruction or system failures. Typical examples are the post-earthquake response requirements in Pakistan (2011) and Haiti (2010), both of which caused enormous infrastructure loss and were followed by disease outbreaks [9,10]. Resource-rich countries are not exempt from needing a rapid and effective international response to acute events. The Tohoku earthquake followed by a tsunami and the Fukishima Daiichi Nuclear Power plant disaster in Japan are an example of a cascading series of events requiring an international response in a wealthy nation [11].

In these situations, health and well-being can be affected by many conditions, some of which may have existed prior to the event itself. Workers may have to live and work while exposed to the effects of harsh climatic conditions, endure severe limits in available or surviving infrastructure (e.g., accommodation, transportation, food, civil security, medical and public health resources) and may be exposed to endemic and outbreak disease risks that are different from those in their normal place of residence or employment. The social, political, legal, and ethical environments in which the workers will operate can have direct effects on their health in terms of violence, injury, and other harms. These "gaps" in the workers pre-departure and working environments need to be assessed before, during, and on return from deployment.

Practice points:
- Changing needs for operatives in the field due to changing circumstances need to be planned for and are best done prior to departure; including evacuation planning. Humanitarian workers destined to events of this type may require referral for specialized training and counseling in dealing with the consequences [12].
- Prospective humanitarian and aid workers should be evaluated in terms of latent or other diseases that may be uncommon or novel in the geographic area of the future activities. Pre-departure treatment or preventive measures may be indicated and should be discussed with the workers.

Response activities can frequently place providers in situations where they experience or witness illness, injury, and death. Some studies have indicated that the risk of death from violence and the need for medical evacuations and hospitalizations in humanitarian workers is about 6/10,000 person-years of deployment [13]. Humanitarian worker deaths due to violence involve both inexperienced and veteran workers. Many deaths occur early in a deployment, perhaps before threats have been fully assessed and risks recognized [14].

Since the end of the Cold War, conflict situations that create humanitarian need more frequently involve disrupted states rather than wars between nations [15]. In these situations, the risks to civilians and workers may be greater than those involving "traditional" warfare between states. Humanitarian and faith-based workers may also find themselves the direct targets of kidnapping, violence, or death [16].

For the past several years the majority of the attacks on humanitarian workers resulting in fatalities have involved a small number of nations experiencing active armed conflict and low levels of rule of law: Afghanistan, Somalia, Sudan, Pakistan, and Syria are recently reported to have the largest number of incidences of violence against humanitarian workers [17].

Practice point:
- Workers destined to locations with high risks of personal violence should be referred for specialized security briefings and counseling.

The purpose

A detailed assessment of the role and function of the worker is an essential part of the risk assessment. In acute events or rapidly evolving emergencies, the actual activities of the worker may end up being different from those originally anticipated. Preparedness for variability in both the work and social pressures during an event response are important.

Practice point:

- The health risk assessment includes medical issues but goes beyond that to factors of response and adaptability to changes in environment, behavior, social, and ethical contexts. Identification of many of these impacts requires pre-deployment, during-deployment, and post-deployment evaluation.

The processes

Whether institutionally sponsored (NGO, government, or faith-based organization) or individually engaged, there are processes to be aware of in worker's deployment to the field. Some of these are official and regulatory (e.g., passports, visas, travel permits, and health requirements such as yellow fever vaccination under the International Health Regulations). Others are organizational requirements or guidelines (e.g., health kits, insurance) including specific medical examination and/or immunizations required by the employing agency or organization.

Practice points:

- Contingency plans should be developed for those workers with specific needs or concerns (e.g., diabetic diets or food intolerances, maintenance medical therapy) including communication capacity and access to the tools for communication.
- It is suggested that workers prepare and carry personal health and support kits during their deployments [18]. Descriptions of the nature and contents of these kits are available [19].
- Routine travel or medical insurance may not provide cover in areas of conflict or to regions where travel advisories or warnings have been issued. Workers should be aware of the cover available and provided by their employer or agency, and the limitations and exclusions in any policies. Those without organizational cover should obtain adequate cover elsewhere. Medical evacuation cover should be taken.

Field operations are physically and mentally stressful. Burnout, anxiety, stress, depression, and post-traumatic stress disorder (PTSD) can occur in up to 30% of some humanitarian workers [20]. Periodic assessment of the worker in the field, and periods of leave, need to be part of the sustainability and continuity planning for the worker and the response efforts.

Practice points:

- Travel medicine providers should review risk factors for stress and depression, including adverse outcomes following previous deployments and history of alcohol or substance dependence. Advice on recognizing the signs and symptoms of stress-related illness and the importance of adequate social support networks during and following deployment should be provided [21].

- Some humanitarian and aid workers are involved in the direct provision of medical care. These activities may be associated with the risk of blood-borne or hospital-acquired infections [22].
- Humanitarian workers involved in healthcare should be considered for pre-deployment baseline serology for blood-borne infections such as HBV, HCV, and HIV and have baseline two-step tuberculin skin testing (TST) undertaken.
- Those working in locations where antiretroviral post-exposure preventive therapy may not be easily available may wish to add these agents to their personal effects.
- Rapid diagnostic test kits (e.g., malaria) may be appropriate for some workers in resource-poor areas.

Missionaries, although experiencing the same risks and travel health considerations as other humanitarian and disaster response workers, may have additional issues that require attention [23].

Practice points:

- The duration of missions can be many years, creating the need to review the implications of long-term residence in areas of potential health risk. Examples include the practicality of long-term therapy for tropical diseases such as malaria and periodic screening for diseases (e.g., routine health screening for hypertension, cervical, breast, and colonic cancer screening; viral hepatidities, tuberculosis, schistosomiasis, HIV).
- Missionaries are often accompanied by family members, raising issues ranging from planning for pregnancy and childbirth, raising children abroad, and managing family health emergencies, including death abroad. These populations differ from routine travelers and from humanitarian and disaster responders, and specific references and guidelines for them should be considered [24].

Post-deployment review

Workers, particularly those who have been involved in acute events or those returning from long (greater than 3 month) deployments should receive a detailed debriefing and medical review. Attention should be given to any disease, illness, or injury acquired or experienced during the deployment.

Practice points:

- Humanitarian workers involved in dealing with mass casualties or fatalities, conflict, violence, and trauma should be considered for referral for critical incident counseling [25].
- Those working in medical or healthcare fields or those exposed to blood and body fluids or respiratory secretions should have repeat serologic examination and repeat TST carried out at clinically appropriate intervals.
- Those with signs or symptoms of new or increased levels of anxiety, stress, or depression or those with any symptoms of PTSD should be referred for more detailed evaluation and counseling.

References

1 Forsythe DP. *The Humanitarians – The International Committee of the Red Cross.* New York: Cambridge University Press, 2005.

2 Neill S, Chadwick O. *A History of Christian Missions,* 2nd edn. London: Penguin Books. 1991.

3 Global Humanitarian Assistance. *GHA Report 2012.* Wells: Development Initiatives, 2013. http://www.globalhumanitarianassistance.org/wp-content/uploads/2012/07/GHA_Report _2012-Websingle.pdf (accessed 18 June 2013).

4 Harvey P, Stoddard A, Harmer A, et al. *The State of the Humanitarian System: Assessing Performance and Progress. A Pilot Study.* London: ALNAP, Overseas Development Institute, 2010. http://www.alnap.org/pool/files/alnap-sohs-final.pdf (accessed June 17 2013).

5 Taylor G, Stoddard A, Harmer A, et al. *The State of the Humanitarian System, 2012 Edition.* London: ALNAP, Overseas Development Institute, 2012. http://www.alnap.org/pool/files/alnap-sohs-2012-lo-res.pdf (accessed 18 June 2013).

6 Johnson TM, Barrett DB, Crossing PF. Christianity 2012: the 200th anniversary of American foreign missions. *Int Bull Missionary Res* 2012; **36**: 28–29.

7 Fhogartaigh CN, Sanford C, Behrens RH. Preparing young travellers for low resource destinations. *BMJ* 2012; **345**: e7179.

8 Eriksson CB, Bjorck J, Abernethy A. Occupational stress, trauma, and adjustment in expatriate humanitarian aid workers. In: Fawcett J (ed.) *Stress and Trauma Handbook: Strategies for Flourishing in Demanding Environments.* Monrovia, CA: World Vision International, 2003, pp. 68–100.

9 Gushulak BD, MacPherson DW. The basic principles of migration health: population mobility and gaps in disease prevalence. *Emerg Themes Epidemiol* 2006; **3**: 3.

10 Lantagne D, Balakrish Nair G, Lanata CF, Cravioto A. The cholera Outbreak in Haiti: where and how did it begin? *Curr Top Microbiol Immunol* 2014; **379**: 145–164.

11 Christodouleas JP, Forrest RD, Ainsley CG, et al. Short-term and long-term health risks of nuclear-power-plant accidents. *N Engl J Med* 2011; **364**: 2334–2341.

12 Elsharkawi H, Sandbladh H, Aloudat T, et al. Preparing humanitarian workers for disaster response: a Red Cross/Red Crescent field training model. *Humanit Exch* 2010; **46**: 45–47. http://www.odihpn.org/humanitarian-exchange-magazine/issue-46/preparing-humanitarian-workers-for-disaster-response-a-red-cross/red-crescent-field-training-model (accessed 29 July 2013).

13 Rowley EA, Crape BL, Burnham GM. Violence-related mortality and morbidity of humanitarian workers. *Am J Disaster Med* 2008; **3**: 39–45.

14 Sheik M, Gutierrez MI, Bolton P, et al. Deaths among humanitarian workers. *BMJ* 2000; **321**: 166–168.

15 Burkle FM. Lessons learnt and future expectations of complex emergencies. *BMJ* 1999; **319**: 422–426.

16 Kofi AF. Humanitarian action under fire: reflections on the role of NGOs in conflict and post-conflict situations. *Int Peacekeeping* 2012; **19**: 203–216.

17 Humanitarian Outcomes. *The Aid Worker Security Database,* 2012. https://aidworkersecurity .org/ (accessed 3 July 2013).

18 Aitken P, Leggat P, Robertson A, et al. Health and safety aspects of deployment of Australian disaster medical assistance team members: results of a national survey. *Travel Med Infect Dis* 2009; **7**: 284–290.

19 Gushulak BD. Humanitarian aid workers. In: Brunette G (ed.) CDC Health Information for International Travel 2012: *The Yellow Book*. New York: Oxford University Press, 2012, Chapter 8.

20 Antares Foundation. Managing stress in humanitarian workers. In: *Guidelines for Good Practice*, 3rd edn. http://www.antaresfoundation.org/download/managing_stress_in_ humanitarian_aid_workers_guidelines_for_good_practice.pdf (accessed 3 July 2013).

21 Lopes Cardozo B, Gotway Crawford C, Eriksson C, et al. Psychological distress, depression, anxiety, and burnout among international humanitarian aid workers: a longitudinal study. *PLoS One* 2012; **7**(9): e44948.

22 Kortepeter MG, Seaworth BJ, Tasker SA, et al. Health care workers and researchers traveling to developing-world clinical settings: disease transmission risk and mitigation. *Clin Infect Dis* 2010; **51**: 1298–1305.

23 Doty DB. Missionary health preparation. *Ensign* 2007; (March): 62–67. http://www.lds.org/ ensign/print/2007/03/missionary-health-preparation?lang=eng&clang=eng (accessed 4 June 2013).

24 McArthy AE. Long term travellers and expatriates. In: *Yellow Book 2012 – Health Information for International Travel* 2012. New York: Oxford University Press, 2012, Chapter 8. http://wwwnc.cdc.gov/travel/yellowbook/2012/chapter-8-advising-travelers-with-specific -needs/long-term-travelers-and-expatriates (accessed 12 June 2013).

25 Flannery RB, Jr., Everly GS, Jr. Crisis intervention: a review. *Int J Emerg Ment Health* 2000; **2**: 119–125.

CHAPTER 23

Long-term travelers

Claire Davies & Ted Lankester

InterHealth Worldwide, London, UK

Introduction

Long-term travelers form a diverse group including missionaries, aid workers, military, corporate employees, and backpackers away for an extended period. These patients pose particular conundrums to the travel medicine practitioner. The need to cope with a variety of challenges, such as disconnection from good health services, adverse living conditions, adjustment to weather extremes, cultural differences (particularly for women), uncertainty about the future, and high levels of exposure to the local population mean that these travelers are exposed to particular risks. Psychiatric problems, chronic diarrhea, and infectious diseases such as schistosomiasis are all more common [1], as is hepatitis B [2], while the risk of malaria rises exponentially with the period of exposure [3]. Despite these risks, only one-third may seek pre-travel advice. Many will also indulge in risk behavior [4]. This group therefore merits careful attention pre-trip, in addition to planning for support during the assignment and mid- or post-trip screening for a variety of physical and psychologic issues.

The pre-travel consultation

Sufficient time should be allowed for the pre-travel consultation, preferably a minimum of 30 minutes, paying careful attention to the following areas:
- Planning ahead for vaccinations as far as possible to allow time to complete courses of multi-dose vaccinations such as for rabies, Japanese encephalitis, and hepatitis B.
- Consideration of access to any booster vaccinations, particularly for those planning to be away for extended periods. Fallout from follow-up is common; electronic systems that send email reminders for overdue vaccinations may alleviate this.
- For children, consideration should be given to whether they will be following the vaccine schedule of their country of origin or that of their destination.
- Those who will be remote from good healthcare should receive education in the use of standby treatments for common conditions such as travelers' diarrhea.

Essential Travel Medicine, First Edition.
Edited by Jane N. Zuckerman, Gary W. Brunette and Peter A. Leggat.
© 2015 John Wiley & Sons, Ltd. Published 2015 by John Wiley & Sons, Ltd.

- It is worth remembering that less than one episode of illness in ten when traveling is vaccine preventable, so it is essential to prioritize health promotion and advice about other key health issues, including vehicle accidents.

Other matters pertinent to the individual and destination, such as malaria prevention, are considered in further detail below.

Malaria prevention in long-term travelers

Many travelers are averse to taking long-term medications and compliance with malaria prophylaxis has been shown to be poor [5,6]; nevertheless this area needs careful evaluation and should therefore be offered along with careful communication of the risks from malaria.

It is worth seeking advice from any official sources of information regarding long-term malaria prophylaxis endorsed by one's own government's health department, as these may vary between countries. However, there is increasing evidence of lack of harm from the use of long-term malaria prophylaxis and for many individuals this possibility may be outweighed by the risk of malaria. Those using chloroquine for longer than 5 years should be recommended to have an annual ophthalmic examination to screen for retinal toxicity. Rotation between different forms of prophylaxis is also an option where patients or clinicians are concerned about the risks.

In spite of this, many travelers decide to discontinue their prophylaxis. Such decisions carry differing levels of risk dependent upon the length of stay, seasonality of malaria, capability of local healthcare facilities, and the patient's medical background. If the traveler makes a decision to discontinue, then the travel medicine practitioner should offer other avenues of assistance in minimizing the risk:

- Careful education about symptoms and signs of malaria, including written information and access to remote high-quality advice.
- Consideration of seasonal prophylaxis for areas where there are periods of high transmission.
- Provision of standby treatment obtained from a reputable source with written instructions on its use.
- Reiteration of the need for personal protective measures.
- Reiteration of the need to retreat bednets with permethrin (often forgotten) or use long-lasting insecticide-impregnated nets.

Those traveling to their location for the first time should be strongly encouraged to be on malaria prophylaxis for a long enough period before they can be safely judged to have made an assessment of the risk in their locality with the support of an experienced travel medicine practitioner.

Patients often request rapid diagnostic tests, but these have not been shown to be reliable when used by non-clinicians. In addition, false negatives are common and they are unable to provide information on levels of parasitemia or parasite clearance following treatment [7].

Pre-travel medical assessment

Many sending employers insist on a medical examination for fitness, particularly when traveling to high-risk regions or where access to healthcare may be suboptimal. Pre-trip screening may take the form of a questionnaire or a face-to-face medical examination. Recent recordings of blood pressure, weight, and height should be included on questionnaires. Face-to-face medical examinations probably reduce the risk of non-disclosure in addition to allowing the clinician to assess the individual's knowledge of self-management of any chronic conditions and to offer tailored advice according to the individual and destination. A full blood count may be performed for those traveling to resource-poor areas. Those at increased cardiovascular risk should have further testing to include lipids, renal and liver function, and screening for diabetes.

Those with newly diagnosed significant chronic conditions, with a lack of knowledge of self-management, or with poorly controlled chronic conditions should defer travel until the issues have been addressed.

Psychological considerations

Mental health issues are common reasons for medical evacuation; therefore, this area needs careful attention [8,9]. Psychologists can usefully be involved pre-long-term travel by assessing psychologic resilience for the role and location and by providing self-help tools to increase resilience. Medical advisors may need to identify pre-existing psychologic health issues that may impact on the individual (or others), and advise employers on management support and adaptations if the advisor acts in an occupational health capacity.

Important areas to be explored include:
• a history of any psychiatric illness, especially those with current, recent, or recurrent symptoms
• a history of substance abuse: alcohol, drugs
• recent bereavement, separation, or life crises
• ability to have coped with previous stress
• psycho-social support networks.

If in doubt, a psychiatric opinion should be sought.

Individuals can be supported pre-travel to build resilience either individually with a psychologist or within a group setting, with the discussion targeted on supporting the traveler to manage stress levels with increased confidence and understanding.

Access to healthcare

It is important to discuss with travelers plans for how they might access healthcare while away. There are a few important differences to take into account:

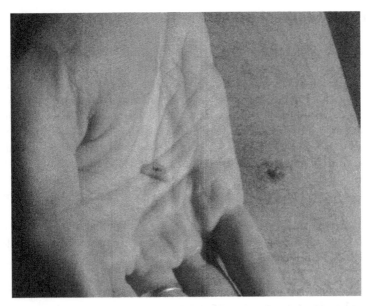

Figure 23.1 A tumbu fly diagnosed via telemedicine after emerging from a lesion in a patient previously treated for a skin abscess.

- Preparation for different healthcare "cultures." Some centers may have a tendency to over-investigate whereas others may lack resources to implement a minimum level of care.
- Adequate health insurance should be in place. It is usually possible to obtain cover for pre-existing conditions but at a higher premium. Travelers should be advised always to disclose any health conditions to their insurers.
- Those traveling to resource-poor areas should have access to some form of remote advice, preferably with a combination of an emergency telephone line and use of telemedicine. Figure 23.1 shows a tumbu fly diagnosed via telemedicine after emerging from a lesion in a patient previously treated for a skin abscess.
- Loss of a formal linkage to a health system means that individuals may fall out of screening programs, such as cervical screening. Use of electronic health records with reminder systems may help; otherwise, these issues can be managed by implementing a process of routine medical checks, usually instigated by employers.
- Travelers with chronic diseases need to consider how to access follow-up and monitoring and also a reliable source of medications. Arrangements should be in place for ongoing monitoring, including remote access to support from their specialist if needed.

Pregnancy and delivery

Those who choose to reside and deliver away from their country of origin need to consider whether the local antenatal care and facilities for delivery are of a sufficient standard with which the woman feels comfortable. Important differences may manifest as variability in the level of antenatal screening offered and local antenatal policies unsuitable for expatriates, such as intermittent preventive prophylaxis of malaria. Medical facilities in resource-poor areas may be less well resourced to cope with obstetric emergencies and lack the technology needed to deal with neonatal complications. Women should be encouraged to plan in advance for any pregnancy and base themselves near medical facilities that they have confidence in to offer both routine and emergency support. Moving to their nominated place of delivery is recommended early in the third trimester. For many, this means coming back their country of origin and has the added advantage of accessing family support.

The decision about when to return abroad with a new baby is individual and will depend on many factors, such as availability of health facilities in the country of travel, family issues, and work requirements of the spouse. It is wise at least to complete the 6-week postnatal check for mother and baby and the first set of immunizations before departure. Travelers residing in countries highly endemic for TB and/or hepatitis B should ask their doctor for a BCG vaccination at 6 weeks and hepatitis B vaccine to be given with the first three sets of immunizations if not included in their home country's health program. BCG vaccination is rarely used in the United States.

Post-travel support

Those who have been away for an extended period, particularly in a resource-poor area or where there are particular risks, should be offered a medical check at the end of their time abroad. Attention should be paid to:
- Review of any chronic disease management.
- Targeted screening for infectious diseases such as schistosomiasis, sexually transmitted infections, and blood-borne viruses as appropriate.
- Education about the potential for malaria to present after return.
- Investigation and management of any ongoing symptoms, e.g., chronic diarrhea.
- A full blood count should be taken, paying attention to eosinophilia plus a stool sample for parasitology. Diets rich in saturated fat are common in many parts of the world and a review of cardiovascular risk, including cholesterol measurement, may be indicated.
- The incidence of TB is higher in long-term travelers [10] and screening may be offered as either a Mantoux test or a blood test for an interferon-gamma-based assay, particularly for healthcare workers or those working in high-risk environments such as prisons. However, many travelers opt for no action unless symptoms start to develop.

"Reverse culture shock" is common and a medical check provides an opportunity for travelers to discuss their experiences. Spending time on enjoyable activities and ensuring time is spent with friends and family while maintaining links and relationships in connection with the country of travel can all promote reintegration. Children who have spent long periods in a variety of cultures (so-called "third culture kids") may benefit from organized activities with similar groups of children in their home country, so they do not feel too "different" or isolated.

Psychologic problems are common, especially depression and anxiety, but are often understated in the context of a rushed consultation [10]. Making time to listen

Table 23.1 Some suggestions for carrying out a post-trip psychologic evaluation.

- It can be done by an experienced physician or psychologist
- It is carried out over 90 minutes in a semi-structured discussion
- Establish personal empathy based on rapport and trust
- Explore and share the client's issues and feelings
- Hold and manage distress and pain
- Recognize signs of PTSD
- Discuss meanings or apparently lost meanings
- Agree on an action plan for further support

and engage is essential. Post-traumatic stress disorder may present or re-trigger years after the incident. Those with any significant symptoms should be offered psychologic support, but preferably from professionals who understand the context and conditions to which they have been exposed and the challenges of reintegration. Table 23.1 gives some suggestions for how to carry out a post-travel psychologic evaluation.

Those returning from long-term assignments or from any international travel that has been intense, remote, or dangerous will often have symptoms that are a mixture of the physical and the psychologic. In order to meet these needs effectively and to reduce the risk of chronic health problems developing, physicians need time, empathy, and training to listen, examine, investigate, and advise long-term travelers effectively.

References

1 Chen LH, Wilson ME, Davis X, et al. Illness in long-term travelers visiting GeoSentinel clinics. *Emerg Infect Dis* 2009; **11**: 1773–1782.
2 Smalligan RD, Lange WR, Frame JD, et al. The risk of viral hepatitis A, B, C and E among North American missionaries. *Am J Trop Med Hyg* 1995; **53**: 233–236.
3 Phillips-Howard PA, Radalowicz A, Mitchell J, Bradley DJ. Risk of malaria in British residents returning from malarious areas. *BMJ* 1990; **300**: 499–503.
4 Dahlgren AL, DeRoo L, Avril J, et al. Health risks and risk-taking behaviors among International Committee of the Red Cross expatriates returning from humanitarian missions. *J Travel Med* 2009; **16**: 382–390.
5 Hamer DH, Ruffing R, Callahan MV, et al. Knowledge and use of measures to reduce health risks by corporate expatriate employees in western Ghana. *J Travel Med* 2008; **15**: 237–242.
6 Burdon J. Use of malarial prophylaxis amongst a population of expatriate church workers in northeast Zaire. *J Travel Med* 1998; **5**: 36–38.
7 Whitty CJM, Armstrong M, Behrens RH. Self-testing for falciparum malaria with antigen-capture cards by travelers with symptoms of malaria. *Am J Trop Med Hyg* 2000; **63**: 295–297.
8 Patel D, Easmon CJ, Dow C, et al. Medical repatriation of British diplomats resident overseas. *J Travel Med* 2000; **7**: 64–69.
9 Foyle MF, Beer MD, Watson JP. Expatriate mental health. *Acta Psychiatr Scand* 1998; **97**: 278–283.
10 Cobelens FG, van Deutekom H, Draayer-Jansen IW, et al. Risk of infection with Mycobacterium tuberculosis in travellers to areas of high tuberculosis endemicity. *Lancet* 2000; **356**: 461–465.

SECTION IV
Environmental travel health risks

CHAPTER 24

Aviation and travel medicine

Michael Bagshaw[1], Ian C. Cheng[2], & Robert Bor[3]

[1] Cranfield University, Cranfield, UK
[2] James Cook University, Townsville, Queensland, Australia
[3] Royal Free London NHS Foundation Trust, London, UK

Physics of the flight environment

Atmospheric pressure

Total gas pressure falls with altitude in a regular manner, halving every 18,000 ft (5500 m), with the 21% oxygen proportion remaining constant to very high altitudes.

Atmospheric temperature

The atmospheric temperature reduces by 1.98 °C per 1000 ft (300 m) to the tropopause [40,000 ft (12,200 m)] [1,2].

Atmospheric ozone

The ozonosphere normally exists between 40,000 and 140,000 ft (12,200 and 42,700 m), with ozone concentrations up to 10 parts per million (ppm). Significant amounts of ozone do not form below 40,000 ft (12,200 m). Modern passenger jet aircraft are fitted with catalytic converters in the Environmental Control System (ECS), which break down ozone before it enters the pressurized cabin [1,3].

Cosmic radiation

Aircraft occupants are exposed to elevated levels of cosmic radiation of galactic and solar origin. The Earth's magnetic field provides protection from cosmic radiation approaching the atmosphere, with the protective effect greatest at the equator and least at the magnetic poles. The Earth's surface is shielded from cosmic radiation by the atmosphere, the ambient radiation increasing with altitude by approximately 15% for each increase of around 2000 ft (dependent on latitude).

Cosmic radiation doses

Doses are well within the limits recommended by the International Commission on Radiological Protection (ICRP). For occupational exposure these are a 5-year average

Essential Travel Medicine, First Edition.
Edited by Jane N. Zuckerman, Gary W. Brunette and Peter A. Leggat.
© 2015 John Wiley & Sons, Ltd. Published 2015 by John Wiley & Sons, Ltd.

effective dose of 20 mSv (millisieverts) per year, with no more than 50 mSv in a single year. The annual limit for the general public is 1 mSv.

Health risks of cosmic radiation
Although there is no level of ionizing radiation exposure below which effects may not occur, epidemiologic evidence indicates that the probability of airliner occupants suffering any abnormality or disease as a result of exposure to cosmic radiation is very low [1,4,5].

Physiology of flight

Because exposures are relatively rapid, brief, and not cumulative, flyers do not adapt to the hypoxic environment, unlike inhabitants of terrestrial high altitudes. However, the aircraft can be a means of transporting an individual to a high-altitude destination.

Hypoxia
This is a lack of sufficient oxygen to meet the needs of the body tissues. With increasing altitude, the air pressure decreases and above about 10,000 ft (3000 m) there is insufficient oxygen available to maintain adequate cerebral function. Flyers ascend to altitude in a matter of minutes and adapt to hypoxia by an increase in blood flow and a modest hyperventilation, limiting the effects of hypoxia. Individuals abruptly exposed to altitudes of 10,000 ft (3000 m) and above suffer mental and physical effects; above this altitude, supplementary oxygen must be used.

To allow a margin of safety, the maximum certified cabin altitude in pressurized passenger aircraft is 8000 ft (2440 m), at which barometric pressure is 565 mmHg and arterial oxygen pressure is around 55 mmHg (see the oxyhemoglobin dissociation curve in Figure 24.1), and venous oxygen pressures have only fallen by 1–2 mmHg.

The minimum cabin pressure of 565 mmHg (75.1 kPa) [8000 ft (2440 m)] will bring a healthy individual's arterial PaO_2 along the plateau of the oxyhemoglobin dissociation curve at the top of the steep part (Figure 24.1), still saturated. However, people with respiratory disease may have arterial oxygen pressures at ground level as low as 55–60 mmHg. Their further fall in arterial PaO_2 can be reversed completely by the administration of oxygen, 30% oxygen at 8000 ft (2440 m) being equivalent to breathing air at ground level. Given prior notice, most airlines can provide a personal oxygen supply for such passengers.

Aircraft pressurization
Aircraft operating below 10,000 ft (3000 m) do not require oxygen equipment. Most commercial passenger aircraft fly higher and maintain the cabin pressure above 565 mmHg [8000 ft (2440 m)], providing an environment in which the occupants breathe cabin air.

The cabin air supply is bled from the outside air entering the aircraft engine, or may be supplied via electrically driven compressors. The mixed conditioned air is distributed via overhead ducts and grills, circulated around the cabin, and extracted

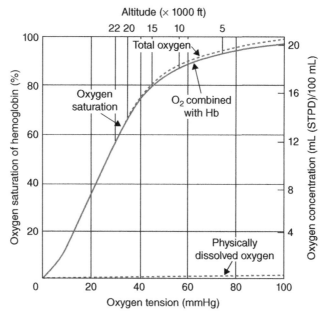

Figure 24.1 Oxygen dissociation curve for blood. Source: Zuckerman 2013 [35]. Reproduced with permission of Wiley.

through vents at floor level. Recirculated air is passed through high-efficiency particulate air (HEPA) filters of the same specification as used in hospital operating theaters; they are 99.99% efficient in the removal of physical contaminants and the product air is bacteriologically cleaner than the air in buildings, trains, or buses.

Although clean, the aircraft cabin air remains dry. During flight, moisture is derived from the activities of the cabin occupants and from the galleys and washrooms, giving a maximum relative humidity of 10–20%. These levels are associated with surface drying of the skin, mucous membranes, and cornea, which may cause discomfort. Normal homeostatic mechanisms prevent dehydration and there is no harm to health [2,6–10].

An emergency oxygen supply is provided in the event of failure of the pressurization system.

Mechanical effects of pressure change

The climb to cruise altitude takes about 30 minutes and involves a maximum fall of about 200 mmHg (26.6 kPa) in cabin pressure [to the equivalent of 8000 ft (2440 m)]. Descent to landing takes much the same time. Body fluids and tissues generally are virtually incompressible and do not alter shape to any important extent when such pressures changes are applied. The same is true of cavities such as the lungs, gut, middle ear, and facial sinuses that contain air, provided that they can vent easily. Gas-containing spaces that cannot vent easily behave differently.

Gas within will usually be at a pressure very close to that outside, and must follow Boyle's law. Ascent from ground level (760 mmHg) to 8000 ft (2440 m) (565 mmHg) will expand a given volume of trapped gas by about 35%. This may cause slightly uncomfortable gut distension in healthy people but it is not an important problem.

The cavity of the middle ear vents easily, but sometimes fails to fill because the lower part of the Eustachian tube behaves as a non-return valve, especially when it is inflamed. As a result, the cavity equilibrates easily on ascent but does not refill on descent, and the ear-drum bows inwards, causing pain that can be severe (otic barotrauma) [2,6,8–10].

Altitude-induced decompression illness

If ambient pressure falls quickly to less than half of its original value, the gas dissolved in blood and tissue fluids may come out of solution precipitously, forming bubbles and obstructing flow in small blood vessels.

Atmospheric pressure halves by 18,000 ft and decompression illness occurs rarely, if at all, below this altitude. It is very rare below 25,000 ft (7600 m) and therefore is normally of no concern at passenger aircraft cabin altitudes, which normally do not exceed 8000 m. However, it does occasionally occur in those passengers who have been exposed to a hyperbaric environment prior to flight, such as divers and tunnel workers. Sub-aqua divers can be at risk and are advised to allow a minimum of 12 hours to elapse between diving and flight, or 24 hours if the dive required decompression stops [10,11].

Clinical aspects of aviation medicine

Travel by air is a safe means of transport. However, from the physiologic point of view, flying is a means of putting susceptible people at risk, in addition to being a potential means of spreading infectious disease.

Jet lag

Apart from the homeostatic drive for sleep, the major influence on performance and alertness is the internal circadian clock. Circadian rhythms fluctuate on a regular cycle, which lasts something over 24 hours. Many body functions have their own circadian rhythm and they are synchronized to a 24-hour pattern by "zeitgebers" (time givers), light being among the most powerful.

Moving to a new light/dark schedule (as in time zone changes) leads to a discrepancy between internal body timing and external environmental cues. The internal clock can take days or weeks to readjust, depending on the number of time zones crossed (desynchronosis).

Fatigue is defined as the likelihood of falling asleep. Therefore, in practical terms, there is little difference between chronic fatigue and acute tiredness. Fatigue can be caused by sleep loss and circadian desynchronosis, but it can also result from low motivation and low levels of external stimulation.

Preventive measures

Preventive measures include the following:

- Sleep scheduling:
  - At home, the best possible sleep should be obtained before a trip.
  - On a trip, as much sleep per 24 hours should be obtained as at home.
  - Feelings should be trusted – if the individual feels sleepy and circumstances permit, then they should sleep.
- Good sleep habits:
  - A regular pre-sleep routine should be developed.
  - Sleep time should be kept protected.
  - The individual should avoid going to bed hungry, but should not eat or drink heavily before going to bed.
  - Alcohol and caffeine should be avoided before bedtime.

Bright light (more than 2500 lux), used at the appropriate time in the circadian cycle, can help to reset the circadian clock.

The best times for light exposure and light avoidance are dependent on the direction of travel and number of time zones crossed. The ideal is to make the best use of the natural zeitgebers in resetting the body clock.

Some people find drugs such as short-acting benzodiazepines helpful in promoting sleep and, if used for 2–3 days after travel, can assist in resetting the sleep cycle.

Melatonin is secreted by the pineal gland with a rhythm linked to the light/dark cycle through the suprachiasmatic nucleus. It is effective in inducing sleep when taken at the appropriate stage in the circadian cycle. However, if taken at the wrong stage, it can disrupt the sleep/wake cycle and destabilize sleep patterns. This limits its usefulness in treating jet lag.

There is no simple or single solution for combating the effects of jet lag. The individual has to evolve the strategies to suit his or her particular needs [12–15].

Travelers' thrombosis [deep venous thrombosis/venous thromboembolism (DVT/VTE)]

Long-haul travel is associated with prolonged periods of immobility, a recognized risk factor for deep venous thrombosis (DVT) first described by Virchow in 1856. However, there have been concerns as to whether there are other factors specific to air travel that further increase the risk.

In the general population, DVT occurs in 1–3 per 1000 people per year, of which 20% give rise to pulmonary embolism. The pathogenesis of thrombosis still relies on the basic premise of Virchow, who identified circulatory stasis, hypercoagulability, and endothelial injury as the risk factors.

Several clinical studies have shown an association between air travel and the risk of DVT, with the risk in travelers increasing with the distance traveled. A recent case–control study showed that all modes of travel increased the risk of DVT about twofold, with an absolute risk of one thrombosis per 6000 journeys; most cases of DVT are asymptomatic.

It has been found that combinations of risk factors synergistically increase the risk of thrombosis. In people with factor V Leiden, the risk of thrombosis after flying was increased about 14-fold, and in women using oral contraceptives, it was increased around 20-fold.

It has also been shown that the risk increases with the number of flights taken in a short time-frame and also with the duration of the flight. The majority of these clots are asymptomatic and disperse naturally.

Thus, even though the overall risk of DVT after air travel is only moderately increased, clear subgroups can be identified in whom the risk is higher.

The low humidity of the aircraft cabin does not in itself lead to dehydration. Excessive alcohol consumption may cause dehydration, but there is no evidence that this is a significant risk factor leading to DVT.

Two recent studies of reduced oxygen partial pressure with non-hypoxic control groups found no evidence of coagulation. There is no evidence that hypoxia or the hypobaric environment of an aircraft cabin is a significant risk factor for the development of DVT.

Although there is good evidence for the value of aspirin in preventing arterial thromboembolic disease, its role in the prevention of venous thromboembolic disease is much less clear. The side-effect profile is significant.

There is no evidence to support the use of aspirin in preventing the development of DVT during flight.

For those travelers at medium to high risk of DVT, there is evidence that the use of compression stockings appears to substantially lower the risk of asymptomatic DVT, but it remains unclear as to whether this reduction is clinically significant.

One study has shown that for 20–40% of travelers, the commercially available stockings do not fit adequately. It is essential for stockings to be correctly fitted so as to provide adequate compression to stimulate venous return.

Although the use of low molecular weight heparin for the prevention of DVT in the aviation setting is not supported by direct evidence, in a high-risk traveler consideration may be given to a single prophylactic dose prior to flying.

Although the relative risk of developing venous thrombosis when flying is significant, the absolute risk of developing symptomatic DVT is very low. The absolute risk of developing a pulmonary embolus during or after a flight between the United Kingdom and the east coast of the United States has been calculated as less than one in one million [2,16–18].

Medical practitioners need to be circumspect in advising any preventive measures, taking careful account of efficacy and risk profile of the preventive method.

Motion sickness

Motion sickness is a normal human response to unfamiliar motion and affects different individuals in different ways.

Causes

The causes are complex and there is no doubt that the vestibular apparatus in the inner ear plays an essential role.

Motion during travel may generate patterns of sensory input conflicting with those based on terrestrial experience, leading to central effects and motion sickness. Some people appear to have more sensitive vestibular systems than others.

Anxiety and hyperventilation may play a part in the development of motion sickness. Anxiety and tension increase the sensitivity of the whole nervous system, and if the vestibular system is already sensitive, the anxiety can take it above the critical level. Hyperventilation acts in a similar way by increasing nerve sensitivity, making motion sickness more likely in a susceptible individual.

Alcohol increases the sensitivity of the vestibular system and the after-effects may play a role in some cases.

Prevention

The human body has a remarkable ability to adapt to new sensations. With continued exposure to a provocative environment, such as flying, new sensory patterns become accepted as the norm and motion sickness occurs less easily.

To avoid motion sickness, stimulation of the semicircular canals should be minimized by limiting head movement. For an individual known to be susceptible to motion sickness, this advice should be followed *before* the onset of symptoms.

Vision is powerful and it is good practice to fix the gaze on a stable, distant horizon. If there is no horizon, for example when flying in cloud, it helps to rest the head on the back of the seat and keep the eyes closed. Bending the head forward to read induces motion sickness in the susceptible individual and should be avoided.

It makes little difference whether one eats before a flight. Motion sickness originates in the vestibular system, not the stomach, so one should eat as normal, maintaining the blood sugar level. Similarly, smells and heat are not causes.

An effective drug is hyoscine. Cinnarizine is effective for longer but must be taken at least 30 minutes before exposure to provocative motion. Both have side effects, including drowsiness.

It helps to avoid alcohol and, in the case of people who are prone to motion sickness, this should be for at least 24 hours prior to flying [9,19].

Passenger fitness to fly

Medical clearance is required when:
- fitness to travel is in doubt as a result of recent illness, hospitalization, injury, surgery. or instability of an acute or chronic medical condition;
- special services are required (e.g., oxygen, stretcher, or authority to carry or use medical equipment).

Medical clearance is not required for carriage of a disabled passenger outside these categories, although special needs (such as a wheelchair) must be reported to the airline at the time of booking.

It is vital that passengers carry essential medication with them, and not pack it in their checked baggage.

Deterioration on holiday or on a business trip of a previously stable condition, or an accident, can require medical clearance for the return journey. A stretcher may be needed, together with medical support, which can incur considerable cost. Travel insurance is always essential.

Assessment criteria

The passenger's exercise tolerance can provide a useful guide on fitness to fly; if unable to walk a distance greater than about 50 m without developing dyspnea, the passenger is unlikely to tolerate the relative hypoxia of the pressurized cabin. Guidance is provided on the web sites of the Aerospace Medical Association and the British Thoracic Society [2,9,20–22].

Most airlines require information to be submitted via a standard medical information form (MEDIF) available on the web site of the airline or the International Air Transport Association (IATA). Table 24.1 summarizes the guidelines recommended by one international carrier. This list is not exhaustive, and it should be remembered that individual cases might require individual assessment by the attending physician. Table 24.2 summarizes the web sites providing medical information for fitness to fly assessment.

Spread of infectious disease

There is no evidence that the pressurized cabin makes transmission of disease any more likely. The risk of disease transmission to susceptible passengers, by person-to-person droplet spread within the aircraft cabin, is associated with sitting within two rows of a contagious passenger for a flight time of more than 8 hours [2,23–27]. Obviously, individuals should not travel with a febrile illness.

Mental health issues in aviation

Air travel can exacerbate existing psychologic disorders in airline passengers; it can also trigger psychologic problems and abnormal behavior in otherwise healthy people. Motion sickness, stress associated with travel generally, claustrophobia, disrupted sleep and eating routines, and being brought into close physical proximity with strangers, can challenge even the most resilient flyers [28,29]. Crowds at airports and aircraft noise, hunger, unusual food, and language and communication difficulties are common sources of stress for passengers, as is anticipation or apprehension about what lies ahead at the end of the journey.

When denied their usual routines, some people exhibit primitive distress, which may manifest as anger, withdrawal, expression of a sense of entitlement, or inability to cope. Although this is not mental illness *per se*, it may reflect personal stress and distress [30].

Fear of flying

Given high accident rates in the very early years of flying, often leading to injury or death, a fear of flying in the first part of the twentieth century could be considered a rational reaction to a dangerous activity. Since that time, civil aviation has become so safe that flying may even be safer than staying at home, driving, or taking a train. Consequently, in the modern era, a fear of flying is no longer viewed as rational [31].

Fear of flying is defined as "A specific phobia characterized by a marked, persistent, excessive fear that is precipitated by the experience or immediate prospect of air travel" [32]. Exposure to the phobic stimulus almost invariably provokes an anxiety response, which the individual may experience as uncomfortable and unwelcome, and which produces significant interference or psychologic distress. There are

Table 24.1 Guidelines for medical clearance.

Category	Do not accept	Remarks
Cardiovascular disorders	Uncomplicated myocardial infarction within 7 days	Myocardial infarction less than 21 days requires MEDIF assessment
	Uncontrolled heart failure	This includes CABG and valve surgery.
	Open heart surgery within 10 days	MEDIF assessment required up to 21 days postoperatively. Transpositions, ASD/VSD, transplants, etc., will require discussion with airline medical advisor
,	Angioplasty: No stenting 3 days With stenting 5 days	
Circulatory disorders	Active thrombophlebitis of lower limbs	Recently commenced anticoagulation therapy requires assessment
	Bleeding/clotting conditions	
Blood disorders	Hb <7.5 g/dL	MEDIF assessment required for Hb less than 10 g/dL
	History of sickling crisis within 10 days	
Respiratory disorders	Pneumothorax that is not fully inflated, or within 7 days after full inflation	
	Major chest surgery within 10 days	MEDIF assessment required up to 21 days post-surgery
	If breathless after walking 50 m on ground, or on continuous oxygen therapy on ground	Consider mobility and all aspects of total journey, interlining, etc.
Gastrointestinal disorders	General surgery within 10 days	Laparoscopic investigation may travel after 24 hours if all gas absorbed. Laparoscopic surgery requires MEDIF up to 10 days
	GI tract bleeding within 24 hours	MEDIF required up to 10 days

(continued overleaf)

Table 24.1 (*continued*)

Category	Do not accept	Remarks
CNS disorders	Stroke, including subarachnoid hemorrhage, within 3 days	Consider mobility/oxygenation aspects. MEDIF up to 10 days
	Epileptic fit (grand mal) within 24 hours	Petit mal or minor twitching – common sense prevails
	Brain surgery within 10 days	Cranium must be free from air
ENT disorders	Otitis media and sinusitis	
	Middle-ear surgery within 10 days	
	Tonsillectomy within 1 week	
	Wired jaw, unless escorted and with wire cutters	If fitted with self quick-release wiring may be acceptable without escort
Eye disorders	Penetrating eye injury/intraocular surgery within 1 week	If gas in globe, total absorption necessary – may be up to 6 weeks, specialist check necessary
Psychiatric disorders	Unless escorted, with appropriate medication carried by escort, competent to administer such	MEDIF required. Medical, nursing, or highly competent companion/relative escort
Pregnancy	After end of 36th week for single uncomplicated. After end of 32nd week for multiple uncomplicated	Passenger advised to carry medical certificate
Neonates	Within 48 hours	Accept after 48 hours if no complications present
Infectious disease	If in infective stage: International Health Regulations prohibit travel if suffering from an infectious disease while it is still contagious	As defined by American Public Health Association [36]

Table 24.2 Fitness to fly assessment.

General medical advice	Aerospace Medical Association: http://www.asma.org/asma/media/asma/Travel-Publications/medguid.pdf
General medical advice	Civil Aviation Authority – UK: http://www.caa.co.uk/default.aspx?catid=2497&pagetype=90
Respiratory system	British Thoracic Society: https://www.brit-thoracic.org.uk/document-library/clinical-information/air-travel/bts-air-travel-recommendations-2011/
Cardiovascular system	British Cardiovascular Society: http://www.bcs.com/documents/BCS_FITNESS_TO_FLY_REPORT.pdf
Communicable diseases	Communicable Diseases Network Australia: http://www.health.gov.au/internet/main/publishing.nsf/Content/412C1D90C7B1B06DCA257BF0001DE862/$File/aeroplane%20communicable%20disease%20update%202006.pdf

secondary fears often associated with a fear of flying, which include claustrophobia (a fear of enclosed spaces), agoraphobia (a fear of being in open spaces or in the outside world), or general panic disorder, which may stem from a range of different causes. It is important to recognize that a fear of flying can also be associated with comorbid psychologic factors such as low mood, excessive alcohol intake, significant life changes (loss of a job, ill health, difficulties in interpersonal relationships, etc.). Among many other causes, a fear of flying can also be triggered as a side-effect of prescribed medication or the ill effects of recreational drug use [33].

The most obvious behavioral response to a fear of flying is avoidance. Anxious flyers may exhibit a number of safety behaviors, such as having a preference for a specific seat (aisle or exit seats for quick escapes, or window seats to facilitate avoiding interaction with others). Such individuals may question airline staff about the weather, delays, technical problems, or the pilot's qualifications. Belligerent or aggressive behavior among certain passengers may also be fueled by anxiety. There is also some evidence that fearful flyers have an increased tendency to use medication and alcohol when flying.

People who exhibit fear of flying also tend to fear somatic symptoms of anxiety. They find distractibility, increased heart rate, hyperventilation, sweating, nausea, and associated symptoms unbearable, and this gives rise to a secondary anxiety, namely a fear of fear itself.

It is important to distinguish between those who are apprehensive about flying but can complete an air journey successfully and those who have an incapacitating fear that prevents them from ever traveling by air. Approximately 2.5% of the general adult population are considered to be truly phobic.

Factors considered most relevant to the etiology include conditioning and learning pathways, individual differences, physiologic factors, cognitive biases and distortions, and traumatic reactions to actual incidents or accidents [31,34].

A "one size fits all" approach to treatment will fail to help a significant number of fearful flyers, as their unique and specific problem may not be completely addressed.

This may not reflect the extremely high positive outcomes reported by many airlines and group interventions. Self-reported anxiety immediately after treatment is often positive, but may wane as individuals confront their anxieties on their own, away from a structured, supportive, and therapeutic context.

In vivo exposure has demonstrated the best results in terms of acute treatment gains. Relaxation training, distraction, visualization, exposure, cognitive reappraisal, and other methods have been demonstrated to be effective, particularly with fear of flying that has not responded to simple education around aircraft systems and flight safety [34].

Fear of flying is not a unitary clinical phenomenon and each fearful flyer experiences their problems in a different way. Consequently, interventions need to be tailored to the individual.

Conclusion

- Although the partial pressure of oxygen in a pressurized aircraft cabin is less than that at sea level, it is more than adequate for normal healthy individuals.
- The probability of airliner occupants suffering any abnormality or disease from exposure to cosmic radiation is very low.
- The individual must evolve personal strategies for combating the effects of jet lag.
- The absolute risk of developing symptomatic DVT when flying is very low.
- Motion sickness is a normal response to unfamiliar motion but rare in commercial air travel.
- Medical clearance is required when fitness to travel is in doubt.
- Air travel can exacerbate existing medical and psychologic disorders.
- Treatment of fear of flying should be tailored to the individual.
- Travelers should ensure they have adequate insurance cover.

References

1 Gradwell DJ. The Earth's atmosphere. In: Rainford DJ, Gradwell DP (eds.) *Ernsting's Aviation Medicine*, 4th edn. London: Hodder Arnold, 2006, pp. 3–8.
2 Ahmedzai S, Balfour-Lynn IM, Bewick T, et al. Managing passengers with stable respiratory disease planning air travel: British Thoracic Society recommendations. *Thorax* 2011; **66**(Suppl 1): i1–i30.
3 Committee on Air Quality in Passenger Cabins of Commercial Aircraft, Board on Environmental Studies and Toxicology, Division on Earth and Life Studies National Research Council. *The Airliner Cabin Environment and the Health of Passengers and Crew*. Washington, DC: National Academies Press, 2002, p. 57.
4 Bagshaw M. Cosmic radiation in commercial aviation. *Travel Med Infect Dis* 2008; **6**: 125–127.
5 International Air Transport Association. *Medical Manual*, 5th edn. Montreal: IATA, 2012, pp. 31–38.
6 Ernsting JK, Ward J, Rutherford OM. Cardiovascular and respiratory physiology. In: Rainford DJ, Gradwell DP (eds.) *Ernsting's Aviation Medicine*, 4th edn. London: Hodder Arnold, 2006, pp. 30–31.

7 Bull K. Cabin air filtration: helping to protect occupants from infectious diseases. *Travel Med Infect Dis* 2008; **6**: 142–144.

8 Committee on Air Quality in Passenger Cabins of Commercial Aircraft, Board on Environmental Studies and Toxicology, Division on Earth and Life Studies National Research Council. *The Airliner Cabin Environment and the Health of Passengers and Crew.* Washington, DC: National Academies Press, 2002, pp. 183–190.

9 Aerospace Medical Association Medical Guidelines Task Force. Medical Guidelines for Airline Travel, 2nd edn. *Aviat Space Environ Med* 2003;**74**(Suppl): A1–A20.

10 Macmillan AJF. Principles of the pressure cabin and the effects of pressure change on body cavities containing gas. In: Rainford DJ, Gradwell DP (eds.) *Ernsting's Aviation Medicine*, 4th edn. London: Hodder Arnold, 2006, pp. 109–127.

11 Risdall J. Clinical management of decompression illness. In: Rainford DJ, Gradwell DP (eds.) *Ernsting's Aviation Medicine*, 4th edn. London: Hodder Arnold, 2006, pp. 757–766.

12 Caldwell JA. Aviator fatigue and relevant fatigue countermeasures. In: Rainford DJ, Gradwell DP (eds.) *Ernsting's Aviation Medicine*, 4th edn. London: Hodder Arnold, 2006, pp. 773–784.

13 Waterhouse J, Reilly T, Atkinson G, Edwards B. Jet lag: trends and coping strategies. *Lancet* 2007; **369**: 1117–1129.

14 Sack RL. Jet lag. *N Engl J Med* 2010; **362**: 440–447.

15 Herxheimer A, Waterhouse J. The prevention and treatment of jet lag. *BMJ* 2003; **326**: 296–297.

16 World Health Organization. *WHO Research Into Global Hazards of Travel (WRIGHT) Project.* Geneva: WHO Press, 2007.

17 Giangrande P. Haematology. In: Rainford DJ, Gradwell DP (eds.) Ernsting's Aviation Medicine, 4th edn. London: Hodder Arnold, 2006, pp. 659–664.

18 Kahn SR, Lim W, Dunn A, et al. Prevention of VTE in nonsurgical patients: Antithrombotic Therapy and Prevention of Thrombosis, 9th edn: American College of Chest Physicians Evidence-Based Clinical Practice Guidelines. *Chest* 2012; **41**(2 Suppl): e195S–e226S.

19 Benson AJ, Rollin Stott JR. Motion sickness. In: Rainford DJ, Gradwell DP (eds.) *Ernsting's Aviation Medicine*, 4th edn. London: Hodder Arnold, 2006, pp. 459–475.

20 Bagshaw M. Commercial passenger fitness to fly. In: Rainford DJ, Gradwell DP (eds.) Ernsting's Aviation Medicine, 4th edn. London: Hodder Arnold, 2006, pp. 791–799.

21 International Air Transport Association. *Medical Manual*, 5th edn. Montreal: IATA, 2012, pp. 1–2.

22 Smith D, Toff W, Joy M, et al. Fitness to fly for passengers with cardiovascular disease. *Heart* 2010; **96**(Suppl 2): ii1–ii16.

23 Committee on Air Quality in Passenger Cabins of Commercial Aircraft, Board on Environmental Studies and Toxicology, Division on Earth and Life Studies National Research Council. *The Airliner Cabin Environment and the Health of Passengers and Crew.* Washington, DC: National Academies Press, 2002, pp. 152–170.

24 Australian Transport Safety Bureau. *Passenger Health – the Risk Posed by Infectious Disease in the Aircraft Cabin.* Canberra: Commonwealth of Australia, 2008.

25 Mangili A, Gendreau MA. Transmission of infectious diseases during commercial air travel. *Lancet* 2005; **365**: 989–996.

26 Leder K, Newman D. Respiratory infections during air travel. *Intern Med J* 2005; **35**: 50–55.

27 World Health Organization. *Tuberculosis and Air Travel: Guidelines for Prevention and Control,* 3rd edn. Geneva: WHO Press, 2008.

28 Bor R, Hubbard T (eds.) *Aviation Mental Health.* Farnham: Ashgate Publishing, 2006.

29 Bor R. *Anxiety at 35,000 Feet: an Introduction to Clinical Aerospace Psychology.* London: Karnac, 2004.

30 Bor R (ed.) *Passenger Behaviour.* Farnham: Ashgate Publishing, 2003.

31 Oakes M, Bor R. The psychology of fear of flying (part 1): a critical evaluation of current perspectives on the nature, prevalence and aetiology of fear of flying. *Travel Med Infect Dis* 2010; **8**: 327–338.

32 American Psychiatric Association. *Diagnostic and Statistical Manual of Mental Disorders*, 4th edn. (DSM-IV). Washington, DC: American Psychiatric Press, 1994.

33 Bor R, van Gerwen L (eds.) *Psychological Perspectives on Fear of Flying.* Farnham: Ashgate Publishing.

34 –Oakes M, Bor R The psychology of fear of flying (part 2): a critical evaluation of current perspectives on approaches to treatment. *Travel Med Infect Dis* 2010; **8**, 339–363.

35 Zuckerman JN (ed.) *Principles and Practice of Travel Medicine*, 2nd edn. Oxford: Wiley-Blackwell, 2013.

36 Benenson AS (ed.) *Control of Communicable Diseases in Man*, 15th edn. Washington, DC: American Public Health Association, 1990.

CHAPTER 25

Expedition and wilderness medicine

Sean T. Hudson[1], Will Smith[2], David R. Shlim[3], Caroline J. Knox[4], &
Karen J. Marienau[5]

[1] Maryport Health Centre, West Cumberland Hospital, Maryport, Cumbria, UK
[2] St. John's Medical Center, Jackson, WY, USA
[3] Jackson Hole Travel and Tropical Medicine, Wilson, WY, USA
[4] Castlegate Surgery, Cockermouth, Cumbria, UK
[5] St. Paul, MN; formerly US Centers for Disease Control and Prevention, Atlanta, GA, USA

Traveling at extremes

The human body was not designed to function in the extreme regions of this world. It has only been through quite profound adaptations and behavioral changes that we are able to survive in the austere environment. This does mean, however, that these regions represent a challenging and exciting working environment for remote medical practitioners.

Altitude

Since populations have lived and especially as explorers began traveling to higher and higher altitudes, the human body has attempted to adapt to the hypobaric hypoxia that ensues. The body is able to adapt to these altitudes over 2500 m in a limited fashion [1], but at some point the individual's altitude threshold is reached and they can quickly develop life-threatening illness, and if not reversed the condition can lead to death. Some individuals and populations are able to adapt impressively whereas others have maladaptive physiologic responses that can cause life-threatening illness at much lower altitudes that others tolerate well [2,3].

Each person seems to have an individual altitude threshold that is thought to be somewhat genetic, but may have other associated factors such as concurrent viral infection, hydration status, underlying physical fitness, etc. Hence an individual's altitude threshold may change based on each altitude exposure. There are many reports of individuals with no prior problems at a given altitude, but who develop reentrant problems when they return to the same altitude. Conversely, a patient may have experienced significant problems at altitude in the past but later returns and has no problems. All of the physiologic, genetic, and other parameters related to altitude illness remain a multifactorial process.

Essential Travel Medicine, First Edition.
Edited by Jane N. Zuckerman, Gary W. Brunette and Peter A. Leggat.
© 2015 John Wiley & Sons, Ltd. Published 2015 by John Wiley & Sons, Ltd.

The most obvious curative treatment to altitude illness is descent. This is some-times an easy treatment option, but often descent is hindered by resources, weather, terrain, or simply poor decisions by the individual and/or group involved.

Acclimatization

Acclimatization is the process by which the body adapts its physiology to respond to a hypoxic environment. Principally, the changes allow increased delivery and more efficient cellular oxygen utilization.

The capacity to acclimatize varies considerably between individuals and species and is unrelated to physical fitness, gender, or age. Some have the ability to adjust quickly without discomfort, whereas others develop altitude illness and recover; some, however, never adjust despite gradual ascent. Genetic factors are important to the ability to acclimatize, which has confounded many elite athletes who incorrectly presumed that their fitness would allow them to ascend without attention to acclimatization guidelines. Even the most genetically advanced altitude dweller can succumb if the rate of ascent is too rapid.

The body undergoes a number of changes that allow the body to operate in a hypoxic environment. At altitude, the rate and depth of respiration increase (hyper-ventilation), driven by the hypoxic ventilatory response (HVR) in response to the lower oxygen levels. The resulting respiratory alkalosis caused by the reduced carbon dioxide is buffered and compensated by the increased renal excretion of bicarbon-ate in the proximal tubules of the kidneys, a process known as metabolic alkalosis. This compensatory process allows a rate of respiration sufficient to provide enough oxygen. Similarly, the cardiovascular system also develops a compensatory mecha-nism and the heart rate and cardiac output increase in order to increase the amount of oxygen supplied to the body tissues. An associated mild elevation in blood pres-sure occurs. Hematologically, the compensatory mechanism involves an increase in erythropoietin with a concomitant increase in red blood cell production.

The subsequent increased production of 2,3-diphosphoglycerate (2,3-DPG) in the red blood cells, which controls the movement of oxygen from red blood cells to body tissues, causes left-shifting of the oxygen dissociation curve, facilitating the release of oxygen from hemoglobin to cells. The adaptations that occur can result in changes to the physiology which may last for 2 weeks or sometimes longer once the individual descends.

Incidence and background

The incidence of altitude illness is difficult to predict accurately as there are many factors involved. However, several studies have been published and have been well summarized [1,2]. In general, the incidence of acute mountain sickness (AMS) with sleeping altitudes of 2000 m ranges from 20 to 30%. Faster ascents or higher ele-vation gains have been shown to increase the incidence of AMS. At sleeping alti-tudes up to 5000 m, the incidence of AMS can approach 80%, especially with rapid ascent profiles. The incidence of more severe illness (HACE/HAPE – see the following descriptions of these conditions) is much less and has been listed at 2–3% once one approaches very high altitudes of 3500–5500 m. At high altitude (1500–3500 m), the incidence is generally well under 1% [1,2].

The human body has an amazing ability to adapt when exposed to hypobaric hypoxia. At the point where the body fails to compensate further or other maladaptive factors come into play, many body systems become affected. The two most profoundly affected are the neurologic and pulmonary systems. As with any medical condition, one must always consider other possible etiologies in a differential diagnosis. At altitude this must also be considered, as any medical condition can also occur at altitude (e.g., myocardial infarction, pulmonary embolism, gastrointestinal illness) [4].

High-altitude neurologic problems

Neurologic problems at altitude are common and can range from a simple headache to a host of other problems, including ataxia and altered mental status, and cumulating in death. Often these progress from the high-altitude headache (HAH), which is a hallmark of the Lake Louise Acute Mountain Sickness scoring scale [5]. This scale is commonly used by looking at headache above 2500 m plus one or more of the following: gastrointestinal symptoms (anorexia, nausea, or vomiting), insomnia, dizziness, and lassitude or fatigue. Symptoms can occur after a few hours or may take several days to develop. The pathophysiology is complex and end-stage high-altitude cerebral edema (HACE) does have elevated intracranial pressures due to vasogenic edema, but many other factors are also now being considered, such as inflammatory and other cellular-mediated factors induced by altitude. The key clinical pearl for all altitude illness is never to continue ascending with any significant neurologic or pulmonary symptoms. If symptoms are worsening, then immediate descent is warranted. Medications and other treatments are only temporizing and descent is therefore the only curative treatment before irreversible impairment occurs in the body [1–3].

High-altitude headache (HAH)

- Can have multifactorial causes (dehydration, sleep problems, exertion, etc.), but occurs without the constellation of other AMS/HAPE symptoms.

Acute mountain sickness (AMS)

- HAH with addition of other symptoms: gastrointestinal symptoms (anorexia, nausea, or vomiting), insomnia, dizziness, and lassitude or fatigue as described in the Lake Louise AMS Scoring Scale [5].

High-altitude cerebral edema (HACE)

- Progression along the continuum from AMS to the development of more profound neurologic dysfunction to include ataxia, altered mental status, seizure, unresponsive/coma, death.

High-altitude pulmonary edema (HAPE)

HAPE is responsible for the greatest number of altitude deaths [2]. Although the absolute number of cases remains small, HAPE is often overlooked in its early stages and can be misdiagnosed as "high-altitude cough" or bronchitis/pneumonia. As symptoms progress, there is a marked increase in pulmonary hypertension and uneven hypoxic pulmonary vasoconstriction, leading to focal areas of capillary leak. This non-cardiogenic pulmonary edema has seen some benefit with some of the newer agents used for pulmonary hypertension seen at lower elevations (e.g., tidalafil). Several other cellular mechanisms are being investigated to develop further therapies (e.g., nitrous oxide, alveolar Na^+ channels). HAPE can occur alone or in combination with other neurologic symptoms experienced at altitude. When they do occur together, they contribute to significant patient deterioration and death [1–3].

Prevention/treatment of high-altitude problems

The prevention and treatment of all the above conditions (HAH, AMS, HACE, HAPE) often overlap and therefore will be discussed together. Prevention can be derived from pre-planning gradual ascent profiles, pharmaceutical aids, and other less commonly used tools such as altitude sleep chambers. Often travelers have the ability to modify their acclimatization schedule and, if done appropriately, most of the severe symptoms from altitude can be avoided. Sometimes rescue and military scenarios necessitate a rapid ascent profile and the risk to benefit of the mission and therapies available must be evaluated. Many treatment modalities cross over between the neurologic (HAH/AMS/HACE), pulmonary (HAPE), and other altitude maladies [1–3]. A few topics are discussed briefly in the text and Table 25.1 provides a summary of many of the prevention and treatment strategies used for high-altitude illness.

Ascent profile

Above 2500 m, there are no definitive studies but many experts recommend gaining a sleeping altitude of only 500 m per day. "Sleep low, work high" is also a common mantra when exerting at higher altitudes [1]. If minor symptoms are present or worsening, often a descent of only 500–1000 m and a few days of rest may allow the travel itinerary to continue [1–3].

Oxygen

Oxygen is probably the most beneficial in HAPE prevention and treatment, but is also helpful for AMS/HACE. Often limited supplies are available at high altitudes. In altitude communities, a home oxygen concentrator can often do remarkable things for a few days with great success. Doses will generally be limited to the supply of oxygen available; slow, continuous, prolonged use of a low flow is advantageous over a high flow for a short time frame. Titration to oxygen saturations greater than 90% is reasonable at moderate altitudes, but may be difficult to sustain at higher altitudes with limited oxygen [1–3].

Acetazolamide (Diamox)

Multiple trials have established the benefit of acetazolamide in prevention and a limited number also suggest that it can be used for treatment in conjunction with other modalities. A dose level of 125 mg twice daily is usually sufficient. Higher dose ranges seem to be associated with increased side-effects (paresthesias, diuresis)

Table 25.1 The most common prevention and treatment strategies for altitude illness.

Medication	Indication	Route	Dosage
Acetazolamide (Diamox)	AMS, HACE, HACE prevention	Oral	125 mg every 12 h; pediatrics 2.5 mg/kg every 12 h
	AMS treatment (possibly HACE treatment adjunct)	Oral	125–250 mg every 12 h; pediatrics 2.5 mg/kg every 12 h
	Periodic breathing	Oral	62.5 mg at bedtime
Dexamethasone (Decadron)	AMS, HACE (possibly HAPE) prevention	Oral	2 mg every 6 h or 4 mg every 12 h
	AMS, HACE treatment	Oral, IV, IM	4 mg every 6 h (8 mg initial dose for severe symptoms)
		Oral, IV, IM	Pediatrics (for treatment only) 0.15 mg/kg every 6 hr
Nifedipine (Procardia)	HAPE prevention	Oral	30 mg SR every 12 hours
Tadalafil (Cialis)	HAPE prevention (possibly HAPE treatment adjunct)	Oral	10 mg every 12 h – longer half-life than sildenafil
Sildenafil (Viagra)	HAPE prevention (possibly HAPE treatment adjunct)	Oral	50 mg every 8 h
Oxygen	AMS, HACE, HAPE prevention and treatment	Inhaled	2–4 L/min (or titrated to effect)
			Consider lower flow (1 L/min) due to limited supply to sustain treatment
Salmeterol	HAPE prevention and possibly as HAPE adjunct treatment	Inhaled	125 µg inhaled every 12 h (albuterol could be considered every 4 h if available)
Ondansetron (Zofran)	Nausea/vomiting from altitude or other illness	ODT	4–8 mg every 12 h

Treatment	Indication		Comments
Hydration	HAH, AMS prevention and treatment		1 L of hydration should be one of the first treatments of HAH
Stop ascent, rest, descent if not improving	AMS treatment		Descend 500–1000 m and reassess over 1–3 days
Immediate descent	HACE, HAPE treatment		
Portable hyperbaric chamber	HACE, HAPE treatment		If unable to descend immediately, must continuously pump to clear CO_2
Ibuprofen (and other NSAIDs)	AMS prevention and treatment		Ibuprofen 600 mg every 8 h

IM, intramuscular; IV, intravenous; ODT, orally disintegrating tablet; SR, sustained release.

without added benefit. Once acclimatization has been facilitated at a given altitude, acetazolamide can be stopped without any harmful effects (unlike steroids) [1–3].

Steroids

Most commonly dexamethasone is used for the prevention and treatment of HACE, but newer studies are also showing some possible benefit for HAPE prevention and possibly treatment. This probably is multifactorial and related to its action on cellular membrane stability and inflammatory responses. Caution should be exercised to avoid abruptly stopping steroids once taken at altitude and if taken for the past several days [1–3].

Nifedepine

As a calcium channel blocker, nifedepine is thought to help with prevention and even treatment of HAPE with its effects on pulmonary hypertension. As with many drugs, there is only a single study [6] that showed a definitive improvement, but many experts that feel it is reasonable to use it in conjunction with other modalities. The newer phosphodiesterase (PDE-5) inhibitors are beginning to show some superiority for HAPE treatment and may actually be more beneficial. Dual treatment with both agents requires significant clinical judgment as there is the possibility of significant hypotension [1–3].

Phosphodiesterase (PDE-5) inhibitors

Tadalafil (Cialis) and sildenafil (Viagra) are used primarily in the prevention and treatment for HAPE as they cause pulmonary vasodilation and decrease pulmonary artery pressure. A single study showed that tadalafil had benefit in preventing HAPE [7]. This drug class is also considered a reasonable treatment option once HAPE has developed. Although they are starting to be more commonly used, no large systematic study has confirmed their benefit [8]. Like many treatments in wilderness/remote medicine. much of what is done is extrapolated. Tadalafil seems to be slightly more commonly used as it has a longer half life [1–3].

Portable hyperbaric chambers

These reinforced bags can be used for all altitude problems. However, they not only have limitations due to their cost, weight, and need for transport to remote locations – placing a critical patient inside and then continuing medical care and monitoring are difficult. Continuous pumping of the bag (10–20 pumps per minute) is required to flush carbon dioxide out continuously and to maintain the elevated pressure necessary to simulate temporary descent. Although the bag can be life saving, if a patient can actually be transported to lower elevations, a delay should generally not be introduced in order to use a portable chamber [1–3].

Ibuprofen and other NSAIDs

There has been some suggested benefit from ibuprofen and other non-steroidal anti-inflammatory drugs (NSAIDs) in the prevention and treatment of AMS [9]. Definitive studies are still lacking, but given no contraindications it would reasonable to add an NSAID to acetazolamide in the prevention of AMS.

Dietary/herbal supplements

Ginkgo biloba has been found to have variable results in multiple studies, thought possibly due to the different Ginkgo biloba preparations versus multiple other possible confounders [2]. There are a multitude of other supplements (coca leaves, etc.) with some regional anecdotal benefit, but further evaluation needs to be performed before any formal recommendations can be made [1].

Other high-altitude conditions

- **UV keratitis (snow blindness)** – Appropriate eyewear is crucial when traveling at altitude. Once a patient has been exposed, generally symptomatic pain control is warranted until the cornea can heal, which may be delayed at altitude. Limited use of topical ocular anesthetics can be made, but prolonged use can be harmful [1–3],
- **High-altitude retinal hemorrhage (HARH)** – Generally this is not problematic unless involving central visual fields. Limited treatment is available at altitude and even with appropriate sub-specialty care, most resolve with descent and time [1–3].
- **Periodic breathing** – This condition is still not fully understood, but is thought to relate from the baseline feedback mechanisms of the body to maintain a normal oxygen, carbon dioxide, and acid–base status. Breathing patterns that can sometimes lead to difficulty in sleeping can be normalized with small doses of acetazolamide 62.5 mg orally at night. Some patients are more susceptible than others, and the condition may resolve or improve with acclimatization [1–3].
- **High-altitude deterioration** – Above 5500 m, the body is unable to acclimatize further and begins a variable rate of deterioration. Injuries are difficult or impossible to heal and other non-altitude illnesses are nearly impossible to treat. Sustained exposure above 8,000 m leads to rapid deterioration such that death will occur in a matter of days [2,3].

Hot environment
Thermoregulation

Behavioral changes and vasodilation initially control body temperature in the heat. Surface blood flow can increase up to 20-fold and increases heart rate and stroke volume. If the body temperature continues to rise, sweating commences, heat being absorbed from the skin as the liquid evaporates. High humidity reduces efficiency. Pale, wicking clothing with a wide-brimmed hat or scarf helps heat reduction [10–12].

Body temperature depends on

Metabolic heat produced

　　　　　+　　　　　　　　　vs　　　　　　　　Heat dissipated

Environmental heat load

Hydration and dehydration

There is a large interpersonal variation in fluid needed to maintain hydration in the heat. Starting each day well hydrated is important, with regular drinking during the day. If sterilizing drinking water, adding neutralizing tablets or flavor *after* full sterilization improves palatability and encourages drinking. Dehydration leads to nausea, headache, tiredness, malaise, irritability, reduced urine output, and thirst, along with a raised heart rate, raised respiratory rate, reduced skin turgor, and an inability to spit on the ground. Darkness of urine has been shown to equate to levels of dehydration; self-monitoring aims for pale urine. Heat syncope due to gravitational pooling can occur before acclimatization [13–15].

For mild dehydration, plain water is usually sufficient provided that the person is also eating. With significant dehydration, with coexisting diarrhea or anorexia, oral rehydration sachets (ORSs) are quick to use. An equivalent fluid can be simply made up with 1 L of clean water, half a teaspoon of salt, and four teaspoons of sugar [16].

Hyponatremia

This can sometimes be difficult to distinguish from heat-related illnesses. Ingestion of large volumes of fluid without electrolytes leads to low plasma sodium. Risk factors include being female, low body weight, taking NSAIDs, high motivation, and missed meals. Symptoms and signs are similar to those of dehydration, namely nausea, headache, and fatigue, but often with bloating, pale urine, and polyuria. If not rectified, confusion, coma, seizures, and death may follow. If high volumes of fluid are needed for high-intensity activity but no meals are taken, fluid with electrolytes is recommended. In the early stages, supporting the patient and withholding further fluid are usually enough to ensure recovery. Heat cramps – painful spasms of muscles that have been working hard – are linked to mild hyponatremia and the cooling of muscles. Treatment involves stretching and massage, along with replacing sodium [17–19].

Acclimatization

This usually takes 7–10 days and is mostly lost again within a few weeks of returning to temperate climes. The temperature threshold for initiating heat-loss mechanisms becomes lowered with vasodilation and sweating each beginning earlier. Sweat rates increase but the amount of sodium in the sweat becomes lower, allowing faster evaporation and preservation of body sodium. Plasma volume is also increased. The best way to prepare for the heat is to do regular moderate- to high-intensity exercise in temperate conditions (activating heat loss mechanisms). Once in the hot environment, gentle to moderate exercise accelerates acclimatization. Heart rate can be a sensitive reflection of heat stress and reduces with acclimatization. Initial peripheral edema is common [13,20].

Minor conditions
Sunburn

This is often underestimated but impairs vasomotor control and sweating for up to 1 week after the burn. Long-term risks of increased sun exposure include malignant melanomas, squamous and basal cell carcinomas, and cataracts. Sunscreen needs to be highly protective against UVA and UVB, applied *before* any sun exposure and reapplied regularly [21].

Solar keratitis

Sand and snow can reflect sunlight and exposure of the eyes to solar radiation can damage the outer layer of the cornea. This gives painful, photophobic, red eyes. Good-quality sunglasses, ideally with side protection, prevent this. Treatment includes cycloplegics to reduce ciliary muscle spasm and topical antibiotics to prevent infection.

Miliaria rubra

Sweat glands block and fluid builds up below the blockage, giving the miliaria or prickly heat. It can cause intense irritation to the skin and impairs sweating. Prevention includes regular washing of skin and ventilation where possible. Antihistamines help the itching [11].

Skin problems and foot care

Humid environments increase the risk of infection; cuts or abrasions should be treated early with antiseptic. Boots should be well fitted, allowing a little room for swelling. Emollients and pumicing can help with cracked heels and superglue can be used for large, difficult cracks. Blisters can also be a huge problem, particularly in sandy conditions. Reddened tender areas (hot spots) should be treated early with a gel dressing such as Compeed and/or zinc oxide tape. Blisters should not be burst unless very tense or over a joint.

In wet conditions, particularly in the jungle, feet can become macerated and overrun by fungal infections. Feet should be kept dry at night, and topical antifungals applied. Pitting keratolysis is caused by corynebacteria and gives a distinct set of black "pits" on the soles of the feet along with an unpleasant smell; it is successfully treated with clindamycin lotion.

Heat-related illnesses

Heat exhaustion or exertional heat illness (EHI)

If the amount of heat gained is greater than that dissipated, the body temperature will continue to rise. Dehydration is common and if venous return is beginning to be compromised, the body will shift fluid back from the periphery to the core, with subsequent reduced effectiveness of heat loss.

Risk factors and medications that increase the risk of heat-related illness are listed in Tables 25.2 and 25.3.

Signs and symptoms of heat exhaustion

Fatigue, thirst, malaise, nausea, vomiting, diarrhea, muscle aches or cramps, headache, and dizziness can all occur. Casualties will have a normal conscious level but there may be subtle changes such as poor coordination and reduced mental sharpness. Skin will be hot and sweating, mucosa dry, and heart rate and respiratory rate raised. Hematuria may reflect rhabdomyolysis [25,26].

Table 25.2 Risk factors for heat-related illness [12,22,23].

Individual	Environmental	Situational
Poor fitness	High temperature	Dehydration
Obesity	High humidity	Poor acclimatization
Diabetes mellitus	High solar load and little shade	Inappropriate clothing
Thyroid disease	High temperature and humidity	High exertion
Extremes of age	the previous day	Weight of pack carried
Skin disorders, e.g., scleroderma		Fatigue
or ectodermal dysplasia		Missed meals
Previous or family history of		Sleep deprivation
heat-related illness		Alcohol or drug intake
Certain medications (see list)		Peer pressure
		High motivation
		Sunburn or miliaria rubra
		Intercurrent illness, e.g., fever,
		diarrhea

Table 25.3 Medications that increase the risk of heat-related illness.

Drug	Effect
Diuretics	Dehydrate
ACE inhibitors	
Alcohol	
Sedatives	
Haloperiodol	
Beta-blockers	Alter vasomotor response
Vasodilators	
Antidepressants (TCAs, MAOIs, SSRIs)	Increase metabolic heat
Thyroxine	generated
Amphetamines, cocaine, ecstasy	
Neuroleptics	Reduce sweating
Anticholinergics	[20,24]
Antihistamines	

ACE, acetylcholinesterase; MAOIs, monoamine oxidase inhibitors; SSRIs, selective seratonin reuptake inhibitors; TCAs, tricyclic antidepressants.

Heat stroke

If heat exhaustion is not recognized and treated properly, body temperature will continue to rise and progression to full heat stroke will occur. There is significant risk of neurologic damage or death. Signs and symptoms will be similar to those of heat exhaustion plus a reduction in conscious level. This may develop insidiously, with confusion, disorientation moving on to coma ± seizures, or may present with sudden loss of consciousness. Body temperature will be above 40 °C and the skin will be hot, but sweating may well have stopped as fluid will be needed to maintain cardiac venous return.

Above approximately 42 °C, cellular derangement begins, with autonomic and hypothalamic dysfunction, leading to possible loss of vasodilation, shivering, or pinpoint pupils. Disseminated intravascular coagulation, rhabdomyolysis, renal failure, and compartment syndrome can follow if the initial event is survived [25,26].

Treatment of heat exhaustion or heat stroke

The risk of neurologic damage or death is directly related to the time spent with extremely high body temperatures – the area under the curve with temperature over 40 °C and time on the axes.

Treatment steps are as follows:
- Lie the casualty in the shade, stripped to underwear, ideally off hot ground.
- Use history and examination to distinguish between a heat-related illness and dehydration or hyponatremia.
- Reduce the body temperature as quickly as possible:
  ◦ spray with water and fan;
  ◦ if ice is available, place it around the head, neck, groin, and axillae;
  ◦ ice- or water-soaked towels can be laid over the body;
  ◦ ice immersion is used in some military establishments.
- If dehydrated, rehydrate with ORSs if fully conscious or intravenous normal saline if not. Dextrose may be helpful to combat any hypoglycemia.
- Antiemetics will reduce nausea and vomiting.
- Evacuate, assess others at risk [27–29].

Classic heat stroke

This heat-related illness occurs more slowly and without particular exertion, for example, while in a non-air-conditioned vehicle or a tent. At highest risk are those at the extremes of age or with pre-existing medical conditions. Signs and symptoms are similar to those of EHI, although there is rarely profuse sweating, or rhabdomyolysis. Treatment is similar [13,28].

Cold environment

Thermoregulation

Thermoregulation is the maintenance of a steady core temperature and is the balance of heat gain and heat loss [30]. Heat is produced as a result of metabolic activity and of exercising or shivering. Heat loss is a result of radiation, convection, conduction, evaporation, and respiration.

The hypothalamus processes information from thermoreceptors in the core and the periphery. This stimulus then impacts on the core temperature by generating vasoconstriction, vasodilatation, and thermogenesis. Behavioral components will affect heat loss by stimulating the person to change clothing or seek shelter.

Hypothermia classification

Hypothermia is defined as a core temperature of <35 °C, although measuring a core temperature in the field is very difficult.

Mild hypothermia (35–32 °C)

- Shivering thermogenesis begins before the victim is hypothermic.
- Victim develops amnesia/dysarthria/ataxia.
- Generally normotensive, a degree of tachycardia, and tachypnea.
- Shivering comes in waves before stopping.

Moderate hypothermia (32–28 °C)

- Sometimes referred to as stumbles, fumbles, mumbles, and grumbles.
- Shivering stops below 32 °C and consequently inexperienced assessors can be misled into underestimating the severity of hypothermia.
- As the core temperature falls the subject becomes bradycardic (refractory to atropine below 28 °C) and is at risk of developing atrial fibrillation.
- Blood pressure and respiratory rate fall and pupils become dilated (<30 °C).

Severe hypothermia (<28 °C)

- Subject becomes comatose and has absent corneal and oculocephalic reflexes.
- Profoundly hypotensive.
- High likelihood of developing ventricular fibrillation (maximum risk: 22 °C).
- Subject becomes apneic, asystolic, and areflexic with fixed pupils.
- The EEG is flat at 19 °C.

Management of mild and moderate hypothermia

- Stop and seek shelter.
- Wet clothing should be removed carefully and replaced with warm, dry clothing.
- Insulate the individual from the ground to prevent further heat loss.
- If available, getting into a warm sleeping bag with a warm person.
- It is important that others in the group are protected from further heat loss.
- Warm sugary fluids should be given by mouth. The sugar provides energy that allows the patient to continue shivering and generating heat. The presence of a warm fluid in the esophagus and stomach my help to stabilize cardiac tissue.

Management of severe hypothermia

- Treat as above, gently removing wet clothing and replacing with warm, dry clothing.
- Victims should be transported as soon as possible to a center where monitored rewarming, preferably cardiopulmonary bypass, is possible [31].
- Sudden movements should be kept to a minimum in an attempt to reduce the risk of developing a cardiac arrhythmia.
- Remember to manage the victim's other injuries when the environment allows. If the environment is particularly harsh, then only manage life-threatening injuries until you can find or create shelter for the patient.

Frostbite

Introduction

Frostbite occurs when the local temperature in an extremity falls low enough for ice crystals to form [32]. Predisposing factors are poor insulation, restrictive clothing, hypothermia, and exhaustion. Physiologic factors such as dehydration and hypoxia also appear to increase the risk of developing frostbite. Certain medical conditions such as diabetes, peripheral vascular disease (PVD), Raynaud's phenomenon, psychiatric illness, and previous frostbite predispose to the condition.

Any part of the body can be affected by frostbite. However, typically exposed areas or those that are subject to wet or restrictive conditions are predominantly affected. The face, ears, cheeks, nose, fingers/hands, toes/feet, buttocks, thighs, and genitalia are the commonest sites.

Pathophysiology

As the skin cools, cold-induced vasoconstriction is followed by cold-induced vasodilation. This is known as the hunting response and protects the extremities from cold injury. It occurs in approximately 5-minute cycles. As the extremity cools further, vasodilation terminates, which results in a significant reduction in blood flow but does protect the core from further heat loss [33]. With further cooling, the blood become increasingly viscous, and below <0 °C ice crystal formation occurs. Blisters may develop and prostaglandin $F_{2\alpha}$ and thromboxane A_2 cause platelet aggregation and thrombosis, which results in ischemia.

Clinical presentation

Generally, people describe the affected extremity as feeling numb and cold to the touch, often like a piece of wood [34]. The tissue may appear blistered or dusky. The blisters can be clear or blood filled, depending on the extent of the frostbite.

Thawing and reperfusion lead to an intense throbbing pain. The subsequent clinical course is variable but usually frostbite victims experience some degree of sensory loss for many years after injury, perhaps indefinitely [35].

Good prognostic indicators are retained sensation, normal skin color, and clear rather than cloudy fluid in any blisters present. Early formation of edema and clear blisters that extend to the tips of the digits are a good sign. Poor prognostic signs include non-blanching cyanosis, firm skin, lack of edema, and small, proximal, dark hemorrhagic vesicles [36]. However, no prognostic features are entirely predictive and weeks or months may pass before the demarcation between viable and non-viable tissue becomes clear.

Frostnip and frostbite

Frostnip is reversible and is the very early stage of frostbite. If the cold extremity is rapidly warmed it should return to normal within 10 minutes and should result in no long-term damage. The cause of the frostnip must be explored and corrected, otherwise it will recur and perhaps develop into frostbite.

Frostbite can be subdivided into superficial and deep [35,37,38]:
- Superficial
  - Partial skin freezing (first degree): erythema and edema but no blisters.

- Full-thickness skin freezing (second degree): erythema, edema, clear blisters, desquamation and black eschar formation.
- Deep
  - Full-thickness skin and subcutaneous tissue (third degree): hemorrhagic blisters, skin necrosis and purple discoloration.
  - Full-thickness skin to bone (fourth degree): often little edema, mottled and cyanotic, then dry, black and mummified.

Treatment in the field

- Seek shelter.
- Drink warm, sugary fluids.
- Remove wet gloves and socks and replace with dry ones, warm the cold extremity by placing in companion's armpit or groin for 10 minutes only. Do not rub.
- Loosen any restrictive clothing and remove and rings or bracelets.
- Take aspirin (75 mg) for its antiplatelet effect and ibuprofen (800 mg) for its antiprostaglandin effect.
- If sensation returns, one can continue to walk. If there is no return of sensation, go to the nearest warm shelter where treatment can commence if there is no chance of further freezing. If at high altitude, consider supplementary oxygen.

Field rewarming should only be attempted if there is no further risk of refreezing [35]. Tissue that is thawed and then refrozen almost always dies. Consequently, the decision to thaw the frostbitten tissue in the field commits the provider to a course of action that may involve pain control, maintaining warm water baths at a constant temperature, and protecting tissue from further injury during rewarming and eventual transport. Once rewarmed in the field, frostbitten extremities cannot be used for ambulation.

Treatment in hospital [39]

1 Admit frostbite patient to specialist unit if possible.
2 Evaluate for hypothermia and concomitant injury.
3 On admission, rapidly rewarm the affected areas in warm water at 37–39°C (99–102°F) for 15–30 minutes or until thawing is complete.
4 Debride clear or white blisters and apply topical aloe vera every 6 hours.
5 Leave hemorrhagic blisters intact and apply topical aloe vera every 6 hours.
6 Splint and elevate the extremity.
7 Administer antitetanus prophylaxis.
8 Analgesia as indicated.
9 Administer ibuprofen 400 mg orally every 12 hours.
10 Administer benzylpenicillin 500,000 U every 6 hours for 48–72 hours if the skin is edematous.
11 Administer daily hydrotherapy in 40 C water for 30–45 minutes. Do not towel dry the affected tissue.
12 Consider thrombolysis with tissue plasminogen activator and vasodilation with iloprost.

Surgery should be delayed and if necessary should be undertaken by a surgeon with appropriate experience, usually 6–12 weeks after the injury. The exceptions are fasciotomy for compartment syndrome and occasionally early amputation, which is indicated if liquefaction, moist gangrene, or overwhelming infection and sepsis develop. However, some clinicians are now advocating a more aggressive approach. The recent introduction of technetium-99 scintigraphy [40–42] and magnetic resonance imaging scanning [43] allows very early assessment of tissue viability, which permits early planning of interventions.

Non-freezing cold injuries

When individuals are exposed to a cold, wet environment, they are at risk of developing a non-freezing cold injury (NFCI). The environmental temperature is above freezing but the combination of cold and wet causes increased conductive heat loss and sometimes profound neuropathic injury. The tissue appears pale, desensitized, and loose. When rewarmed slowly, there is a short period of pale cyanosis, followed by hyperemia, with redness, swelling, and pain [44]. NFCI pain is often severe and the early use of tricyclic antidepressants has been demonstrated to be effective in both the short and long term.

Scuba and diving medicine

Recreational scuba (self-contained underwater breathing apparatus) diving is an increasingly popular sport [45]. Although a high-risk activity, most people will have enjoyable diving experiences provided that they have proper training and follow safe diving practices.

Physiologic changes from exposure to ambient pressure during and after dives can result in dive-related disorders. The most common triggers leading to death are air supply problems, emergency ascent, cardiac health issues, entrapment or entanglement, and buoyancy issues, underscoring the importance of proper training and physical and psychologic fitness for diving [46]. A basic understanding of the unique characteristics of the underwater environment, causes of diving-related disorders, and familiarity with recommendations for the diving-related medical evaluation can provide the practitioner with skills for assessing an individual's fitness for diving and recommending safe diving behavior [45,47–54].

Diving physics and physiologic changes related to diving [45,47]

- Boyle's law: at constant temperature, the volume of gas in an enclosed space changes inversely with changes in pressure.
  - Barotrauma is tissue damage that occurs when a diver fails to equalize pressure in a gas-filled space with the pressure of the surrounding water during descent (compression) or ascent (decompression).
- Henry's law: at constant temperature, the partial pressure of inspired gases changes with changes in ambient pressure.

- During compressed air dives, inspired nitrogen is dissolved in the blood and tissues; how much depends on depth and time at depth.
- As ambient pressure decreases during ascent, nitrogen is gradually eliminated from the body.

Diving disorders
Barotrauma (non-pulmonary) [45,48]
Middle ear barotrauma (middle ear squeeze) and sinus barotrauma are the most common sites of barotrauma.

- Middle ear barotrauma:
  - Caused by inability to equalize pressure in the middle ear with ambient pressure due to Eustachian tube dysfunction from descending faster than equalization can occur; acute or chronic inflammation; nasal congestion or obstruction; anatomic abnormalities; tympanic membrane (TM) scarring; prolonged decongestant use; excessive smoking.
  - Potentially serious consequences can occur if a diver continues to descend without equalizing pressure or forcefully attempts to equalize without ascending: TM deformation and rupture (vertigo, nausea, vomiting, and disorientation secondary to caloric stimulation may occur), hearing loss, and tinnitus.
- Inner ear barotrauma:
  - Caused by difficulties equalizing middle ear pressure, particularly if forceful Valsalva maneuvers were used.
  - Relatively rare.
  - Potential consequences range from round or oval window rupture with perilymph fistula to cochlear hemorrhage with sensorineural hearing loss and vestibular dysfunction.
  - Requires referral to an otolaryngologist.
  - Manifestations can mimic those of inner ear decompression sickness – treatments are very different.
- Sinus barotrauma:
  - Caused by inability to equalize pressure between the sinuses and surrounding water, usually due to transient nasal pathology or chronic sinusitis.
  - Palliative treatment is usually sufficient.

Ear and sinus barotrauma can usually be prevented by careful attention to pressure equalization during descent (or ascent), descending or ascending slowly in a feet-down position, and avoiding diving with significant nasal, otic, or sinus congestion. Systemic or topical nasal decongestants before a dive can be helpful, but should be used with caution owing to the potential for a rebound effect.

Pulmonary barotrauma [45,48,51–54]
During ascent, if the expanding compressed air inside a diver's lungs is not allowed to escape by exhaling, or is trapped in a lung segment by local obstruction, the expanding gas may lead to pulmonary overinflation and alveolar rupture. Arterial gas embolism (AGE), the most serious consequence of pulmonary overinflation, is life threatening and requires immediate recompression in a hyperbaric chamber.

Arterial gas embolism (AGE)

AGE occurs when air bubbles enter the arterial circulation via the pulmonary veins and left heart, and lodge in arterioles and capillaries. The brain is especially susceptible, but AGE may occur in the heart and other organs. Manifestations almost always occur within 5–10 minutes of surfacing:

- Central nervous system AGE – gross neurologic deficits, most commonly stupor or confusion, unconsciousness, seizures, motor or sensory deficits, visual disturbances.

  Major risk factors for pulmonary overinflation and AGE include the following:
- Breath holding during ascent or shooting to the surface too rapidly for exhalation to compensate for the degree of gas expansion.
  - Often results from panic associated with running out of air, equipment dysfunction, or loss of buoyancy control.
  - Can occur from very shallow or brief dives if a diver breath-holds with lungs maximally expanded during ascent.
- Chronic or acute lung conditions causing local obstruction.

Decompression sickness [45,48,51–54]

Decompression sickness (DCS), or "the bends," caused by formation of bubbles in blood (primarily venous) and tissues, ranges from mild to life threatening. Clinical manifestations result from direct and indirect effects of bubbles in the tissues or bloodstream. The complicated pathophysiology includes the rates of inert nitrogen gas absorption (saturation) and elimination by tissues. Dive depth and time at depth are major determinants of nitrogen saturation. Nitrogen is eliminated through the lungs during ascent, but equilibrium is not reached until several hours after surfacing.

Dive tables and dive computers provide guidelines for safe diving depth and time to minimize the risk of DCS. However, one can dive within recommended limits and still develop DCS.

DCS risk factors [51,54,55]

- Ascending faster than the recommended rate.
- Deep, long dives.
- Approaching or diving beyond no-decompression limits.
- Diving in cold water and hard exercise at depth.
- Possible risk factors (inconclusive evidence):
  - Dehydration, obesity, poor physical condition, hard exercise after surfacing, alcohol use before or after diving, unidentified individual risk factors.

DCS Type I and Type II

These may occur simultaneously.

- DCS Type I (non-systemic or musculoskeletal)
  - Characterized by the absence of neurologic and other systemic signs/symptoms.
  - Usually manifests as musculoskeletal pain that is dull or throbbing, and poorly localized around a joint
    - 95% have onset within 6 hours of surfacing
    - requires recompression treatment.

- Skin rash and pruritus are common cutaneous manifestations; usually resolve spontaneously within 12–24 hours.
- Cutis marmorata or skin marbling may be a harbinger of more serious symptoms; may require recompression treatment.
- DCS Type II (neurologic or systemic)
  Generally, the sooner the onset of signs or symptoms after a dive, the more severe is the case, more rapid the progression, and more urgent the treatment.
  Clinical manifestations:
  - Central nervous system (most common):
    - low back or abdominal pain, hypoesthesia, weakness, gait abnormality, paralysis, visual deficits, impaired/loss of consciousness, seizures.
  - Vestibular (inner ear DCS):
    - tinnitus, hearing loss, vertigo, dizziness, and nausea or vomiting
    - dive profile and timing of symptom onset help differentiate from inner ear barotrauma; if unclear, treat for DCS.
  - Pulmonary (rare):
    - chest pain aggravated by inspiration, cough, increased respiratory rate
    - pulmonary congestion, respiratory failure, shock, and death may rapidly ensue without immediate recompression.

Decompression illness [45,51,52]

Decompression illness (DCI) encompasses both DCS and AGE. Treatment is the same, but causes differ. Distinguishing between the two conditions is important for future diving implications.

DCI treatment [51–53]

- Primary first aid: 100% oxygen (O_2) and medical stabilization, followed by recompression in a hyperbaric chamber, breathing 100% O_2.
  - Treatment is usually successful unless excessively delayed.
  - Repeat treatments over days to weeks maybe required for some patients; a smaller percentage may have permanent, residual deficits, including death.
    Advice for preventing, or minimizing the consequences, of DCI:
- Proper training and certification.
- Diving equipment in good working order.
- Diving within one's physical, psychologic, and skill limitations.
- Avoiding diving if feeling unwell.
- Adhering to dive table or dive computer recommendations.
- Following recommendations for repetitive dives, flying or ascending to altitude after diving.
- Familiarity with signs and symptoms of DCI *and* seeking evaluation promptly should they develop.
  - Treatment delays may be due to denial, rationalization, embarrassment, or cost.
- Purchasing dive accident insurance.
  - Costs of emergency transport to, and treatment in, a hyperbaric chamber can be thousands of dollars and should not be deterrents.

Fitness to dive
Medical evaluation for diving [49,50,56,57]
Certain levels of physical and psychologic fitness are necessary for safe diving. A physically or mentally unstable diver will endanger at least two lives – his or her own and the dive buddy. A medical evaluation that focuses on the heart, lung, ears, sinuses, and psychologic status and identifies chronic conditions is recommended for anyone who wants to dive. Periodic re-evaluations are recommended to determine continued fitness for diving. The World Recreational Scuba Training Council's physical examination guidelines for determining fitness to dive includes a comprehensive discussion of conditions that are relative or absolute contraindications [50].

Medications and diving [50,58]
Many conditions are treated with medications. Many drugs are considered to be safe, but others are considered absolute contraindications to diving. Seizures, respiratory or cardiac compromise, hypoglycemia, impaired cognition, and panic attacks can be catastrophic events under water. When evaluating the safety of a drug related to diving, several factors must be considered:
- The condition being treated.
- How long the person has been on the drug.
- Intended and unintended effects of the drug:
  ◦ the increased partial pressure of nitrogen can be expected to increase the drowsiness effect of many drugs.
- Most antimalarial drugs are considered to be safe for diving, with the exception of mefloquine.

  Articles on classes of medications and diving are available at http://www.diver salertnetwork.org/medical/faq/.

Flying after diving [45,53]
Flying too soon after diving increases DCS risk because of the decrease in atmospheric pressure. Guidelines apply to recreational air dives followed by flights at cabin altitudes of 2000–8000 feet for divers *without* symptoms of DCS. They also apply to other modes of ascending to higher altitudes after diving, such as by driving or hiking.
- Single no-decompression dive: wait at least 12 hours.
- Multiple dives per day or multiple days of diving: wait at least 18 hours.
- Dives requiring decompression stops (decompression dives): wait "substantially longer than 18 hours."

Diving at altitude [59]
Diving at elevations above 1000 feet is considered altitude diving. Certification is highly recommended because of the increased risk of DCS and other hazards. Different tables and algorithms from those used at sea level are required.

Returning to diving following diving trauma or illness [52]
Diving-related conditions should have resolved before resuming diving. There should be no increased risk of recurrence or worsening of tissue damage.

Other diving hazards

Nitrogen narcosis [48]

The narcotic effects of dissolved nitrogen under pressure cause nitrogen narcosis. This can lead to disregard for personal safety, such as removing the regulator mouthpiece or swimming to unsafe depths. During air dives, narcosis usually appears at around 130 feet of seawater, but susceptibility varies among divers.

Marine trauma

Divers should be familiar with the local dangerous marine life and other physical hazards such as strong currents, rocks, or reefs.

Diving resources

- Divers Alert Network (DAN): http://www.diversalertnetwork.org:
  - Diving safety tips and diving medicine articles for divers and health practitioners.
  - 24-hour emergency hotline.
  - Dive accident insurance.
- http://en.wikipedia.org/wiki:
  - Comprehensive list of international diving organizations.

References

1 Luks AM, McIntosh SE, Grissom CK, et al. Wilderness Medical Society consensus guidelines for the prevention and treatment of acute altitude illness. *Wilderness Environ Med* 2010; **21**: 146–155.

2 Hacket PH, Roach, RC. High-altitude medicine and physiology. In: Auerbach PS (ed.) *Wilderness Medicine*, 6th edn. Philadelphia, PA: Mosby Elsevier, 2012, pp. 2–32.

3 Freer L, Hacket PH. High-altitude medicine. In: Bledsoe GH, Manyak MJ, Townes DA (eds.) Expedition and Wilderness Medicine. Cambridge: Cambridge University Press, 2009, pp. 240–263.

4 Hacket PH, Roach RC. High-atitude illness. *N Engl J Med* 2001; **345**: 107–114.

5 Roach RC, Bartsch P, Oelz O, Hacket PH. Lake Louise AMS Scoring Consensus Committee. The Lake Louise acute mountain sickness scoring system. In: Sutton JR, Houston CS, Coats G (eds.) *Hypoxia and Molecular Medicine*. Burlington, VT: Charles S Houston, 1993, pp. 272–274.

6 Oelz O, Maggiorini M, Ritter M, et al. Nifedipine for high altitude pulomary oedema. Lancet 1989; **ii**: 1241–1244.

7 Maggiorini M, Brunner-La Rocca HP, Perth S, et al. Both tadalafil and dexamethasone may reduce the incidence of high-altitude pulmonary edema. *N Engl J Med* 2002; **346**: 1631–1636.

8 Fagenholz PJ, Gutman JA, Murray AF, Harris NS. Treatment of high altitude pulmonary edema at 4240 m in Nepal. *High Alt Med Biol* 2007; **8**: 139–146.

9 Lipman GS, Kanaan NC, Holck PS, et al. Ibuprofen prevents altitude illness: a randomized controlled trial for prevention of altitude illness with nonsteroidal anti-inflammatories. *Ann Emerg Med* 2012; **59**: 484–490.

10 Casa DJ, Clarkson PM, Roberts WO. American College of Sports Medicine roundtable on hydration and physical activity: consensus statements. *Curr Sports Med Rep* 2005, **4**: 115–127.

11 Bledsloe GH, Manyak MJ, Townes DA (eds.) *Expedition and Wilderness Medicine*. Cambridge: Cambridge University Press, 2009, pp. 349, 479–491, 590–591.

12 Charkoudian N. Skin blood flow in adult human thermoregulation: how it works, when it does not, and why. *Mayo Clin Proc* 2003; **78**: 603–612.

13 McKardle WD, Katch FI, Katch VL. *Essentials of Exercise Physiology*, 2nd edn. Philadelphia, PA: Lippincott Willliams & Wilkins, 2000, pp. 61–62, 219–225, 429–449.

14 Armstrong LE, Maresh CM, Castellani JW, et al. Urinary indices of hydration status. *Int J Sport Nutr* 1994; **4**: 265–279.

15 Murray R. The effects of consuming carbohydrate-electrolyte beverages on gastric emptying and fluid absorption during and following exercise. *Sports Med* 1987; **4**: 322–351.

16 WHO, UNICEF. *Oral Rehydration Salts. Production of the New ORS*. WHO/FCH/CAH/06.1. Geneva: World Health Organization. http://www.who.int/child_adolescent_health/docum ents/fch_cah_06_1/en/index.html (accessed 7 February 2015).

17 Rogers IR, Hew-Butler T. Exercise-associated hyponatremia: overzealous fluid consumption. *Wilderness Environ Med* 2009; **20**: 139–143.

18 Sawka MN, Burke LM, Eichner ER, et al. American College of Sports Medicine position stand. Exercise and fluid replacement. *Med Sci Sports Exerc* 2007; **39**: 377–390.

19 Rehrer NJ. Fluid and electrolyte balance in ultra-endurance sport. *Sports Med* 2001; **31**: 701–715.

20 Auerbach PS (ed.) *Wilderness Medicine*, 5th edn. St, Louis, MO: Mosby, 2007, pp. 117–124, 228–283.

21 Wang SQ, Stanfield JW, Osterwalder U. In vitro assessments of UVA protection by popular sunscreens available in the United States. *J Am Acad Dermatol* 2008; **59**: 934–942.

22 Costil DL, Branam G, Fink W, Nelson R. Exercise induced sodium conservation: changes in plasma renin and aldosterone. *Med Sci Sports* 1976; **8**: 209–213.

23 Wallace RF, Kriebel D, Punnett L, et al. The effects of continuous hot weather training on risk of exertional heat illness. *Med Sci Sports Exerc* 2005; **37**: 84–90.

24 Joint Formulary Committee. British National Formulary 65, March-September 2013. London: *Pharmaceutical Press*, 2013.

25 Harries M, Williams C, Stanish W, Micheli L. *Oxford Textbook of Sports Medicine*, 2nd edn. Oxford: Oxford Medical Publications, 1998, pp. 97–109, 272–279.

26 Moran DS, Pandolf KB, Shapiro Y, et al. Evaluation of environmental stress index for physiological variables. *J Therm Biol* 2003; **28**: 43–49.

27 Roberts WO. Exertional heat stroke: life-saving recognition and onsite treatment in athletic settings. *Rev Bras Med Esporte* 2005; **11**: 329e–332e.

28 Bouchama A, Dehbi M, Chaves-Carballo E. Cooling and hemodynamic management in heatstroke: practical recommendations. *Crit Care* 2007, **11**(3): R54.

29 Smith JE. Cooling methods used in the treatment of exertional heat illness. *Br J Sports Med* 2005; **39**: 503–507.

30 Guyton AC, Hall JE. *Textbook of Medical Physiology*, 11th edn. Philadelphia, PA: Saunders Elsevier2005.

31 American Heart Association. 2005 *American Heart Association Guidelines for Cardiopulmonary Resuscitation and Emergency Cardiovascular Care. Part 10.4: Hypothermia. Circulation* 2005; **112**(Suppl IV): IV-136–IV-138.

32 Murphy JV, Banwell PE, Roberts AHN, McGrouther AD. Frostbite: pathogenesis and treatment. *J Trauma* 2000; **48**: 171–178.

33 Mills WJ. Clinical aspects of freezing cold injury. In: Pandolf KB, Burr RE (eds.) *Textbooks of Military Medicine: Medical Aspects of Harsh Environments*, Vol. 1. Rockville, MD: Office of the Surgeon General, US Army, 2002, pp. 429–467.

34 Reamy BV. Frostbite: review and current concepts. *J Am Board Fam Prac* 1998; **11**: 34–40.

35 West JB, Schoene RB, Luks AM, Milledge JS. *High Altitude Medicine and Physiology*, 5th edn. Boca Raton, FL: CRC Press, 2013.

36 Pollard AJ, Murdoch DR. *The High Altitude Medicine Handbook*. Abingdon: Radcliffe Medical Press, 2003.

37 McCauley RL, Smith DJ, Robson MC, Heggers JP. Frostbite. In: Auerbach PS (ed.) Wilderness Medicine, 4th edn. St. Louis, MO: Mosby, 2001, pp. 178–206.

38 Biem J, Koehncke N, Classen D, Dosman J. Out of the cold: management of hypothermia and frostbite. *CMAJ* 2003; **168**: 305–311.

39 McCauley RL, Hing DN, Robson MC, Heggers JP. Frostbite injuries: a rational approach based on the pathophysiology. *J Trauma* 1983; **23**: 143–147.

40 Cauchy E, Chetaille E, Marchand V, Marsigny B. Retrospective study of 70 cases of severe frostbite lesions: a proposed new classification scheme. *Wild Environ Med* 2001; **12**: 248–255.

41 Greenwald D, Cooper B, Gottlieb L. An algorithm for early aggressive treatment of frostbite with limb salvage directed by triple-phase scanning. *Plast Reconstr Surg* 1998; **102**: 1069–1074.

42 Imray C, Grieve A, Dhillon S, The Caudwell Xtreme Everest Research Group. Cold damage to the extremities: frostbite and non-freezing cold injuries. *Postgrad Med J* 2009; **85**: 481–488.

43 Barker JR, Haws MJ, Brown RE, et al. Magnetic resonance imaging of severe frostbite injuries. *Ann Plast Surg* 1997; **38**: 275–279.

44 Ungley CC, Blackwood W. Peripheral vasoneuropathy after chilling. 'Immersion foot and immersion hand.' *Lancet* 1942; **ii**: 447–451.

45 Lynch JH, Bove AA. Diving medicine: a review of current evidence. *J Am Board Fam Med* 2009; **22**: 399–407.

46 Denoble PJ, Caruso JL, Dear Gde L, et al. Common causes of open-circuit recreational diving fatalities. *Undersea Hyperb Med* 2008; **35**: 393–406.

47 Spira A. Diving and marine medicine review. Part I: diving physics and physiology. *J Travel Med* 1999; **6**: 32–44.

48 Spira A. Diving and marine medicine review. Part II: diving diseases. *J Travel Med* 1999; **6**: 180–198.

49 Bove AA. Medical evaluation in sport diving. In: Bove AA, Davis JC (eds.) *Diving Medicine*, 4th edn. Philadelphia, PA: Saunders, 2004, pp. 519–533.

50 Recreational Scuba Training Council. *Medical Statement. http://www.wrstc.com/downloads/10%20-%20Medical%20Guidelines.pdf* (accessed 28 August 2013).

51 Vann RD, Butler FK, Mitchell SJ, Moon RE. Decompression illness. *Lancet* 2010; **377**: 153–164.

52 Thalmann ED. Decompression illness: what is it and what is the treatment? *Alert Diver* March/April 2004. Durham, NC: Divers Alert Network. http://www.diversalertnetwork.org/medical/articles/article.asp?articleid=65 (accessed 28 August 2013).

53 Department of the Navy. Diagnosis and treatment of decompression sickness and arterial gas embolism. In: *US Navy Diving Manual*, Vol. 5, Revision 6, SS521-AG-PRO-010. Washington, DC: Naval Sea Systems Command, Chapter 20. www.usu.edu/scuba/navy_manual6.pdf (accessed 7 February 2015).

54 Vann RD. Mechanisms and risks of decompression. In: Bove AA, Davis JC (eds.) *Diving Medicine*, 4th edn. Philadelphia, PA: Saunders, 2004, pp. 127–164.

55 Scubadoc. *Obesity and Scuba Diving*. Diving Medicine Online. http://www.scuba-doc.com/obesity.html (accessed 28 August 2013).

56 Pollock NW, Uguccioni DM, Dear Gde L (eds.) *Diabetes and Recreational Diving: Guidelines for the Future: Workshop Proceedings June 19, 2005*. Durham, NC: Divers Alert Network, 2005. www.danasiapacific.org/main/diving_safety/DAN_Doc/pdfs/diabetes_guidelines.pdf (accessed 7 February 2015).

57 Godden D, Currie G, Denison D, et al. British Thoracic Society guidelines on respiratory aspects of fitness for diving. *Thorax* 2003; **58**: 3–13.

58 St Leger Dowse M, Cridge C, Smerdon G. The use of drugs by UK recreational divers: prescribed and over-the-counter medications. *Diving Hyperb Med* 2011; **41**: 16–21.

59 Ware J. *Diving at Altitude*. Diving Medicine Online. Scuba Clinic Forum. http://www.scuba-doc.com/divealt.html (accessed 28 August 2013).

CHAPTER 26

Venomous poisonous animals and toxins

Mark A. Read

Expedition and Wilderness Medicine, Thuringowa Central Queensland, Australia

Introduction

Injuries caused by venomous and poisonous animals are a major cause of morbidity worldwide and can be a significant public health concern. Although most injuries are non-fatal, treatment by healthcare providers and hospitalization for those more seriously affected incur a significant burden on healthcare systems [1], particularly in developing countries [2].

The animals responsible for these illnesses and injuries can be found in a great diversity of habitats, including urban and rural landscapes, arid deserts, tropical rainforests, and the marine environment. The huge variety of species range in size from tiny ants (<5 mm long) to stingrays weighing more than 200 kg. They include those species that we are familiar with, such as bees, wasps, and jellyfish, to lesser known species such as the highly venomous caterpillars of the South American moth *Lonomia* [3] and poisonous birds of the genus *Pitohui* from Papua New Guinea [4].

It is often difficult to associate the minor injury inflicted by a small, often non-threatening, animal with the subsequent profound and sometimes devastating effect of being envenomated or poisoned. Evolutionary selection pressure and inter-specific competition have meant that some animals have developed sophisticated and effective mechanisms for delivering their toxins via some form of traumatizing apparatus (venomous animals), whereas others have developed toxins that need to be ingested or absorbed to be effective (poisonous animals).

Venom serves multiple functions, but is most commonly used as a defensive mechanism and an efficient way to incapacitate/immobilize (and in some cases start digesting) potential prey [5]. Similarly, poisonous animals utilize toxins to protect themselves from predators; in some cases they do not even produce the compounds themselves – they ingest, store, and sequester the toxins produced by other organisms [6]. This complex relationship between predators and their prey has been taking place for millions of years, in what has been dubbed an "evolutionary arms race" [5].

Venoms and poisons are some of the most complex biologically active compounds found in the animal kingdom. Some compounds, such as tetrodotoxin, may be found in an identical form in as many as five different phyla (Annelida, Chaetognatha,

Essential Travel Medicine, First Edition.
Edited by Jane N. Zuckerman, Gary W. Brunette and Peter A. Leggat.
© 2015 John Wiley & Sons, Ltd. Published 2015 by John Wiley & Sons, Ltd.

Nemertea, Mollusca, Chordata) and from some 20–30 different species [7]. Defensive venoms, when acting in isolation, are rarely fatal to humans, but can cause immediate, extreme localized pain. These defensive venoms are often aided by the presence of hyaluronidase, which acts to break down the extracellular cell-cementing substance hyaluronic acid [8], allowing the toxin to infiltrate the tissues more rapidly. The offensive or predatory venoms are more complex and can be highly variable in composition and physiologic effects [9]. They can also be very prey specific. The mangrove catsnake, *Boiga dendrophila*, a tree-dwelling species from South-East Asia that preys primarily on birds, has a component in its venom, denmotoxin, that acts as a bird-specific post-synaptic neuromuscular blocker [10]. Some species can choose to deploy either defensive or predatory venom depending on the level of threat or size of prey. The Transvaal thick-tailed scorpion, *Parabuthus transvaalicus*, from southern Africa has a pain-inducing pre-venom, which appears to be utilized in defense and to immobilize small prey, whereas in high-threat situations or when targeting large prey, a more energetically expensive, protein-rich main venom is injected [11].

Poisonous animals also possess an impressive chemical arsenal. For example, many poison arrow frogs from Central and South America secrete a range of neurotoxins in their skin [7], which serve as a chemical defense against predation. These toxins are sequestered from the frogs' diet, and can come from a range of sources, including ants, beetles, and millipedes [6].

Nature of human envenomation

Despite these toxins being developed to dissuade attack by predators or to target prey other than humans [7], the complexity of some of these compounds means that venoms or poisons can affect multiple physiological pathways and organ systems within the human body. The venom of many species of venomous snakes, for example, can contain pre- and post-synaptic neurotoxins, myotoxins, nephrotoxins, and hemorrhagic toxins [12]. These toxins act on most major physiologic pathways and tissue types accessible by the bloodstream, hence successful treatment of snakebite usually requires thorough supportive care to maintain cardiovascular, respiratory, and renal function while definitive treatment (antivenom) is given.

There are a range of complicating factors that often compound the effects of envenomation and poisoning on humans. In some cases, the initial interaction may go unnoticed, such as some bites from venomous snakes, or be unrecognized because the immediate effects are very minor, such as the often painless sting from irukandji jellyfish (*Carukia barnesi*) in Australia [13]. This may lead to a delay in treatment, which can cause complications. There is a poor understanding of the mode of action for many animal-derived toxins [5] and limited antivenoms to provide definitive treatment. In many cases, venomous and poisonous animals are also encountered in remote locations or resource-poor settings where access to adequate healthcare facilities is limited [12]. An emerging issue in more developed countries is envenomations from exotic pets [14]. A study in the United Kingdom indicated that medical professionals needed to treat 760 patients over a 6-year period who had been bitten or stung by venomous reptiles, spiders, centipedes, or scorpions kept as pets [14].

Relevant statistics for human envenomations and poisonings

There is a distinctive pattern in the human behaviors that increases the risk of being envenomated or poisoned by an animal. In developed nations, envenomation or poisoning usually occurs around the home or during recreational activities, whereas in developing countries, it also occurs around the home but is more likely to affect people involved in subsistence farming activities [15]. Poisoning from ingesting or handling an animal is less common and most likely to occur as a result of eating an unfamiliar poisonous animal, such as one of the xanthid crabs [16] or one of the many species of pufferfish [17].

Statistics for envenomations and poisonings are regionally specific, with some locations having higher presentation rates than others. Envenomations accounted for an estimated 2.5% of 7981 emergency department injury presentations in Queensland, Australia, between 1998 and 2005 [18]. The majority of those envenomations were spider bites (27%), whereas snakebites accounted for 6% [18]. In comparison, in the United States, between 2006 and 2008 there was an average of 261,149 presentations per year to emergency departments caused by envenomations, with stings from hornets, bees, or wasps accounting for 15%, followed by spider bites at 3.5% and snakebites only 0.8% [1].

Statistics from field-based expeditions support the data from hospital presentations – that the real risk of being envenomated or poisoned is very low [19]. Of 10,499 travelers presenting at the Canadian International Water and Energy Consultants (CIWEC) clinic in Kathmandu, Nepal, between 1998 and 2005, bites from venomous and non-venomous insects, ticks, and spiders accounted for only 0.7% of the diagnoses [20]. For the marine environment, quantitative data on injuries from venomous animals are poor. A study examining the cause of death in 112 Divers Alert Network Europe scuba fatalities indicated that interactions with marine life (from envenomations, poisoning, and attacks) contributed to <3% of these [21].

Preparedness for treating envenomation and poisoning

Despite all the challenges associated with the epidemiology of envenomations and poisonings caused by animals, death and serious sequelae can be prevented in almost all cases by appropriate first aid and rapid attendance at a healthcare facility [18]. Although the incidences of envenomations or poisonings are low, the risk can be further minimized by:

1 Completing comprehensive and informed risk assessments specific for the travel destination [19].
2 Undertaking comprehensive travel pre-planning, including familiarization with the venomous and poisonous animals at the destination, ascertaining what antivenoms may be required and whether they are available in-country, and ensuring that the medical kit contains specific drugs/antivenoms and equipment.

3 Implementing standard protocols and procedures while at the destination, with particular emphasis on those procedures that reduce the risks from venomous and poisonous animals.

References

1 Langley RL. Animal-related injuries resulting in emergency department visits and hospitalizations in the United States, 2006–2008. *Hum Wildlife Interact* 2012; **6**: 123–136.

2 Konings M, Maharajh HD, Gopeesingh S. Injuries from arthropod, reptile and marine bites and stings in South Trinidad. *J Rural Trop Public Health* 2007; **6**: 1–5.

3 Kowacs PA, Cardoso J, Entres M, et al. Fatal intracerebral hemorrhage secondary to *Lonomia obliqua* caterpillar envenoming. *Arq Neuropsiquiatr* 2006; **64**: 1030–1032.

4 Dumbacher JP, Beehler BM, Spande TF, et al. Homobatrachotoxin in the genus *Pitohui*: chemical defense in birds? *Science* 1992; **258**: 799–801.

5 Casewell NR, Wüster W, Vonk FJ, et al. Complex cocktails: the evolutionary novelty of venoms, *Trends Ecol Evol* 2013; **28**: 219–229.

6 Savitzky AH, Mori A, Hutchinson DA, et al. Sequestered defensive toxins in tetrapod vertebrates: principles, patterns, and prospects for future studies. *Chemoecology* 2012; **22**: 141–158.

7 Brodie ED, III,. Toxins and venoms. *Curr Biol* 2009; **19**: R932.

8 Markovic-Housley Z, Miglierini G, Soldatova L, et al. Crystal structure of hyaluronidase, a major allergen of bee venom. *Structure* 2000; **8**: 1025–1035.

9 Fry BG, Roelants K, Champagne DE, et al. The toxicogenomic multiverse: convergent recruitment of proteins into animal venoms. *Annu Rev Genomics Hum Genet* 2009; **10**: 483–511.

10 Pawlak J, Mackessy SP, Fry BG, et al. Denmotoxin, a three-finger toxin from the colubrid snake *Boiga dendrophila* (mangrove catsnake) with bird-specific activity. *J Biol Chem* 2006; **281**: 29030–29041.

11 Inceoglu B, Lango J, Jing J, et al. One scorpion, two venoms: prevenom of *Parabuthus transvaalicus* acts as an alternative type of venom with distinct mechanism of action. *Proc Natl Acad Sci U S A* 2003; **100**: 922–927.

12 Cheng AC, Currie BJ. Venomous snakebites worldwide with a focus on the Australia–Pacific region: current management and controversies. *J Intensive Care Med* 2004; **19**: 259–269.

13 Murray L, Daly F, Little M, et al. *Toxicology Handbook*, 2nd edn. Sydney: Elsevier Australia, 2011.

14 Warwick C, Steedman C. Injuries, envenomations and stings from exotic pets. *J R Soc Med.* 2012; **105**: 296–299.

15 Cruz LS, Vargas R, Lopes AA. Snakebite envenomation and death in the developing world. *Ethn Dis* 2009; **19**(Suppl 1): S1-42–S1-46.

16 Llewellyn LE, Dodd MJ, Robertson A, et al. Post-mortem analysis of samples from a human victim of a fatal poisoning caused by the xanthid crab, *Zosimus aeneus*. *Toxicon* 2002; **40**: 1463–1469.

17 Arakawa O, Hwang D-F, Taniyama S, et al. Toxins of pufferfish that cause human intoxications. In: Ishimatsu A, Lie H-J (eds.) *Coastal Environmental and Ecosystem Issues of the East China Sea*. Tokyo: Terrapub and Nagasaki University, 2010, pp. 227–244.

18 Krahn D, Barker R, Pandie Z, et al. Envenomation. *Injury Bull Qld Injury Surveill Unit* 2007; **(95)**: 1–6.

19 Anderson SR, Johnson CJH. Expedition health and safety: a risk assessment. *J R Soc Med* 2000; **93**: 557–562.

20 Boggild AK, Costiniuk C, Kain KC, et al. Environmental hazards in Nepal: altitude illness, environmental exposures, injuries, and bites in travelers and expatriates. *J Travel Med* 2007; **14**: 361–368.

21 Denoble PJ, Marroni A, Vann RD. Annual fatality rates and associated risk factors for recreational scuba diving. In: Vann R, Lang M (eds.) *Recreational Diving Fatalities. Proceedings of the Divers Alert Network 2010 April 8–10 Workshop*. Durham, NC: Divers Alert Network, 2011, pp. 73–85.

CHAPTER 27

Cruise ships and travel medicine

Sally S.J. Bell[1] & Eilif Dahl[2]

[1] *Clinical Quality Consultant, London, UK*
[2] *Haukeland University Hospital, Bergen, Norway*

Introduction

Although many hazards and concerns relevant to cruise ship travel are covered in other chapters, cruising is viewed separately, since the environment, facilities, mode of travel, and risks specific to cruise ships differ from those for other modes of travel.

Background

The cruise industry is growing, with over 20 million passengers annually on nearly 300 ships. The ships are also growing, with many over 100,000 tons and some exceeding 200,000 tons. They can carry over 6000 passengers, although 2000–3000 is more usual, with a passenger-to-crew ratio of 2:1 or 3:1. Voyage length varies from hours to months. On some ships passengers will be of the same nationality, on others many nations are represented, with resultant difficulties in understanding language and customs. Crew come from over 100 different countries, although all will be expected to understand the ship's operating language, usually English, for safety reasons.

International regulations, such as the WHO International Health Regulations (2005) [1], address most health requirements for ship operations. The Maritime Labour Convention 2006 [2] relates to crew health and welfare and states that ships carrying 100 or more persons must have a qualified doctor.

The size of ship and route will influence the passenger demographics, and also the challenges that might be encountered and the ability of staff to cope with them. They may call frequently at ports with excellent medical facilities as in Alaska, or have many days at sea between remote ports in the South Pacific with less sophisticated medical facilities than on the ship itself.

Whereas all crew must pass a medical examination, no such requirement exists for passengers, with an average age of over 50 years. Often those in the poorest health will choose the remotest itineraries without considering the risk and discomfort engendered by possible disembarkation.

Essential Travel Medicine, First Edition.
Edited by Jane N. Zuckerman, Gary W. Brunette and Peter A. Leggat.
© 2015 John Wiley & Sons, Ltd. Published 2015 by John Wiley & Sons, Ltd.

Staff and facilities on-board

Although all cruise ships have medical centers, cruising is not risk free. Facilities on board vary greatly. The best may have international accreditation, and most will comply with the American College of Emergency Physicians minimum standards [3], which are regularly updated to reflect international guidelines and expectations. Less well set-up ships may have a single employed nurse, with a doctor traveling on a free cruise who is present only to comply with regulations.

Facilities on top cruise ships

- International accreditation (ISO or healthcare specific).
- Modern resuscitation and monitoring equipment.
- Laboratory.
- X-ray.
- Ultrasound.
- Comprehensive pharmacy.
- Medical staff qualified and experienced in emergency and family practice, with training including:
  - advanced cardiac life support
  - advanced trauma life support
  - pediatric life support
  - use of all equipment
  - regular maritime medicine updates.

Medical disembarkations and evacuation

Patients may be referred ashore when appropriate facilities are available. When a patient's health deteriorates, the ship's doctor might decide to evacuate them, after discussion with Captain, shoreside Medical Director, evacuation provider, and next of kin.

Factors to consider include
- Distance to nearest port.
- Medical facilities ashore.
- Weather conditions.
- Suitability of patient for evacuation.
- The possibility of evacuation by boat.
- Availability of helicopter if within range (about 1 day's sailing from port).
- Risk of evacuation procedure.
- Need for air ambulance evacuation to a higher level of care elsewhere.
- Financial impact of deviation, such as extra fuel and berthing fees.
- Possible liability for compensation to passengers.

Crew health

Crew are required to have a valid medical certificate (for details, see ILO/IMO guidelines [4]) and usually receive travel health advice during an examination performed by a doctor experienced in maritime health (Table 27.1). Crew with specific conditions (e.g., cardiovascular disease, diabetes, epilepsy) may have restricted certificates or be "unfit for sea service." Should a crew member fall ill during their leave, fitness to return to sea must be reassessed.

Dental fitness is important, as only basic dental care is possible on board. Although the company must cover emergency dental treatment ashore, other treatment will be billed to the crew member. All crew are therefore advised to visit the dentist at home.

Passenger health

Although passengers require a medical certificate only in some specific cases, their general fitness to travel should always be considered, in addition to the risks of exacerbation of any pre-existing condition. All should be strongly advised to take out travel insurance covering cancellation pre-travel, care on board and ashore, and repatriation. Pre-travel advice is summarized in Table 27.2.

A passenger capable of walking short distances at home may be challenged by walking from their cabin to the restaurant on ships over 1000 feet long. The ship's movement increases the challenge. The frail and elderly often find they need a wheelchair, but need a companion to push it.

Apart from weight gain, increased food intake raises salt intake. This commonly leads to ankle edema, frequently with an alarming purpuric rash. It usually responds

Table 27.1 Pre-travel advice for crew requesting a travel medicine consultation[a].

Consider:
- Childhood vaccinations up-to-date
- Vaccinations with respect to full possible itinerary:
  - Yellow fever vaccination (or exemption) required for all
  - Hepatitis B for medical staff
  - Hepatitis A for sewage workers
  - Influenza vaccine (offered to all crew on most ships)
- Advice for worldwide risks as destinations may change at short notice:
  - Food hygiene
  - Endemic diseases
  - Sexually transmitted diseases
  - Diet and exercise
- Visit dentist

[a]This advice is usually given by the doctor issuing the medical certificate, but a change in itinerary may occur afterwards.

Table 27.2 Pre-travel advice for passengers.

- Review itinerary for relevant local travel advice
- Check vaccines and other prophylaxis required for area of travel
- Update childhood vaccination status
- Ensure full travel insurance coverage, including cancellation, medical disembarkation and repatriation
- Obtain doctor's report for any medical conditions including all medications taken and allergies
- Pack a supply of regular medications, to allow for unexpected travel delays, loss, or damage
- Pack medications in hand baggage
- Prepare a first-aid kit, with motion sickness medication, insect repellent, sun screen, alcohol hand gel and simple painkillers
- Where relevant:
  - Doctor's letter regarding travel with controlled substances, syringes, and needles
  - Copy of recent ECG
  - Check availability of refrigeration on-board for medicines such as insulin
  - Check both voltage and frequency (Hz) of electricity supply on board for medical equipment (e.g., nebulizers, oxygen concentrators)
  - Ensure suitable storage is available for oxygen cylinders

to elevation, easily done by inserting a spare lifejacket below the foot of the mattress. Others with reflux or respiratory difficulty can use a lifejacket below the head of the mattress.

The combination of change in diet and exercise habits may lead to atrial fibrillation ("holiday heart").

Those who are fit to travel but not to fly often cruise from a home port, but should they need to be disembarked en route, travel home can be difficult.

Pregnancy

The safety of both mother and baby should be considered carefully at any gestation. Since there will be no facilities for neonatal intensive care, passengers and crew are not permitted to travel beyond the gestational age when the fetus is viable (usually 24 weeks).

Motion sickness

Prevention is the mainstay of management. Any passenger totally dependent on oral medications (e.g., transplant recipients) should be carefully advised with respect to motion sickness and its prevention. Passengers prone to motion sickness should take medication prior to sailing, since absorption is reduced in those already affected. Extremely susceptible persons should continue medication throughout the trip. Antihistamines are commonly used, but scopolamine patches are not prescribed on most cruise vessels because of side-effects in the elderly such as confusion. Passengers already unwell may consult the ship's doctor for intramuscular medication, usually promethazine. The provision of oral medication will vary between cruise lines, so passengers are well advised to bring their own supplies.

Land sickness is a sensation of continuing motion noted for 1–2 hours after disembarkation. Mal de débarquement syndrome, however, is a rare disorder of perceived motion that may persist for years after a voyage. More common in women than men, the persistent and treatment-resistant symptoms include a sensation of motion usually associated with fatigue, imbalance, and impaired cognition. The cause is unknown.

Infectious diseases

Written with the cooperation of the cruise industry, the American CDC Vessel Sanitation Program Operations Manual [5] has clear procedures for the management of infectious disease on-board, including food and water safety, and reporting and management of both respiratory and gastrointestinal disease. Passengers and crew are usually screened prior to boarding for both respiratory and gastrointestinal illness.

Norovirus

This common and extremely contagious disease flourishes in close communities such as on cruise ships. As incidence increases ashore, so it increases on-board, often imported by passengers traveling from outbreak areas. Stringent procedures are in place to contain infection, emphasizing hand hygiene and isolation of all cases. Even vague symptoms should be reported immediately to the medical center aboard. Self-medication should not be attempted.

Legionella

Occasional cases of legionella can be traced back to jacuzzis and dead ends in the potable water system. Clear procedures for cleaning, disinfection, inspection, and flushing are therefore in place. All pneumonia cases are tested for legionella on most ships.

Childhood illnesses

Many crew members come from communities where vaccination is poor and diseases such as rubella, varicella, mumps, and measles are not universal, so outbreaks are possible, with a concomitant risk to susceptible passengers. For this reason, some major lines now require pre-employment vaccination of all crew.

Sexually transmitted and blood-borne diseases

Both passengers and crew are at risk of sexually transmitted disease from contacts aboard and ashore. Needle stick injuries are a risk, from either legitimate use or drug abuse. Passengers injecting medications should ask for a sharps bin, and crew members should be alert to evidence of needle use.

Risks ashore

Infectious diseases that may be contracted ashore are covered elsewhere; however, passengers should not develop a false sense of security from the carefully regulated environment on-board. They are advised against indiscriminate eating and drinking ashore, and should be vaccinated and otherwise advised for travel to each port of call. The risk for a traveler visiting a port for just a few hours in the daytime is very different for that of a traveler spending a significant time inland, particularly for malaria. Protection from mosquitoes remains important in both malarial and dengue risk areas.

Other risks include:
- travel in vehicles such as tuk-tuks or taxis with no seatbelts and poor safety features
- mugging and pickpockets
- marine envenomation from jellyfish, sea snakes and fish
- animal bites in areas with rabies.

Mental health

Psychiatric conditions should be assessed very carefully. Even the mildly demented must travel with an able companion. The opportunity for suicide is ever present, and once overboard survival is unlikely. Once suicidal intent is suspected, 24-hour watch is instigated until disembarkation for psychiatric assessment in the next port.

Dentistry

Although few, if any, ships now carry a dentist, simple dental care is possible aboard. The mainstay of treatment is with antibiotics and painkillers, but some ship's doctors can repair dentures, insert temporary fillings, and re-cement crowns.

Dialysis

Passengers on chronic ambulatory peritoneal dialysis should only travel on the advice of their nephrologist and should always carry extra dialysis fluid, suitable antibiotics for peritonitis, and a full medical report including contact details for their nephrologist. Some ships offer specialist hemodialysis cruises.

Sexual assault

Although this is a rare occurrence, ship's medical staff are usually trained to use forensic kits. Management of these cases may involve flagging state police and authorities in the next port and also laboratory services in a third country.

Communications

Modern satellite communications now allow access to telemedical services and Internet sources of information. It is possible to telephone the patient's own physician or the receiving physician ashore for advice. Staff may also update their knowledge online.

Conclusion

The above information, coupled with media inflation of specific incidents, may give the impression that cruise ship travel is hazardous. It is, however, ideal for those wishing to travel in style and safety, with excellent medical care available on-board round the clock, and good links to centers of excellence ashore.

References

1 World Health Organization. *Alert, Response, and Capacity Building Under the International Health Regulations (IHR)*. http://www.who.int/ihr/about/en/ (accessed 4 February 2015).

2 International Labour Organization. *Maritime Labour Convention, 2006*. http://www.ilo.org/global/standards/maritime-labour-convention/lang--en/index.htm (accessed 4 February 2015).

3 American College of Emergency Physicians. *Health Care Guidelines for Cruise Ship Medical Facilities*. http://www.acep.org/Content.aspx?id=29980 (accessed 4 February 2015).

4 International Labour Organization. *Guidelines on the Medical Examinations of Seafarers*. http://www.ilo.org/sector/Resources/codes-of-practice-and-guidelines/WCMS_174794/lang-en/index.htm (accessed 4 February 2015).

5 Centers for Disease Control and Prevention. *Vessel Sanitation Program*. http://www.cdc.gov/nceh/vsp/ (accessed 4 February 2015).

CHAPTER 28

Mass gatherings and travel medicine

Joanna Gaines & Gary W. Brunette

Centers for Disease Control and Prevention, Atlanta, GA, USA

Overview

Travelers attending mass gatherings face unique health risks beyond those typically associated with their destination. Mass gathering medicine has roots in emergency medicine, with a traditional focus on injuries or the provision of on-site medical services [1]. More recently, there has been a recognition of the need for a more proactive research agenda using a multidisciplinary approach that incorporates various aspects of public health and travel medicine, including risk assessments, disease surveillance, sanitation, food and water safety, public works, environment, and risk communication [1,2]. Medical providers should consider the unique health needs of persons who attend mass gatherings, as they attract both novice and experienced travelers. This chapter focuses on travelers to international mass gatherings; however, information provided here may also be applicable to travelers attending domestic mass gatherings.

What is a "mass gathering"?

Mass gatherings are typically defined as a large number of people (ranging from 1000 to >25000) who gather at a specific location, for a specific purpose, for a defined time frame [3]. Practically, a mass gathering can be thought of as any gathering of people that strains local resources. Some mass gatherings are highly structured events that occur on an established time frame, such as the annual Hajj pilgrimage to Mecca that all Muslims are obligated to complete at least once in their lifetime. During this event, Hajj pilgrims journey between multiple sites. Other mass gatherings may involve attendees moving from place to place, such as the 2014 FIFA World Cup, with soccer matches held in 12 different cities across Brazil. Mass gatherings also occur spontaneously, such as the 2005 funeral of Pope John Paul II, which brought together an estimated 4 million mourners in Vatican City [4,5].

Hosts are the country and city or specific site where the mass gathering will be held. Some mass gatherings are held at multiple cities within the same country; for example, the 2006 FIFA World Cup was held in 12 host cities across Germany [6]. Mass gatherings may have event organizers within the host country, such as the 2012 London Olympic Committee. Organizers may be involved in lobbying for their selection as host, in addition to being charged with carrying out a successful event. Mass gathering sports events often involve a governing body that may set requirements for a host site and monitor their ability to prepare for hosting. For the Olympics, an extensive vetting process conducted by the International Olympic Committee (IOC), takes place 9 years before a city hosts the Games. For mass gathering events overseen by a governing body, the host cities must demonstrate that they have sufficient infrastructure, including housing, transportation, and security [7].

Important characteristics

Medical providers should understand the characteristics of the mass gathering that a person will attend. Gatherings can be effectively described by considering their location, health and safety risks, venue, purpose, size, participants, duration, timing, activities, and capacity.

- **Location**: Who is the host? What is the local infrastructure like? What is the environment like?
- **Health and safety risks**: What types of diseases are endemic to the location? Will security be adequate? What type of safety issues are there?
- **Venue**: Where will the mass gathering be held? Indoors or outdoors? Will the venue, including food, water, and sanitation facilities, be adequate? Is the mass gathering mobile or static (i.e., will attendees be moving from one place to another, such as in a pilgrimage)?
- **Purpose**: Why will people attend? Is the event political, religious, social, or athletic? The purpose of an event can affect the activities and mood of participants.
- **Size**: How dense will crowds be? How prepared are organizers to manage large crowds? Consider the density of attendees rather than the number. Densely packed crowds may facilitate disease spread.
- **Participants**: Are attendees primarily male or female, young or old?
- **Duration**: How long does the gathering last? The longer the event lasts, the more likely it is that local resources will become strained.
- **Timing**: When does the mass gathering occur? What will the weather be like? Is the mass gathering during a peak travel time for the host country/city?
- **Activities**: What will participants do? Are attendees likely to be engaged in risky or strenuous behaviors? Will there be alcohol or drug use?
- **Capacity**: What capacity do hosts have to detect, respond, and prevent public health emergencies? For recurring mass gatherings, what health outcomes have been previously associated with them?

Table 28.1 gives the characteristics of example mass gatherings.

Table 28.1 Characteristics of sample mass gatherings.

Mass gathering event	Location	Health and safety risks	Venue	Purpose	Size	Participants	Duration	Timing	Activities	Capacity
2016 Summer Olympic and Paralympic Games	Rio de Janeiro, Brazil	Malaria not endemic to Rio de Janeiro metro area Potential for safety and security risks to travelers	35 venues Some newly constructed	Sporting event	9 million tickets for sale Crowd density varies	>14,000 athletes >200 national committees International spectators	Olympic Games: 5 August 2016 to Paralympic Games: 7 September 2016	Cooler weather due to southern hemisphere location	28 Olympic sports 22 Paralympic sports	International Olympic Committee Host Organizing Committee
Glastonbury Music Festival[a]	Worthy Farm, Pilton, England	History of crime, drug use, violence	Static Dairy farm Housing in RVs, temporary campsites Safe water, handwashing stations provided	Music festival	~175,000 attendees Crowd density varies	Younger adults Mixed gender International attendees	5 days in late June	Summer		Medical care provided by UK's "Festival Medical Services"
Hajj (annual)	Mecca, Kingdom of Saudi Arabia (KSA)	Engineering has improved crowd flow to prevent stampedes, accommodate disabled pilgrims	Mobile Multiple mosques /temples KSA- constructed housing	Religious gathering	>1 million High-density movement of persons High-density housing	Compulsory for all able-bodied Muslims at least once in lifetime. People in poor health may choose to attend. Multiple nationalities in attendance	Annually, 8–12th of the last month of the Islamic calendar Umrah pilgrimage can be taken at any point during year.	Seasonal variation due to lunar calendar Climate may be extremely hot, humid	Rituals include standing, walking for extended periods of time, head shaving, animal sacrifices Access to water and food may be limited at times	KSA publishes required and recommended vaccinations annually[b]

[a] http://www.glastonburyfestivals.co.uk/.
[b] http://saudiembassy.net/services/hajj_requirements.aspx.

Common health problems

Mass gatherings pose a potential risk to attendees in the form of exacerbation of chronic medical conditions, injuries, and the spread of infectious diseases.

Emergency medical services are often incorporated in preparations for mass gatherings and are usually sufficient to address acute medical conditions, such as myocardial infarction, asthma, and minor injuries. Conditions such as heat exhaustion, dehydration, hypothermia, or sunburn can also affect attendees and are usually handled on-site. More than 1000 people were treated for heat-related conditions during the 1996 Olympic Games in the southeastern United States [8].

Safety is of particular concern with mass gatherings because of their size and the possibility of a catastrophic incident [1,4]. A number of examples of mass casualties at events have resulted from poor crowd management, structural collapses, fires, and violence including targeting of the event by groups such as terrorists. Regarded as the deadliest sporting event riots, the football riots in Lima, Peru, in 1964 resulted in 318 people being killed and more than 500 injured [4]. More than 100 people were killed during a stampede at the 2011 Sabarimala pilgrimage in Kerala, India [4]. In 1997, over 300 pilgrims died in a fire during the Hajj in Mecca, Saudi Arabia [9].

Attendees of mass gatherings are at risk for infectious disease. An outbreak of influenza occurred during the 2008 World Youth Day in Sydney, Australia [10]. Meningococcal disease outbreaks followed a 1997 youth football tournament in Belgium [11] and the 2000 Hajj in Saudi Arabia [12]. In 2013, an outbreak of norovirus on a flight affected 26 passengers who had attended World Youth Day in Brazil [13]. Mass gatherings also pose risks to groups due to inadequate food and water safety, poor sanitation, and inadequate facilities [1,4]. In 1987, a strain of antibiotic-resistant *Shigella sonnei* affected thousands of attendees at the Rainbow Family Gathering in North Carolina, who were exposed at the event and infected others after returning home, resulting in a multistate outbreak [14].

Mass gatherings have implications for global health security – attendees may be exposed to infectious diseases in one location and then import the infection into their home country. More than two million pilgrims attended the Hajj in 2009 during the H1N1 pandemic and in 2013 during the outbreak of Middle East respiratory syndrome (MERS) in the Arabian Peninsula [4]. Attendees may import diseases to a host site, and also spread disease upon their return home [15]. In 2010, measles outbreaks in Germany were linked to youth who had attended events in Taizé, France [16].

Guidance for clinicians

Assessing risk

- **Ask about itineraries and activities**. Knowing a patient's destination is the first step, keeping in mind that patients may add side trips or extend travel beyond the mass gathering. Verify the itinerary to identify additional risks beyond those associated with the event. For example, if a patient indicates that they will be attending the 2016 Olympic Games in Rio de Janeiro, malaria prophylaxis would not be a consideration for those who intend to stay within the Rio metro area. However, this traveler may choose to also visit the Amazon rainforest (where malaria is endemic), thus putting them at risk [17]. The CDC's Travelers' Health website (http://www.cdc.gov/travel) posts travel notices to educate travelers and medical providers about health issues associated with specific destinations.

- **Consider your patient's unique characteristics.** Chronic health conditions may be exacerbated by the activities associated with a mass gathering. Patients should ensure that they have adequate supplies of medication for the duration of their trip, and also documentation for any prescriptions. The very old and the very young are more susceptible to extreme environmental conditions such as extreme heat or cold and are more susceptible to many infectious diseases.

Mitigating risk

- **Identify requirements** for mass gathering attendees beyond those normally required for entry to the country. For example, all pilgrims to the Hajj are required to have meningococcal vaccinations; this requirement does not apply to other travelers to Saudi Arabia [18].
- **Identify recommendations** for attendees, as hosts may make additional recommendations on the basis of public health concerns. In response to the emergence in 2013 of the MERS coronavirus, Saudi Arabia recommended that elderly or immunocompromised people delay their pilgrimage [18].
- **Educate travelers on appropriate preventive measures.** These may include choosing safe food and water from vendors or using insect repellents. All attendees to mass gatherings should be educated on the importance of regular handwashing and the use of an alcohol-based sanitizer when soap and water are not available.
- **Visit the CDC's Travelers' Health website at http://www.cdc.gov/travel.** This website is updated regularly with travel health notices; information is also provided on mass gatherings such as the Hajj and Olympic Games. Users can access an electronic copy of CDC's *Health Information for International Travel*, also known as the "Yellow Book."
- **Other useful web sites providing guidance include:** http://www.who.int/ihr/ith_and_mass_gatherings/en/ and http://www.hpa.org.uk/webc/HPAwebFile/HPAweb_C/1317138422305 [19].

Guidance for travelers

- **Consult a travel medicine provider at least 4–6 weeks before the departure date.** This should allow adequate time to receive most vaccinations. Inform the provider of your itinerary and any planned activities: this allows more accurate recommendations to ensure your health and safety.
- **For US travelers, register your travel plans with the US Department of State's Smart Traveler Enrollment Program (STEP)** (https://step.state.gov/step/). Travelers can subscribe to receive notifications on travel warnings, travel alerts, and other information for specific destination(s), and also to ensure that

the Department of State is aware of your presence should you have serious legal, medical, or financial difficulties while traveling. STEP can also help friends and family reach travelers in the event of an emergency at home [20].

- **Ensure that any current medical conditions are well controlled before departure**. These should be discussed with your medical provider during the pre-travel consultation.
- **Visit the CDC's Travelers' Health website at http://www.cdc.gov/travel**. Learn more about specific destinations and view any travel notices for your destination.

References

1 Arbon P. Mass-gathering medicine: a review of the evidence and future directions for research. *Prehosp Disaster Med* 2007; **22**: 131–135.
2 Tam JS, Barbeschi M, Shapovalova N, et al. Research agenda for mass gatherings: a call to action. *Lancet Infect Dis* 2012; **12**: 231–239.
3 WHO. *Communicable Disease Alert and Response for Mass Gatherings – Key Considerations*. Geneva: World Health Organization, 2008, pp. 32–33.
4 Memish ZA, Stephens GM, Steffen R, Ahmed QA. Emergence of medicine for mass gatherings: lessons from the Hajj. *Lancet Infect Dis* 2012; **12**: 56–65.
5 Vatican.com. *The Funeral of Pope John Paul II the Blessed*. http://vatican.com/articles/popes/the_funeral_of_pope_john_paul_ii_the_blessed-a813 (accessed 18 November 2013).
6 FIFA. 2006 *FIFA World Cup Germany*. http://www.fifa.com/worldcup/archive/germany2006/overview.html (accessed 18 November 2013).
7 Olympic.org. *Official Website of the Olympic Movement*. http://www.olympic.org (accessed 18 November 2013).
8 Wetterhall SF, Coulombier DM, Herndon JM, et al. Medical care delivery at the 1996 Olympic Games. *JAMA* 1998; **279**: 1463–1468.
9 Ahmed QA, Arabi YM, Memish ZA. Health risks at the Hajj. *Lancet* 2006; **367**: 1008–1015.
10 Blyth CC, Foo H, van Hal SJ, et al. Influenza outbreaks during World Youth Day 2008 mass gathering. *Emerg Infect Dis* 2010; **16**: 809–815.
11 Reintjes R, Kistemann T, MacLehose L, et al. Detection and response to a meningococcal disease outbreak following a youth football tournament with teams from four European countries. *Int J Hyg Environ Health* 2002; **205**: 291–296.
12 Aguilera J-F, Perrocheau A, Meffre C. Outbreak of serogroup W135 meningococcal disease after the Hajj pilgrimage, Europe, 2000. *Emerg Infect Dis* 2002; **8**: 761–767.
13 CBS/AP. *Norovirus Outbreak Reported on Qantas Flight to Sydney*. http://www.cbsnews.com/8301-204_162-57596531/norovirus-outbreak-reported-on-qantas-flight-to-sydney/ (accessed 13 August 2013).
14 Wharton M, Spiegel RA, Horan JM, et al. A large outbreak of antibiotic-resistant shigellosis at a mass gathering. *J Infect Dis* 1990; **162**: 1324–1328.
15 Abubakar I, Gautret P, Brunette GW, et al. Global perspectives for prevention of infectious diseases associated with mass gatherings. *Lancet Infect Dis* 2012; **12**: 66–74.
16 Pfaff G, Lohr D, Santibanez S, et al. Spotlight on measles 2010: measles outbreak among travellers returning from a mass gathering, Germany, September to October 2010. *Euro Surveill* 2010; **15**: pii=19750.
17 Gershman MD, Jentes ES, Johnson KJ, et al. Travel vaccines and malaria information, by country. In: Brunette G (ed.) *CDC Health Information for International Travel 2014: The Yellow Book*. New York: Oxford University Press, 2014, pp. 347–404.

18 Royal Embassy of Arabia Washington DC. *Saudi Arabia.* http://saudiembassy.net (accessed 23 October 2013).

19 McCloskey B, Endericks T. *Learning from London* 2012. *A Practical Guide to Public Health and Mass Gatherings.* http://www.hpa.org.uk/webc/HPAwebFile/HPAweb_C/1317138422305 (accessed 10 January 2014).

20 US Department of State. *Smart Traveler Enrollment Program.* https://step.state.gov/step/ (accessed 16 October 2013).

CHAPTER 29

Emergency care whilst abroad

Peter A. Leggat & Marc T.M. Shaw
James Cook University, Townsville, Queensland, Australia

Introduction

Conservatively, it is estimated that between 30 and 50% of travelers become ill or injured whilst traveling [1]. Fortunately, few travelers die and those who do tend to die of pre-existing illnesses and accidents, rather than from infectious disease [1,2]. In a Swiss study, accidents constituted about one-third of travel insurance claims [3]. Muggings, theft, and loss also make up a considerable proportion of travel insurance claims [4]. Hence safety and security are a growing topic of interest, not only for intending travelers but also for an increasingly worried world. Travel health advisors need to include safety and security issues on a checklist of itinerary items to be discussed with those travelers full of the excited anticipation of international travel, yet not experienced to witness it directly. In addition, travelers need to take out travel insurance to cover any unexpected medical or dental problems abroad. Medical and dental conditions account for about two-thirds of all travel insurance claims [4]. The most common medical conditions reported for travel insurance claims include respiratory (20%), musculoskeletal (17%), gastrointestinal (14%), ear, nose, and throat (12%), and dental problems (7%) [4].

Although travel insurance is an important recommendation to make to all travelers, in some older studies only about half of general practitioners (GPs) and 39% of travel clinics would recommend travel insurance [5–7]. In addition, about half of GPs in New Zealand usually also advised travelers about how to find medical assistance abroad [5]. Similarly, only about half of travelers reported taking out travel insurance although, importantly, major travel advisories do advise travelers to take out travel insurance [8–11]. The great expense of medical care, hospitalization, or possible aeromedical evacuation (AME) means that travelers cannot afford not to take out travel insurance.

Accessing medical care abroad

Pre-travel health advice is duty bound to minimize health risks specific to the journey and inform travelers on the capability of coping with most minor medical problems. In addition, travel health advisors should also provide guidance on how to identify when

Essential Travel Medicine, First Edition.
Edited by Jane N. Zuckerman, Gary W. Brunette and Peter A. Leggat.
© 2015 John Wiley & Sons, Ltd. Published 2015 by John Wiley & Sons, Ltd.

to seek local medical care either during the trip or upon return. Personal safety needs to be a target topic for travel health advisors to discuss when giving advice to travelers going abroad, yet it is an often neglected issue in travel medicine and has been for many years [12]. The four steps for giving travelers the foundation for healthy and safe journeys are to analyze their itineraries, assess their health, select vaccines and antimalarials, and offer education about the prevention and self-treatment of travel-related diseases [13]. Two further steps need to be added. The first is to guide the traveler to look after themselves medically whilst abroad, both proactively and reactively by advising them on medical managements in response to simple accidents and illnesses that may occur whilst traveling. Second the travel health advisor needs to counsel on the need for travel insurance and how to access emergency assistance. This should include what to do and who to call if and threat-to-self urgency should arise. Providing pre-travel education takes time, and prospective travelers need to leave the clinic with written advice to reinforce important consultation discussions and punch-point information.

In a study of travel insurance claims in Australia, just over one-quarter of claims involved the use of the company's emergency assistance service [14]. About two-thirds (69%) of claims requiring emergency assistance were for medical and dental conditions, with cancellation and curtailment, mostly for medical reasons, making up more than one-eighth of claims (15%) [14]. Emergency assistance provided in this study included policy advice (99%), claiming advice (99%), civil advice or assistance (20%), medical advice or GP referral (6%), hospital emergency room (ER) review (15%), hospital admission (12%), medical or dental follow-up (6%), and aeromedical evacuation (AME) (2.5%) [12]. The most common conditions requiring emergency assistance were musculoskeletal disorders (28%), followed by gastrointestinal disorders (15%), dental conditions (14%), and respiratory problems (12%) [14].

Travelers usually have access to a travel insurance or medical assistance representative, through a 24-hour emergency assistance number, which can advise travelers about finding medical and dental assistance abroad. Nevertheless, apart from travel insurers, there are several possible sources for this information, including travel insurance companies, diplomatic missions, corporate and professional medical networks and emergency medical services, and other sources such as major hotels that may have a hotel doctor on call. It is concerning, however, that only about one-third of British travelers were aware of the emergency services contact numbers for the country that they most recently visited [15]. It is important that travel health advisors discuss the basics of how to deal with medical and other emergencies abroad, including providing advice on the contact numbers for emergency services or how to find this information before they travel.

Emergency assistance companies may have their own network of clinics and AME providers; however, there are a few international organizations that provide international clinic listings, including:
- Clinic Directory the International Society of Travel Medicine [16].
- Directory of the International Association for Medical Assistance to Travelers [17].

In many parts of the world, the promise of payment or having travel insurance may not be sufficient to guarantee treatment, and a cash advance may be required up front, provided by the traveler or the travel insurance company. It follows that travelers should advise their travel insurance company of any significant medical problems and any urgent treatment received through their emergency assistance service whilst traveling. They also need to keep receipts and any medical and dental reports to support any travel insurance claims made on their return [18].

Accessing dental care abroad

Dental treatment abroad, depending on the procedures required, can be expensive. Travel insurance generally provides some coverage against dental expenses incurred while overseas, provided that the conditions treated are not pre-existing [19]. Dental care does not tend to be as accessible in the public health systems of many developing countries; however, once traveling, recommendations concerning suitable dentists available for consultation while overseas may be obtained from embassies/foreign missions, hotels, private hospitals, and travel medicine centers. Emergency assistance companies of travel insurers or local dental societies may be able to make recommendations concerning suitable dental clinics [20], although language barriers can often be a problem if pre-travel planning is not complete. Therefore, before travel, it is worth travelers contacting their dentist for a recommendation for suitable dental treatment services at their destinations, particularly if they are prone to dental problems or if there is need for ongoing care. This needs to be paralleled with a letter for the traveler, outlining their dental history. If is likely that dental treatment will be undertaken abroad, then hepatitis B vaccination should be discussed with the traveler [8]. A "common questions paper on dental care while traveling" has been published by the American Dental Association (ADA) [21]. Although many dental associations remain cautious, medical and dental tourism is booming in many countries [22].

Aeromedical evacuation (AME)

Some travelers may require medical evacuation by road, sea, or air because of the seriousness of their illness or accident. Medical transport, especially AME, can be expensive and it is important that travel insurance covers this for the traveler's destination [17]. AME, whether national or international, is a planned activity, requiring careful assessment and preparation of the patient and liaison with authorities at all stages of the evacuation. Escorts need to be trained health professionals, familiar with equipment on aircraft used for AME [23]. Evacuation is undertaken on a conventional commercial flight or increasingly on a specially fitted out aircraft, either fixed or rotary wing aircraft. The latter are usually maintained by specialized retrieval (air ambulance) companies, emergency services, the military, and occasionally multinational companies [23]. Although travelers may take out appropriate travel insurance, which covers against this contingency, it is important that they also use common sense to ensure that the need for AME is kept to a minimum by minimizing risks and seeking medical advice early, for any medical problems.

Travel and evacuation insurance

Some countries have negotiated reciprocal healthcare agreements, but this generally covers only emergency medical treatment in a hospital, and not in many of the countries where the costs of healthcare are among the highest. Because of the potentially premium costs associated with emergency assistance, travelers need to be advised of the need for comprehensive travel insurance, which includes adequate coverage for medical and dental health care abroad and also AME from the destinations to which they are traveling. Travel insurance policies normally underwrite travel-related, medical, and dental expenses incurred by travelers abroad under conditions specified by the travel insurance policy, in addition to covering other aspects of travel, such as loss/theft insurance and unforeseen cancellation of travel. In addition, travel insurance companies usually provide a direct service, usually through their emergency assistance service contractors, to assist travelers abroad in obtaining medical care, including AME. Almost one in five Australian travelers abroad in one study had been found to have used the travel insurer's emergency assistance service [13].

Exclusions

Travel insurance is the most important safety net for travelers in the event of illness, injury, or unforeseen events, and must be reinforced by GPs and travel health advisers. However, it is important that travelers do not have unrealistic expectations of their travel insurance policies. Excess fees are now common on many aspects of claims with the various types of travel insurance policies available. Even the top-level travel insurance policies usually do not cover travelers against such things as travel to war zones, self-inflicted injuries, unlawful acts, certain infectious diseases such as AIDS and sexually transmitted infections, pregnancy, and participation in professional sports. Those who are expecting to undertake any kind of hazardous pursuit may be required to take out a separate policy that covers them for that activity, or at least they should expect to pay a surcharge on their travel insurance premium, which may be assessed on a case-by-case basis by travel insurance companies. Some sporting organizations, such as those for divers, may recommend a specific travel insurance product. Pregnant travelers need to be especially vigilant, as travel insurers may exclude pregnancy and any complications arising from pregnancy after 26 weeks, or they may either refuse coverage or restrict it even further. For all the disadvantages, however, even in disaster settings, such as with the Bali bombings in 2002 and the Asian tsunami in 2004, travel insurance was able to provide emergency assistance and also to assist in the repatriation of the deceased [24,25].

It is imperative that travel health advisors make travelers, especially elderly travelers, aware that travel insurance does not normally cover any known pre-existing medical or dental problems or disability. In these cases, it may be necessary for travelers to complete further documentation of these conditions and in some cases be clinically assessed by their GP or travel insurance medical representative. It is possible that routine illnesses may also be excluded by the travel insurance policy. It is still important for these travelers to take out a travel insurance policy, since other conditions, not directly linked to their excluded pre-existing condition, are likely to be covered. For those travelers who may be uninsurable because of advanced age or advanced ill health, it is a given that they are advised about destinations where they can travel safely, such as where bilateral government health agreements exist and with the proviso that airlines are prepared to evacuate the traveler. aeromedically A "worst case scenario" discussion gives appropriate focus to risk management with this group of travelers.

All pre-existing illnesses should be fully documented, preferably in a doctor's letter. Emergency documentation, such as medical alert bracelets, can provide emergency responders with pointers to alerting medical conditions such as severe diabetes or asthma, and also allergies. Travel insurance companies will also probably store this medical information for emergency assistance companies.

Third-party insurance

Although travelers can take out travel insurance to cover against illnesses and injuries occurring during their travel, it is important that they do not elect to decline third-party or personal liability insurance from a car rental agency in the event that they are involved in an accident they caused, as many travel insurance policies do not include claims for damage to other persons or property arising from the traveler's operation of cars, boats, jet skis, aircraft, and other motorized devices.

Taking medications abroad

Travelers may be taking medications abroad for several reasons, such as pre-existing conditions or for health and disease prophylaxis and/or for treatment of conditions likely to be encountered abroad. Together with first aid supplies, these may constitute the travelers' medical kit. Any traveler taking medications should be advised to carry these medications on-board the aircraft with them and they need to ensure that they have sufficient medications with them for their entire journey. If medications are lost or stolen during travel, caution is urged with their replacement as counterfeit medication is especially prevalent in developing countries. Travelers should carry separately a copy of their doctor's letter detailing their medications, which when presented to reputable medical sources abroad will assist them in obtaining both appropriate medical care and replacement medications. If travelers need insulin or other injectable drugs, they must carry a doctor's letter noting the same and why they need to have syringes in their luggage. Pre-travel planning should detail this information, together with the need for a traveler's doctor to provide them with a doctor's letter covering their medical conditions and detailing all their medications [26].

Some countries may have special requirements for the importation of large quantities of medications and relevant embassies should be contacted, if in any doubt.

Travel health kits

A well-stocked travelers' medical kit is advisable for anyone going to travel or work overseas. It should include their regular and other personal or travel-related medication. It is also advisable to take a first aid kit as part of the travelers' medical kit, with contents dependent upon both destination and the duration of the journey. A doctor's letter should cover the prescription of any medical kit, although often this is never assessed by authorities. Nevertheless, it is advisable to have it, particularly if the kit contains pain relief and neurologic or psychoactive medication. Customs officials are often very particular about the cross-border transport of such medicines.

If a medical professional issues a medical kit, then they need to ensure that the traveler knows how to use it and its contents. If they are traveling in a group, then they need to assess whether someone in the group has undertaken first aid training. This enables a better response to be made to major and minor medical emergencies whilst traveling [27]. It has been found previously in an Australian study that about one-third of travelers reported possessing a current first aid certificate [28]. Possible contents for a travel medical kit are given in Table 29.1.

Medical equipment kits

There are various equipment kits ranging from basic first aid kits to kits for groups of school children [29] or expeditioners [30], to kits that contain intravenous giving sets, and many have been made commercially available by some organizations. They are designed for the traveler who may be visiting areas where there may not be good access to basic medical equipment and/or where basic medical equipment is reused. Possible contents of a medical equipment kit are listed in Table 29.2.

Dental kits

Dental kits are available for travelers in some countries. These usually contain basic materials and instruments to deal with minor dental problems. It is particularly important for longer term travelers going to work overseas to have a dental check before they leave and to ask their dentist about the availability of dental services at their destination.

Conclusion

Travelers do sometimes encounter significant medical and dental problems abroad. It is important, therefore, that all travelers take out travel insurance appropriate for their destination and activities and also for any pre-existing medical and dental conditions. Travel insurance provides a source of emergency assistance advice, which might include finding medical and dental care abroad, assistance with hospitalization, and arranging for AME in some situations. In the meantime, travelers can benefit from taking a travelers' medical kit appropriate for their destination and activities and for their personal health.

Table 29.1 Contents of a basic travel medical kit.

For all travelers
- First aid kit, including:
  - Items thermometer, adhesive dressings, bandages, tape and antiseptic cream to treat common problems, such as cuts, scratches, burns, strains, and splinters
  - Throat lozenges
  - Eye wash/drops
  - Paracetamol
- Traveler's own medications
- Consider:
  - Minor sedative or melatonin for long-haul travel
  - Insect repellent (e.g., DEET-based product)
  - Sunscreen (best possible sun protection factor)
  - Condoms

Additional items for most destinations
- Antinausea medication
- Broad-spectrum antibiotic for respiratory infections
- Antacids
- Pseudoephedrine/antihistamine
- Laxative

Gastroenteritis kit, especially for developing countries
- Rehydration solution
- Loperamide
- Tinadazole
- Norfloxacin (or azithromycin for children)

Additional items for areas with malaria transmission
- Consider:
  - Insect repellent (e.g., DEET-based product)
  - Permethrin-impregnated bednet
  - Malaria chemoprophylaxis

Additional items for comprehensive kit
- Antihistamines
- Antifungal and antibiotic cream
- Consider:
  - Iodine solution (antiseptic and water disinfection)
  - Permethrin (for bednets/clothing impregnation)
  - Medical equipment kit (see Table 29.2)
  - Acetazolamide (for travel to high altitudes)

Additional items for expedition medical kits
- See Chapter 25

Instructions for use
- Instructions for use (and/or doctor's letter and/or copy of prescription)

Source: Adapted from Shaw et al. 2014 [29], Gherardin 2007 [31], and Leggat and Heydon 2005 [32].

Table 29.2 Basic contents of a medical equipment kit.

- Needles, syringes
- Alcohol swabs
- Cannulas
- Sutures
- Dressings
- Scalpel handle and blades
- Gloves
- Face masks
- Personal data sheet e.g., for name and blood group

Source: Leggat and Heydon 2005 [32]. Reproduced with permission by Elsevier

References

1 WHO. *International Travel and Health*. Geneva: World Health Organization, 2014. http://www.who.int/ith (accessed 29 March 2014).

2 Leggat PA, Wilks J. Overseas visitor deaths in Australia, 2001–2003. *J Travel Med* 2009; **16**: 243–247.

3 Somer Kniestedt RA, Steffen R. Travel health insurance: indicator of serious travel health risks. *J Travel Med* 2003; **10**: 185–189.

4 Leggat PA, Leggat FW. Travel insurance claims made by travelers from Australia. *J Travel Med* 2002; **9**: 59–65.

5 Leggat PA, Heydon JL, Menon A. Safety advice for travelers from New Zealand. *J Travel Med* 1998; **5**: 61–64.

6 Seelan ST, Leggat PA. Health advice given by general practitioners for travellers from Australia. *Travel Med Infect Dis* 2003; **1**: 47–52.

7 Hill DR, Behrens RH. A survey of travel clinics throughout the world. *J Travel Med* 1996; **3**: 46–51.

8 Leggat PA, Zwar NA, Hudson BJ, et al. Hepatitis B risks and immunisation coverage amongst Australians travelling to southeast Asia and east Asia. *Travel Med Infect Dis* 2009; **7**: 344–349.

9 US Department of State, Bureau of Consular Affairs. *US Passports and International Travel*. http://travel.state.gov/content/passports/english/alertswarnings.html (accessed 29 March 2014).

10 UK Government. *Foreign Travel Advice*. https://www.gov.uk/foreign-travel-advice (accessed 29 March 2014).

11 Australian Government Department of Foreign Affairs and Trade. *Smartraveller*. http://smartraveller.gov.au (accessed 29 March 2014).

12 Behrens RH. Protecting the health of the international traveller. *Trans R Soc Trop Med Hyg* 1990; **84**: 611–612.

13 Spira AM. Preparing the traveller. *Lancet* 2003; **361**: 1368–1381.

14 Leggat PA, Griffiths R, Leggat FW. Emergency assistance provided abroad to insured travellers from Australia. *Travel Med Infect Dis* 2005; **3**: 9–17.

15 Hudson KR, Jawad M, Kingdon S, et al. Do members of the British public know how to contact emergency medical services when abroad? *Eur J Emerg Med* 2013; **20**: 214–217.

16 International Society of Travel Medicine. *Global Travel Clinic Directory*. http://www.istm.org/WebForms/SearchClinics/Default.aspx?SearchType=Advanced (accessed 29 March 2014).

17 International Association for Medical Assistance to Travellers. *Medical Directory*. http://www.iamat.org/doctors_clinics.cfm (accessed 29 March 2014).

18 Leggat PA, Carne J, Kedjarune U. Travel insurance and health. *J Travel Med* 1999; **6**: 252–257.

19 Leggat PA, Leggat FW, Kedjarune U. Travel insurance claims made by travellers from Australia for dental conditions. *Int Dent J* 2001; **51**: 267–272.

20 Kedjarune U, Leggat PA. Dental precautions for travelers. *J Travel Med* 1997; **4**: 38–40.

21 American Dental Association, Department of Communications. Dental care while traveling. *JADA* 2006; **137**: 928.

22 Leggat P, Kedjarune U. Dental health, 'dental tourism' and travellers. *Travel Med Infect Dis* 2009; **7**: 123–124.

23 Leggat PA, Aitken P. Travel insurance and aeromedical retrieval. In: Wilks J, Pendergast D, Leggat PA (eds.) *Tourism in Turbulent Times: Towards Safe Experiences for Visitors.* Abingdon: Routledge, 2011, pp. 37–52.

24 Leggat PA, Leggat FW. Emergency assistance provided abroad to insured travellers from Australia following the Bali bombing. *Travel Med Infect Dis* 2004; **2**: 41–45.

25 Leggat PA, Leggat FW. Assistance provided abroad to insured travellers from Australia following the 2004 Asian tsunami. *Travel Med Infect Dis* 2007; **5**: 47–50.

26 Zwar N. Travelling with medicines. *Aust Prescriber* 2006; **29**: 80–82.

27 Leggat PA, Pearn JH, Dürrheim DN. First aid and travellers. *Travel Med Inf Dis* 2003; **1**: 141–143.

28 Leggat PA, Leggat FW. Knowledge and acceptance of first aid and travel insurance by hostelers from north and central Queensland, Australia. *J Travel Med* 2002; **9**: 269–272.

29 Shaw MTM, Harding E, Leggat PA. Illness and injury to students on a school excursion to Peru. *J Travel Med* 2014; **21**: 183–188.

30 Shaw MTM, Dallimore J. The medical preparation of expeditions: the role of the Medical Officer. *Travel Med Infect Dis* 2005; **3**: 213–223.

31 Gherardin T. The pre-travel consultation: an overview. *Aust Fam Physician* 2007; **36**: 300–303.

32 Leggat PA, Heydon JL. Working overseas and medical kits. In: Leggat PA, Goldsmid JM (eds). *Primer of Travel Medicine*, 3rd edn. Brisbane: ACTM Publications, 2005, pp. 128–140.

SECTION V
Post-travel medicine

CHAPTER 30

The returning traveler

Tamar Lachish[1], Alfons Van Gompel[2], & Eli Schwartz[3]
[1]Shaare-Zedek Medical Center, Jerusalem, *Israel*
[2]Institute for Tropical Medicine, Antwerp, *Belgium*
[3]Chaim Sheba Medical Center, Tel-Hashomer, *Israel*

Introduction

According to the World Tourism Organization, there were an estimated 1035 million international tourist arrivals in 2012 throughout the world (http://mkt.unwto.org/en /barometer). Not only are more people traveling, but they are also seeking out new exotic destinations, which means that an increasing number of travelers visit tropical countries. Travel to tropical destinations may expose travelers to pathogens that are hardly encountered in developed countries. Approximately 8% of travelers to the developing world require medical care during or after travel [1]. The majority of health problems reported by these travelers are mild and mostly self-limiting, for example, diarrhea and skin and respiratory disorders [2] (see Figure 30.1). An unknown proportion of travelers who have been exposed to infectious agents may be asymptomatic but may still have the possibility of late sequelae years later. The risk of infection (symptomatic and asymptomatic) depends on personal risk behaviors, implementation of preventive measures, the endemicity of travel-related infectious diseases in the travel area, and the length of travel.

Is there a need for post-travel screening of asymptomatic travelers?

Post-travel screening of asymptomatic travelers is justified if there is a risk of them having acquired occult travel-related infections and there is a potential impact on the traveler's health status. Screening procedures should take into account the behavioral risk patterns, type and length of travel, and the epidemiology of specific diseases in different destinations [3]. Furthermore, the screening depends on available sensitive and specific screening tools.

Bacterial infections [excluding tuberculosis (TB)] usually have a short incubation period and therefore are not the aim of the screening. Many parasites can be carried asymptomatically for years, and most would probably remain inactive for life. A small fraction of parasitic infections may develop late complications years after exposure.

Essential Travel Medicine, First Edition.
Edited by Jane N. Zuckerman, Gary W. Brunette and Peter A. Leggat.
© 2015 John Wiley & Sons, Ltd. Published 2015 by John Wiley & Sons, Ltd.

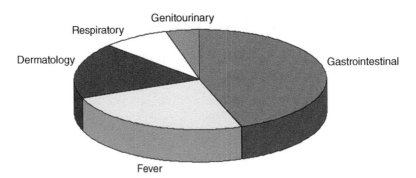

% of ill returned travelers

Genitourinary

Respiratory

Dermatology

Gastrointestinal

Fever

Figure 30.1 Proportion of morbidity per 100 patients. Source: adapted from Freedman et al. (2006) [3].

The problem arising from this possibility is that illness appearing years after exposure may not be linked to past travel and therefore could be difficult to diagnose, and further can result in inadequate treatment. Examples of such parasitic infections are schistosomiasis, which can cause chronic hematuria and colitis or late neurologic complications; *Strongyloides stercoralis* might be complicated with a life-threatening hyperinfection in immunocompromised hosts; *Giardia lamblia* infection could be asymptomatic but yet infective and can cause secondary symptomatic cases; amebiasis can become invasive and form an amebic liver abscess years after inoculation. Of importance is that most parasitic infections are easily treated with a few days' administration of well-tolerated drugs and, as mentioned, the potential consequences of leaving them untreated are in some cases serious or even life threatening.

There have been only a few studies examining the yield from screening asymptomatic returning travelers, and some of these studies were carried out before current diagnostic tools were available. One of the first studies to investigate directly the usefulness of post-travel screening [4], examined 1029 asymptomatic long-term travelers (aged 3 months to 45 years). Stool microscopy for cysts, ova, and parasites showed abnormalities in 207 of 995 patients who were able to produce specimens (18.7%). The commonest abnormal finding was cysts of *Entamoeba histolytica* or *Giardia lamblia*. Full blood counts (FBCs) showed eosinophilia in 67 out of 852 samples (16.1%). Schistosomal serology was positive in 72 out of 676 tests (10.7%). Therefore, the conclusion was that screening long-term travelers according to their relevant history is efficient [4].

In a further study by the same group [5], the utility of history, physical examination, and laboratory tests for screening of long-term travelers returning to Europe from the tropics was examined. A thorough risk factor history in asymptomatic versus symptomatic patients was unable to detect reliably those who would have laboratory evidence of parasitic diseases. For example, schistosomiasis was present in 15% of asymptomatic and 18% of symptomatic individuals [odds ratio (OR) 1.2, $p = 0.46$]; stool microscopy was positive in 14% of both symptomatic and asymptomatic patients, and there was eosinophilia in 9% of symptomatic and 6% of asymptomatic individuals. Furthermore, the risk of schistosomiasis and gastrointestinal parasites did not differ whatever the reported living conditions were. In contrast, targeted laboratory tests (blood count, stool for parasites, and serology for schistosomiasis for those returning from Africa) had a good yield for identifying diseases: positive stool for parasites in 19%, serology for schistosomiasis in 11–17%, and eosinophilia in 8–12% of consecutive patients, regardless of history and symptoms. Some of the positive results had potentially serious long-term implications if left untreated.

In a more recent prospective study, the serology-based attack rates and incidence rates of recent schistosomiasis, strongyloidiasis, filariasis, and toxocariasis in short-term (up to 13 weeks) asymptomatic travelers to endemic areas were low [6]. Diagnosis of parasitic infection was not related to travel duration, the interval between return from travel and blood donation, or eosinophilia. Furthermore, none of travel diary-recorded symptoms (fever, myalgia, skin infection, and gastrointestinal disorders) had any predictive value of seroconversion to any of the aforementioned parasites. The conclusion was that there is no value in screening asymptomatic short-term travelers. The main limitations of this study were that most travelers returned from Asia with a minority returning from Africa, which is far more endemic for *Schistosoma* and *Filaria*, and blood was drawn post-travel at a mean time of 21 days, which might be too early in terms of seroconversion.

Based on the literature considered above, although fairly limited, there is no justification to recommend screening of all asymptomatic short-term returning travelers and instead a risk assessment approach should guide the need for further investigation.

The World Health Organization nevertheless specifies who needs post-travel screening (http://www.who.int/ith/precautions/medical_examination/en/index.html): asymptomatic travelers should be advised to have a medical examination on their return if they:

- suffer from a chronic disease, such as cardiovascular disease, diabetes mellitus, or chronic respiratory disease, or have been taking anticoagulants;
- received treatment for malaria while traveling;
- may have been exposed to a serious infectious disease while traveling;
- have spent more than 3 months in a developing country (long-term traveler or expatriate).

Asymptomatic short-term travelers should rarely be screened, even in cases of self-limiting complaints such as diarrhea or a very short duration fever episode. An exception should be made in patients with a possible exposure to sexually transmitted infections (STIs) or to freshwater. Adventurous travelers frequently adopt lifestyles that put them at greater risk for unusual infections and therefore should be assessed. Travelers who are VFRs rarely seek medical advice and should be assessed thoroughly.

The recommended timing for post-travel screening depends on the specific exposure and the incubation period and time to seroconversion of the possible pathogens. For example, a traveler with a behavioral risk for acquiring an STI should be screened immediately and offered post-exposure prophylaxis and follow-up; a traveler with exposure to freshwater should be counseled about possible clinical manifestations occurring later and schistosoma serology should be deferred until 3 months post-exposure.

Specific exposures and screening

Screening for specific diseases depends on the geographic area visited and on the specific exposures during travel.

Water exposure

Schistosomiasis is caused by helminth parasites of the genus *Schistosoma*. Infection in humans is caused by water contact and transmission occurs via penetration of larval cercariae contaminating freshwater. Schistosomiasis is mainly endemic in the developing world, especially in Africa, where it is hyperendemic in many regions (Figure 30.2).

The clinical manifestations are divided into three stages:
- Cercarial dermatitis (swimmer's itch) pruritus which is caused by penetration of the cercariae and might occur within 24 hours after exposure.
- Acute schistosomiasis (Katayama syndrome), which develops within 2–8 weeks after exposure. The manifestations are due to a hypersensitivity reaction against migration of the schistosomule in the tissues (fever, cough, urticaria, etc.).
- Chronic schistosomiasis is a late reaction (months to years after exposure) that results from granuloma formation around parasite eggs being embedded in the target organ of each schistosoma species.

Diagnosis is based either on the detection of eggs in urine or stool or on serology. Travelers usually have a limited exposure and therefore their burden of infection is low, and looking for eggs has a lower yield than in local populations with recurrent exposures. Furthermore, travelers are more likely to be diagnosed during the acute phase of the disease, that is, before the development of the adult worms that lay eggs. Serology is therefore the method of choice, but seroconversion may take time (6 weeks to 3 months after exposure).

Local populations have recurrent exposure to contaminated freshwater and therefore the chronic phase is the most common presentation of the disease among this group. Only 7–38% of travelers report cercarial dermatitis immediately post-exposure [7,8].

An estimated 85% of the worlds' cases of schistosomiasis are from Africa [9]. In recent decades, schistosomiasis has been gaining attention in the western world owing to the importation of the disease by returning travelers from the tropics. In most cases, the disease was acquired in Sub-Saharan Africa, but in recent years there is cumulative evidence of travel-related schistosomiasis from the Mekong River and its tributaries [10] and South America [11].

Little is known about the risk of infection in travelers. Whitty et al. examined the presentation and outcome of 1107 cases of schistosomiasis acquired in Africa. In their study, 18% of asymptomatic travelers exposed to freshwater in Africa were found to have schistosomiasis [5]. Bierman et al. found that 33% of people asking to be screened for schistosomiasis after a water exposure in an endemic country had schistosomal antibodies [12].

In a study by Meltzer et al. examining the characteristics of schistosomiasis among 137 Israeli travelers, chronic schistosomiasis developed in 26% of patients who were

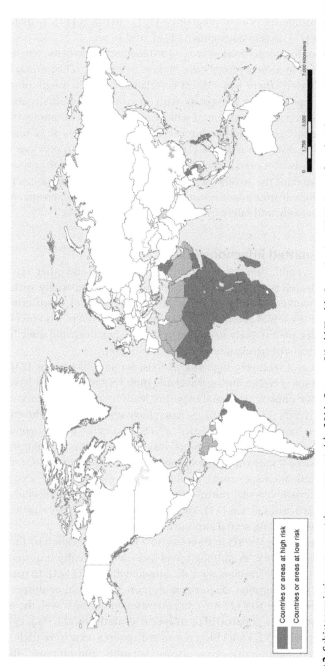

Figure 30.2 Schistosomiasis map: countries or areas at risk, 2011. Source: World Health Organization 2012. Reproduced with permission of the World Health Organization.

initially asymptomatic, i.e. chronic disease can develop in the absence of acute disease [7]. There are several case reports that indicate serious complications of chronic disease in travelers months to several years after exposure, such as female genital schistosomiasis leading to ectopic pregnancy [13], infertility [14], hematospermia, chronic diarrhea [15], myeloradiculopathy [16], and so on.

Screening travelers for schistosomiasis is justified regardless of the length of exposure to fresh water. In a survey from Lake Malawi examining schistosomiasis among non-immune travelers, there was a direct correlation between length of stay at the lakeshore and seropositivity to *Schistosoma*, with up to 90% seropositivity after 10 days of stay [17]. In a recent investigation of schistosomiasis outbreak among travelers to the Crater Lakes in Uganda, despite a mean exposure duration of 22 minutes, the attack rate of acute disease was 100% [18]. This report confirms previous reports of acute schistosomiasis after even a single exposure [8,19]. Based on the presented data and taking into account the possible serious sequel of untreated disease, screening of travelers at risk for schistosomiasis is justified even after a short exposure. Moreover, schistosomiasis is easily and safely treated on an outpatient basis.

Sexually transmitted infections (STIs)

HIV, gonorrhea, syphilis, non-specific urethritis, hepatitis B, and other STIs are a significant risk to travelers who engage in unprotected sex, especially with overseas commercial sex workers [20,21]. It is estimated that 5–50% of short-term travelers engage in casual sex while abroad [22]. Furthermore, travelers who involve themselves in casual sex are less likely to engage in safe sex practices, and these behavioral risks are independent of nationality or travel destination.

Travelers are at a relatively high risk of STIs, for several reasons [23]: the frequency of casual sex is higher during travel and their sporadic partners have a higher prevalence of STIs; unplanned sexual exposure leads to a low adherence of safe sex practices; and travelers (especially males) often have sexual contact with commercial sex workers, who have a higher incidence of STIs than in the general population.

Predictors of an STI risk in an individual traveler are the pattern of travel (alone, with friends versus a family trip), type of travel (for example, a time-out travel after a divorce or a traumatic experience), availability and affordability of sexual services at the travel destination, social norms at the travel destinations, alcohol and illicit drug use, and practice of safe sex [23]. Therefore, when assessing a returned traveler, specific questions regarding sexual exposure should be asked.

Regarding the etiology of STI in travelers, in a recent publication by the GeoSentinel Surveillance Network, examining travel-associated sexually transmitted infections, 0.9% of 112,180 ill travelers were diagnosed with an STI [21]. In patients seen after travel, the most common diagnoses were non-gonococcal or unspecified urethritis (30.2%) and acute HIV (27.6%). In patients seen during travel, the most common diagnoses were non-gonococcal or unspecified urethritis (21.1%), epididymitis (15.2%), and cervicitis (12.3%). Other not rare diagnoses seen were trichomoniasis, gonorrhea, acute inflammatory pelvic disease, balanitis, and phimosis. Ill travelers who had been to south central Asia (the Indian sub-continent) were the least likely to receive a diagnosis of STI, most probably due to local social norms.

The risk of HIV following a single, unprotected, heterosexual and consensual sex act is approximately 0.01% [24] and for hepatitis C after a single sexual exposure it is 0.0–0.6% [25]. Hepatitis B is the only vaccine-preventable STI; the risk of infection following a single act of unprotected sexual intercourse is unknown, and is estimated to be less than the risk following a blood-borne exposure (between 10 and 30%). This risk increases, however, depending on whether an individual has one or more sexual partners [26].

The presence of genital lesions can dramatically increase the risk of acquiring HIV and possibly other sexually transmitted viruses. A single episode of vaginal intercourse gives a risk of 20% and 50% of acquiring gonorrhea in uninfected men and women, respectively [27].

A post-travel STI diagnostic evaluation is indicated when casual sexual activity has occurred during travel, regardless of whether symptoms are present. Treatment (whether definitive or post-exposure prophylaxis) has importance for the individual and also with respect to public health (limiting secondary infection spread).

For pre-exposure prophylaxis, so far hepatitis B is the only STI for which effective vaccination is available. Post-exposure prophylaxis is available for hepatitis B and HIV if given as soon as possible after the exposure (within 72 hours but no longer than 120 hours). A later screening for possible STI should be determined by the nature of sexual exposure and could include an examination of the genitals, appropriate swabs or first-void urine testing, and serologic tests for hepatitis B and C, HIV, and syphilis in patients with exposure to blood products or unsterile needles [28]. The therapy should be guided by serology or culture and by sensitivity tests when possible. Serologic workup can initially be negative, hence in high-risk behavior travelers repeated examinations might be needed according to the relevant incubation periods. Meanwhile, patients should be counseled with respect to the practice of safe sex.

Tuberculosis exposure

The risk of acquiring latent TB is minimal for most travelers, even if they return from popular tourist destinations in high-incidence settings: the duration of stay is usually short, and activities and contacts are such that the risk of acquiring TB infection is minimal. This risk may increase substantially in long-term travelers and expatriates[29].

A study in The Netherlands examined the incidence of tuberculin conversion [measured by the tuberculin skin test (TST)] in several hundred travelers who had spent 3–12 months in one or more countries of high incidence [30]. The results showed a risk of 3.5 per 1000 travel months or an annual risk of approximately 4%. These travelers came into relatively close contact with the local population: 55% traveled for work or as part of their training, and almost all had used local public transport or stayed in "local guesthouses." For people working in the healthcare sector, the risk increased to 7.9 per 1000 travel months compared with 2.8 per 1000 for all others. For long-term travelers, the risk was comparable to that of TB infection among the local population, estimated as 1.0–2.5% per year [30]. For travelers visiting friends and relatives in their home country, the risk of TB acquisition is higher than in others [31].

There is no gold standard for the diagnosis of latent TB infection (LTBI), and the traditional assay, the TST, which has been the mainstay of LTBI diagnosis for over a century, is an imperfect test. In addition to TST, the more recent in vitro blood tests, interferon-gamma (IFN-γ) release assays (IGRAs), are available for the diagnosis of LTBI [32,33]. In fact, both tests assess cell-mediated immunity but they differ in several respects. The TST measures delayed-type hypersensitivity to the multitude of antigens contained in the purified protein derivative (PPD) and hence cross-reacts with BCG and natural infection with other non-tuberculosis mycobacteria. The IGRAs measure IFN-γ release by T-lymphocytes in response to selected antigens that are absent from all BCG strains and from most non-tuberculosis mycobacteria.

The TST has several important limitations:

- Requires reading and interpretation within a 72-hour interval, necessitating two visits, hence possible failure of the patient to return for the test reading.
- False-positive results due to prior BCG vaccination, exposure to non-tuberculosis mycobacteria, or the boosting phenomenon.
- False-negative results can also occur because TST is less sensitive in immunosuppressive conditions, pregnancy, old age, diabetes, and in cases of active TB itself.
- Indeterminate reactions frequently occur.
- The intradermal injection and the reading of the reaction must be performed correctly by experienced personnel and variability in results exists due to operator bias.

IGRAs have at least equal sensitivity to the TST in immunocompetent persons and have potential advantages over the TST:

- Better specificity because IGRAs are unresponsive in persons vaccinated with BCG or infected with non-tuberculous mycobacteria.
- Previous TST has no impact on IGRA results.
- There is no need for a follow-up visit for reading of results.
  - Elimination of technical factors related to measurement of TST induration (the results are numerical, and thus less subject to reader bias).

Although promising as an alternative to TST, IGRAs share similar limitations: they do not discriminate between latent and active TB or between recent, past, and treated TB, and their sensitivity is impaired in immunodeficient persons.

Further important disadvantages of IGRAs are their cost, substantial test–retest variability, and unexpectedly high rates of apparent "conversions" on serial testing of low-risk healthcare worker s[29]. For details on the precise use of these test (TST or IGRA; TST and IGRA, e.g. dual or consecutive testing), we refer to the national policies of each country (e.g., [34–37]).

High risk travelers, such as long-stay travelers or health practitioners, should be encouraged to be examined before and after their trip. Based on the literature [32], IGRAs can be used as a complement test rather than as a replacement for the TST for the diagnosis of latent TB infection in the setting of a travel clinic.

Possible screening tools

The availability of reliable and simple diagnostic laboratory tests for the detection of mainly parasitic infections is pivotal in post-travel screening. Most bacterial infections have a short incubation period and are less likely to be asymptomatic, hence the main purpose of screening is to detect occult parasitic and viral infections. Viral infections are usually associated with STIs (see above) and have easily accessible and reliable diagnostic tools. However, diagnosis of parasitic diseases is more complicated and not always readily accessible. Possible tools that may help in the diagnosis are a complete blood count (CBC) and eosinophil count, ova and parasites in stool (stool microscopy), and serology for *Schistosoma*, *Strongyloides*, and *Filaria*.

CBC

The main interest in a CBC is the eosinophil count. Eosinophilia is defined as the presence of >500 eosinophils per milliliter. Eosinophilia has generally been accepted in clinical practice as a simple, inexpensive, and hence useful general parameter to indicate helminthic infection, especially with nematodes or trematodes.

In different case series, eosinophilia has been documented in 4.8–12% of returned travelers (Table 30.1). In a study by Schulte et al. [38] retrospectively examining 14,298 returning travelers attending an outpatient clinic, 698 (4.8%) had eosinophilia. One-third of these patients were asymptomatic. A definite diagnosis was made for 36% of patients with eosinophilia and the positive predictive value for helminthic disease was 18.9%. The negative predictive value was 98.7%. When the eosinophil count reached more than 16% of the total white blood cell count, the positive predictive value increased to 46.6%. These results are comparable to those of Libman et al. [39], who found that 14% of patients with eosinophilia had a demonstrable parasitic infection.

Similar results were also reported by Meltzer et al. [40]. Of their 955 retrospectively evaluated ill-returning travelers, 82 (8.6%) had eosinophilia and 44 (4.4%) were diagnosed with schistosomiasis. In the remaining 38 cases (4.2%), a definite

Table 30.1 Case series of eosinophilia in returning travelers.

Eosinophils (%)	No. of cases	Type of travelers	Country	Ref.
10	1605	Asymptomatic expatriates	Canada	[39]
8	1029	Asymptomatic returning travelers	United Kingdom	[4]
12	510	Symptomatic and asymptomatic returning travelers.	United Kingdom	[5]
8.6	955	Ill-returning travelers	Israel	[40]
4.8	14,298	Symptomatic and asymptomatic returning travelers	Germany	[38]

Table 30.2 Helminths in patients with eosinophilia (serology and stool microscopy).

Helminths (%)				Clinical features/ pathogen
Israel [31] $n = 82$ Symptomatic	Canada [30] $n = 167$ Asymptomatic	United Kingdom [49] $n = 261$ Symptomatic and asymptomatic	Germany [29] $n = 689$ Symptomatic and asymptomatic	
54	4.7	33	6	Schistosomiasis
0	4.1	7.6	1.9	Filaria
6	0	25	2.1	Strongyloides
1.2	NA	3.4	1.0	Ascaris

diagnosis was achieved in only 23.7%. However, they empirically treated those 38 patients with albendazole and this led to a clinical improvement in 90%. Therefore, they recommend a limited investigation for each returning traveler with eosinophilia and instead implementing a thorough history and physical examination, with stool samples for parasites and then a therapeutic trial of albendazole.

In the above-mentioned studies, a diagnosis was made in a small number of patients who were investigated for eosinophilia. However, response to empiric broad-spectrum anthelmintic treatment could be a marker of helminthic infection, and the screening for eosinophilia might therefore be valuable. Furthermore, similar findings were found in patients with and without eosinophilia (Table 30.2), and this might imply that screening of returning travelers is required regardless of eosinophil count.

The main findings in patients with eosinophilia, either by serology or by direct stool examination, are summarized in Table 30.2. As can be seen, schistosomiasis is the most common pathogen among returning travelers with eosinophilia. However, most of the pathogens mentioned in the table can lead to serious sequelae, including life-threatening disease in case of hyperinfection strongyloidiasis.

More updated prospective studies are required to investigate further the true yield of screening for eosinophilia.

Strongyloides serology

In travelers with a relevant exposure history, especially in those presenting with eosinophilia or elevated immunoglobulin E levels, *Strongyloides stercoralis* should be considered in the differential diagnosis, even if infection is asymptomatic. This approach is even more essential in immunocompromised returning travelers, who are at risk of complications from disseminated disease. The diagnosis of strongyloidiasis is made by detecting rhabditiform larvae in concentrated stool or by serology, or by the combination of both [41]. The enzyme-linked immunosorbent assay (ELISA) kit for *Strongyloides* is sensitive and specific, although the sensitivity changes according to the screened population [42]. In a comparison between immigrants with chronic infection and infected travelers, the sensitivity of serology was 98% in the former and 73% in the latter [43]. ELISA can detect infection in both symptomatic and asymptomatic individuals, and can be positive despite repeated negative stool samples. In a analysis by Nuesch et al., almost one-quarter of all their 31 strongyloidosis cases (travelers and immigrants) were detected by untargeted screening, which points to the risk of missing the diagnosis without screening [42].

Filaria serology

Filarial infection is spread through the developing world, but is rare among travelers and is in general associated with prolonged travel and intense exposure to the mosquito vectors that transmit them. In a survey by the GeoSentinel Surveillance Network, filarial infections comprised 0.62% ($n = 271$) of all medical conditions reported in ill returning travelers; 60% of the infections were reported from immigrants and from those immigrants returning to their county of origin (VFRs) [44]. Filarial infection should be considered in returning symptomatic or asymptomatic travelers with unexplained eosinophilia who returned mainly from a long stay in Sub-Saharan Africa but also from South-East Asia.

The standard method for diagnosing active infection is the identification of microfilariae in a blood smear by microscopic examination. Serologic techniques provide an alternative to microscopic detection, but their availability in many countries is limited.

Stool microscopy

Stool microscopy for ova and parasites is still the main diagnostic method to detect protozoa and helminths. Regarding the latter, concentrated stool microscopy identifies more easily soil-transmitted helminths (*Ascaris lumbricoides*, *Trichuris trichiura*, hookworm species) but has a low sensitivity in detecting *Strongyloides* larvae [43].

Regarding protozoa, the two most common parasites are *Giardia lamblia* and *Entameba*. Unfortunately, stool microscopy does not distinguish the pathogenic *E. histolytica* from the non-pathogenic *E. dispar*. Overall, repeated stool testing may be needed to make the diagnosis, especially in travelers with very slight infections, where there may be only one or a few worms and eggs may be absent.

There are only limited available data examining the utility of stool microscopy in returning travelers. In a study by Whitty et al. [5], stool microscopy was positive in 19% of 1029 screened cases and did not correlate with reported eating habits. In the second phase of their study, stool microscopy was positive in 14% of both symptomatic and asymptomatic 510 patients (the most common finding was *E. histolytica* or *dispar*, *G. lamblia*, and gut helminths).Their conclusion was that potentially serious asymptomatic infection is common in travelers. A detailed history of exposure, symptoms, and physical examination added little to detecting cases. Overall, stool microscopy, schistosomal serology, and eosinophil count all produced a good yield.

The major limitation of conventional stool testing is its low sensitivity, hence testing three samples is a common policy to increasing the yield of positive findings [45]. Applying molecular techniques for stool testing for ova and parasite in the initial stages. ten Hove et al. analyzed daily microscopic examination and antigen detection as compared with a weekly performed multiplex real-time polymerase chain reaction (PCR). Of 2591 stool samples *E. histolytica*, *G. lamblia*, *Cryptosporidium*, and *S. stercoralis* were detected in 0.3, 4.7, 0.5, and 0.1% of cases, respectively. These detection rates were increased using real-time PCR to 0.5, 6.0, 1.3, and 0.8%, respectively [46].

The results justify screening of returning travelers with stool microscopy for parasites; however, further prospective studies are needed to clarify the issue better. Investigations dealing with specific pathogens recommend integrating stool microscopy with serology or molecular biology techniques [43,47,48].

Conclusion

Travel to tropical destinations may expose travelers to pathogens that are rarely encountered in developed countries. These infections could be symptomatic or asymptomatic and may hold a potential risk of late complications. Data regarding screening of returning travelers are limited and partly outdated. With these limitations, the conclusions that can be drawn are as follows: screening of all short-term (<3 months) travelers is not justified, and rather a risk assessment approach according to specific exposures and medical history should be implemented; screening long-term travelers (>3 months) is reasonable. The basic screening tools are a CBC and stool for microscopy. Serology for *Schistosoma* and *Strongyloides* should be examined in patients with clinical suspicion, unexplained eosinophilia, or specific exposures. Prospective studies implementing updated diagnostic tools, including molecular techniques for stool examination, are required to support further these recommendations.

References

1 Steffen R, Rickenbach M, Wilhelm U, et al. Health problems after travel to developing countries. *J Infect Dis* 1987; **156**: 84–91.

2 Schwartz E. *Tropical Diseases in Travelers*. Oxford: Blackwell Publishing, 2009.

3 Freedman DO, Weld LH, Kozarsky PE, et al. Spectrum of disease and relation to place of exposure among ill returned travelers. *N Engl J Med* 2006; **354**: 119–130.

4 Carroll B, Dow C, Snashall D, et al. Post-tropical screening: how useful is it? *BMJ* 1993; **307**: 541.

5 Whitty CJ, Carroll B, Armstrong M, et al. Utility of history, examination and laboratory tests in screening those returning to Europe from the tropics for parasitic infection. *Trop Med Int Health* 2000; **5**: 818–823.

6 Baaten GG, Sonder GJ, van Gool T, et al. Travel-related schistosomiasis, strongyloidiasis, filariasis, and toxocariasis: the risk of infection and the diagnostic relevance of blood eosinophilia. *BMC Infect Dis* 2011; **11**: 84.

7 Meltzer E, Artom G, Marva E, et al. Schistosomiasis among travelers: new aspects of an old disease. *Emerg Infect Dis* 2006; **12**: 1696–1700.

8 Colebunders R, Verstraeten T, Van Gompel A, et al. Acute schistosomiasis in travelers returning from Mali. *J Travel Med* 1995; **2**: 235–238.

9 Brunette G (ed.) *CDC Health Information for International Travel 2012: The Yellow Book*. Oxford: Oxford University Press, 2012.

10 Leshem E, Meltzer E, Marva E, Schwartz E. Travel-related schistosomiasis acquired in Laos. *Emerg Infect Dis* 2009; **15**: 1823–1826.

11 Schneider MC, Aguilera XP, Barbosa da Silva J, Jr., et al. Elimination of neglected diseases in Latin America and the Caribbean: a mapping of selected diseases. *PLoS Negl Trop Dis* 2011; **5**(2): e964.

12 Bierman WF, Wetsteyn JC, van Gool T. Presentation and diagnosis of imported schistoso-miasis: relevance of eosinophilia, microscopy for ova, and serology. *J Travel Med* 2005; **12**: 9–13.

13 Sheorey H, Charles PG, Pyman J. Ectopic schistosomiasis in a returned traveler. *J Travel Med* 2004; **11**: 251–252.

14 Crump JA, Murdoch DR, Chambers ST, et al. Female genital schistosomiasis. *J Travel Med* 2000; **7**: 30–32.

15 Neghina R, Neghina AM, Merkler C, et al. Intestinal schistosomiasis, importation of a neglected tropical disease in Romania. Case report of a traveler to endemic regions. *Travel Med Infect Dis* 2009; **7**: 49–51.

16 Makinson A, Morales RJ, Basset D, et al. Diagnostic approaches to imported schistosomal myeloradiculopathy in travelers. *Neurology* 2008; **71**: 66–67.

17 Cetron MS, Chitsulo L, Sullivan JJ, et al. Schistosomiasis in Lake Malawi. *Lancet* 1996; **348**: 1274–1278.

18 Lachish T, Tandlich M, Grossman T, Schwartz E. High rate of schistosomiasis in travelers after a brief exposure to the high altitude Nyinambuga Crater Lake (1630 m), Uganda. *Clin Infect Dis* 2013; **57**: 1461–1464.

19 Leshem E, Maor Y, Meltzer E, et al. Acute schistosomiasis outbreak: clinical features and economic impact. *Clin Infect Dis* 2008; **47**: 1499–1506.

20 Ansart S, Hochedez P, Perez L, et al. Sexually transmitted diseases diagnosed among travelers returning from the tropics. *J Travel Med* 2009; **16**: 79–83.

21 Matteelli A, Schlagenhauf P, Carvalho AC, et al. Travel-associated sexually transmitted infec-tions: an observational cross-sectional study of the GeoSentinel surveillance database. *Lancet Infect Dis* 2013; **13**: 205–213.

22 Matteelli A, Carosi G. Sexually transmitted diseases in travelers. *Clin Infect Dis* 2001; **32**: 1063–1067.

23 Abdullah AS, Ebrahim SH, Fielding R, Morisky DE. Sexually transmitted infections in trav-elers: implications for prevention and control. *Clin Infect Dis* 2004; **39**: 533–538.

24 Pinkerton SD, Martin JN, Roland ME, et al. Cost-effectiveness of postexposure prophylaxis after sexual or injection-drug exposure to human immunodeficiency virus. *Arch Intern Med* 2004; **164**: 46–54.

25 Terrault NA, Dodge JL, Murphy EL, et al. Sexual transmission of hepatitis C virus among monogamous heterosexual couples: the HCV partners study. *Hepatology (Baltimore, Md).* 2013; **57**: 881–889.

26 Alter MJ, Ahtone J, Weisfuse I, et al. Hepatitis B virus transmission between heterosexuals. *JAMA* 1986; **256**: 1307–1310.

27 Mandell GL, Bennett JE, Dolin R. Mandell, Douglas, and Bennett's Principles and Practice of Infectious Diseases, 7th edn. Philadelphia, PA: Churchill Livingstone Elsevier; 2010, pp. 2242–2258.

28 Ward BJ, Plourde P. Travel and sexually transmitted infections. *J Travel Med* 2006; **13**: 300–317.

29 Schwartzman K. Interferon-gamma release assays for latent tuberculosis infection in trav-elers and migrants. Presented at CISTM 13, Maastricht, 19–23 May 2013. www.ISTM.org (accessed 9 October 2013).

30 Cobelens FG, van Deutekom H, Draayer-Jansen IW, et al. Risk of infection with *Mycobac-terium tuberculosis* in travellers to areas of high tuberculosis endemicity. *Lancet* 2000; **356**: 461–465.

31 Lobato MN, Hopewell PC. *Mycobacterium tuberculosis* infection after travel to or contact with visitors from countries with a high prevalence of tuberculosis. *Am J Respir Crit Care Med* 1998; **158**: 1871–1875.

32 Apers L, Yansouni C, Soentjens P, et al. The use of interferon-gamma release assays for tuberculosis screening in international travelers. *Curr Infect Dis Rep* 2011; **13**: 229–235.

33 Redelman-Sidi G, Sepkowitz KA. IFN-gamma release assays in the diagnosis of latent tuberculosis infection among immunocompromised adults. *Am J Respir Crit Care Med* 2013; **188**: 422–431.

34 Mazurek GH, Jereb J, Vernon A, et al. Updated guidelines for using interferon-γ release assays to detect *Mycobacterium tuberculosis* infection. *MMWR Recomm Rep* 2010; **59**(RR-5): 1–25.

35 European Centre for Disease Prevention and Control (ECDC). *Use of Interferon-gamma Release Assays in Support of TB Diagnosis*. http://ecdc.europa.eu/en/publications/Publications/1103 _GUI_IGRA.pdf (accessed July 2013).

36 NICE. *NICE Clinical Guideline 117. Tuberculosis. Clinical Diagnosis and Management of Tuberculosis, and Measures for Its Prevention and Control*. National Institute for Health and Care Excellence, 2011. http://www.nice.org.uk/guidance/cg117 (accessed 5 February 2014).

37 Canadian Tuberculosis Committee. Interferon-γ release assays for latent tuberculosis infection: an advisory committee statement (ACS). *Can Commun Dis Rep* 2010; **36**: 1–21.

38 Schultc C, Krebs B, Jelinek T, et al. Diagnostic significance of blood eosinophilia in returning travelers. *Clin Infect Dis* 2002; **34**: 407–411.

39 Libman MD, MacLean JD, Gyorkos TW. Screening for schistosomiasis, filariasis, and strongyloidiasis among expatriates returning from the tropics. *Clin Infect Dis* 1993; **17**: 353–359.

40 Meltzer E, Percik R, Shatzkes J, et al. Eosinophilia among returning travelers: a practical approach. *Am J Trop Med Hyg* 2008; **78**: 702–709.

41 Loutfy MR, Wilson M, Keystone JS, Kain KC. Serology and eosinophil count in the diagnosis and management of strongyloidiasis in a non-endemic area. *Am J Trop Med Hyg* 2002; **66**: 749–752.

42 Nuesch R, Zimmerli L, Stockli R, et al. Imported strongyloidosis: a longitudinal analysis of 31 cases. *J Travel Med* 2005; **12**: 80–84.

43 Sudarshi S, Stumpfle R, Armstrong M, et al. Clinical presentation and diagnostic sensitivity of laboratory tests for *Strongyloides stercoralis* in travellers compared with immigrants in a non-endemic country. *Trop Med Int Health* 2003; **8**: 728–732.

44 Lipner EM, Law MA, Barnett E, et al. Filariasis in travelers presenting to the GeoSentinel Surveillance Network. *PLoS Negl Trop Dis* 2007; **1**(3): e88.

45 Hiatt RA, Markell EK, Ng E. How many stool examinations are necessary to detect pathogenic intestinal protozoa? *Am J Trop Med Hyg* 1995; **53**: 36–39.

46 ten Hove RJ, van Esbroeck M, Vervoort T, et al. Molecular diagnostics of intestinal parasites in returning travellers. *Eur J Clin Microbiol Infect Dis* 2009; **28**: 1045–1053.

47 Herbinger KH, Fleischmann E, Weber C, et al. Epidemiological, clinical, and diagnostic data on intestinal infections with *Entamoeba histolytica* and *Entamoeba dispar* among returning travelers. *Infection* 2011; **39**: 527–535.

48 Muller A, Bialek R, Kamper A, et al. Detection of microsporidia in travelers with diarrhea. *J Clin Microbiol* 2001; **39**: 1630–1632.

49 Whetham J, Day JN, Armstrong M, et al. Investigation of tropical eosinophilia; assessing a strategy based on geographical area. *J Infect* 2003; **46**: 180–185.

Index

Page numbers in **bold** represent tables.

Essential Travel Medicine, First Edition.
Edited by Jane N. Zuckerman, Gary W. Brunette and Peter A. Leggat.
© 2015 John Wiley & Sons, Ltd. Published 2015 by John Wiley & Sons, Ltd.

Printed and bound by CPI Group (UK) Ltd, Croydon, CR0 4YY

09/10/2024

14571436-0003